Clinical Practice Guidelines of the American Academy of Pediatrics

A Compilation of Evidence-Based Guidelines for Pediatric Practice

GW00367247

American Academy of Pediatrics
141 Northwest Point Blvd
Elk Grove Village, IL 60007

Third edition
Second edition, 1999
First edition, 1997

First edition of this manual was issued under the title: *Practice Parameters of the American Academy of Pediatrics.*

Library of Congress Catalog Card No.: 00-132835
ISBN: 1-58110-063-9
AC0033

The recommendations in this publication do not indicate an exclusive course of treatment or serve as a standard of medical care. Variations, taking into account individual circumstances, may be appropriate.

Foreword

In response to the growing trend toward the practice of evidence-based medicine, the American Academy of Pediatrics' (AAP) Committee on Quality Improvement developed an organizational process and methodology for developing clinical practice guidelines. These guidelines provide physicians with a scientific-based decision-making tool for managing common pediatric conditions.

The evidence-based approach to developing clinical practice guidelines requires carefully defining the problem and identifying interventions and health outcomes. An extensive literature review and data analysis provide the basis for guideline recommendations. The practice guidelines also are subjected to a thorough peer review process prior to publication and subsequent dissemination, implementation, and evaluation. Clinical practice guidelines are periodically reviewed to ensure that they are based on the most current data available.

Academy guidelines are designed to provide physicians with an analytic framework for evaluating and treating common childhood conditions and are not intended as an exclusive course of treatment or as standards of care. When using AAP practice guidelines, clinicians should continue to consider other sources of information as well as variations in individual circumstances. The Academy recognizes the incompleteness of data and acknowledges the use of expert consensus in cases where data do not exist. Thus, AAP practice guidelines allow for flexibility and adaptability at the local level and should not replace sound clinical judgment.

This compilation contains practice guidelines and summaries of technical reports developed and published by the Academy. The full technical reports are available in the online version of *Pediatrics* and can be accessed at www.pediatrics.org. Full technical reports contain summaries of the data reviewed, results of data analyses, and complete evidence tables and bibliographies that also were used to derive practice guideline recommendations. The compendium also contains evidence-based practice guidelines from other organizations that have been endorsed by the Academy. This compendium will be expanded as new pediatric practice guidelines are developed and endorsed and existing guidelines are updated. We encourage you to look forward to future guidelines and revisions.

If you have any questions about current or future practice guidelines, please contact Carla Herrerias, MPH, at the Academy at 800/433-9016, ext 4317. To order copies of the patient education brochures that accompany each guideline, please call the AAP Division of Publications at 888/227-1770.

Charles J. Homer, MD

Table of Contents

Practical Guide for the Diagnosis and Management of Asthma

The following guideline for diagnosis and management of asthma, developed by the National Heart, Lung, and Blood Institute, has been endorsed by the American Academy of Pediatrics.

Practical Guide for the Diagnosis and Management of Asthma

Based on the *Expert Panel Report 2: Guidelines for the Diagnosis and Management of Asthma*

Second Expert Panel on the Management of Asthma

*Shirley Murphy, M.D., *Chair*
University of New Mexico

Eugene R. Bleecker, M.D.
University of Maryland

*Homer Boushey, M.D.
University of California at
San Francisco

*A. Sonia Buist, M.D.
Oregon Health Sciences University

*William Busse, M.D.
University of Wisconsin

Noreen M. Clark, Ph.D.
University of Michigan

Howard Eigen, M.D.
Riley Hospital for Children

Jean G. Ford, M.D.
Columbia University

*Susan Janson, D.N.Sc., R.N.
University of California,
San Francisco

*H. William Kelly, Pharm.D.
University of New Mexico

Robert F. Lemanske, Jr., M.D.
University of Wisconsin

Carolyn C. Lopez, M.D.
Rush Medical College

Fernando Martinez, M.D.
University of Arizona

*Harold S. Nelson, M.D.
National Jewish Medical and
Research Center

Richard Nowak, M.D., M.B.A.
Henry Ford Hospital

Thomas A.E. Platts-Mills,
M.D., Ph.D.
University of Virginia

Gail G. Shapiro, M.D.
University of Washington

Stuart Stoloff, M.D.
Private Family Practice
and University of Nevada

Kevin Weiss, M.D., M.P.H.
Rush Primary Care Institute

Federal Liaison Representatives
Clive Brown, M.B.B.S., M.P.H.
Centers for Disease Control
and Prevention

Peter J. Gergen, M.D.
(formerly with the National Institute
of Allergy and Infectious Diseases)
Agency for Health Care Policy
and Research

Edward L. Petsonk, M.D.
National Institute for Occupational
Safety and Health

*National Heart, Lung, and
Blood Institute Staff*
Ted Buxton, M.P.H.
Robinson Fulwood, M.S.P.H.
Michele Hindi-Alexander, Ph.D.
Suzanne S. Hurd, Ph.D.
Virginia S. Taggart, M.P.H.

R.O.W. Sciences, Inc., Support Staff
Ruth Clark
Daria Donaldson
Lisa Marcellino
Donna Selig
Keith Stanger
Eileen Zeller, M.P.H.

*Executive Committee Member

National Asthma Education and Prevention Program
Coordinating Committee Organizations

Allergy and Asthma Network/
Mothers of Asthmatics, Inc.

American Academy of Allergy,
Asthma, and Immunology

American Academy of
Family Physicians

American Academy of Pediatrics

American Academy of
Physician Assistants

American Association for
Respiratory Care

American Association of
Occupational Health Nurses

American College of Allergy, Asthma,
and Immunology

American College of Chest Physicians

American College of Emergency
Physicians

American Lung Association

American Medical Association

American Nurses Association, Inc.

American Pharmaceutical Association

American Public Health Association

American School Health Association

American Society of Health-System
Pharmacists

American Thoracic Society

Association of State and Territorial
Directors of Health Promotion
and Public Health Education

Asthma and Allergy Foundation
of America

Centers for Disease Control
and Prevention

National Association of School Nurses

National Black Nurses
Association, Inc.

National Center for
Environmental Health

National Center for Health Statistics

NHLBI Ad Hoc Committee on
Minority Populations

National Heart, Lung, and
Blood Institute

National Institute for Occupational
Safety and Health

National Institute of Allergy and
Infectious Diseases

National Institute of Environmental
Health Sciences

National Medical Association

Society for Public Health Education

U.S. Environmental Protection Agency

U.S. Food and Drug Administration

U.S. Public Health Service

Contents

Introduction

Practical and Effective Asthma Care

This *Practical Guide for the Diagnosis and Management of Asthma* describes how primary care clinicians can improve the asthma care they provide within the time constraints of their current clinical practice. More than 130 primary care professionals reviewed this guide to help assure that it is relevant and practical for primary care practitioners.

The recommendations in the Practical Guide are summarized from the National Asthma Education and Prevention Program, *Expert Panel Report 2: Guidelines for the Diagnosis and Management of Asthma* (EPR-2).[1] See page 13 for a summary of some major recommendations from EPR-2.

Asthma Care in the United States Can Be Improved

Undertreatment and inappropriate therapy are major contributors to asthma morbidity and mortality in the United States. A few examples of data that support this assertion are presented below.

- Hospitalizations due to asthma are preventable or avoidable when patients receive appropriate primary care.[2]
  — Asthma is the third leading cause of preventable hospitalizations in the United States.[2]
  — There are about 470,000 hospitalizations and more than 5,000 deaths a year from asthma.

- Studies from two metropolitan areas of children with asthma who used the emergency department[3] and adults hospitalized with asthma[4] found that:
  — Less than half of these patients were receiving anti-inflammatory therapy as recommended in the EPR-2.[1]
  — Only 28 percent of the adult patients hospitalized for asthma had written action plans that told how to manage their asthma and control an exacerbation.[4]

The Practical Guide will help clinicians improve the asthma care they provide and reduce the hospitalizations and emergency department visits needed by their patients.

Airway Inflammation Plays a Central Role in Asthma and Its Management

The management of asthma needs to be responsive to the characteristics that define asthma. The relationships between these characteristics are illustrated in figure 1.

- **Asthma is a chronic inflammatory disorder of the airways.** Many cells and cellular elements play a role, in particular, mast cells, eosinophils, T-lymphocytes, macrophages, neutrophils, and epithelial cells.

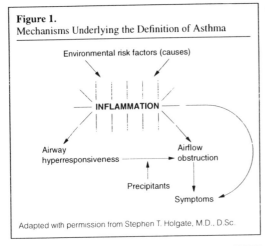

Figure 1.
Mechanisms Underlying the Definition of Asthma

Adapted with permission from Stephen T. Holgate, M.D., D.Sc.

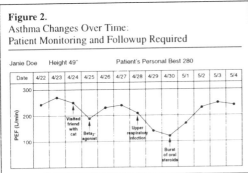

Figure 2.
Asthma Changes Over Time:
Patient Monitoring and Followup Required

- **Environmental and other factors "cause" or provoke the airway inflammation in people with asthma.** Examples of these factors include inhaled allergens to which the patient is sensitive, some irritants, and viruses. This inflammation is always present to some degree, regardless of the level of asthma severity.

- **Airway inflammation causes recurrent episodes** in asthma patients of wheezing, breathlessness, chest tightness, and coughing, particularly at night and in the early morning.

- These episodes of asthma symptoms are usually associated with widespread but **variable airflow obstruction that is often reversible** either spontaneously or with treatment. Airflow obstruction is caused by a variety of changes in the airway, including bronchoconstriction, airway edema, chronic mucus plug formation, and airway remodeling.

- **Inflammation causes an associated increase in the existing airway hyperresponsiveness** to a variety of stimuli, such as allergens, irritants, cold air, and viruses. These stimuli or **precipitants result in airflow obstruction** and asthma symptoms in the patient with asthma.

Asthma Changes Over Time, Requiring Active Management

The condition of a patient's asthma will change depending on the environment, patient activities, management practices, and other factors (see figure 2). Thus, even when patients have their asthma under control, monitoring and treatment are needed to maintain control.

Four Key Components for Long-Term Control of Asthma

The four components of asthma therapy respond to the basic nature of asthma described previously. The four components are listed below and will be described in this guide.

Assessment and monitoring

Pharmacologic therapy

Control of factors contributing to asthma severity

Patient education for a partnership

References

In EPR-2, the Expert Panel cites the scientific literature to support its recommendations or clearly indicates they are "based on the opinion of the Expert Panel." The Panel submitted multiple drafts of EPR-2 for review by more than 140 outside reviewers, including members of the NAEPP Coordinating Committee. This Practical Guide summarizes the recommendations in EPR-2, provides practical information to aid the implementation of those recommendations, and cites selected references from EPR-2. For complete documentation of the recommendations, refer to EPR-2. Copies of the full report can be accessed through the Internet (http://www.nhlbi.nih.gov/nhlbi/lung/asthma/ prof/asthgdln.htm) or purchased from the NHLBI Information Center, P.O. Box 30105, Bethesda, MD 20824-0105 (phone 301-251-1222; fax 301-251-1223).

This guide presents basic recommendations for the diagnosis and management of asthma that will help clinicians and patients make appropriate decisions about asthma care. Of course, the clinician and patient need to develop an individual treatment plan that is tailored to the specific needs of the patient. This report is not an official regulatory document of any Government agency.

Major Recommendations From the *Expert Panel Report 2: Guidelines for the Diagnosis and Management of Asthma* [1]

Diagnose asthma and initiate partnership with patient.

- **Diagnose** asthma by establishing:
  — A history of recurrent symptoms,
  — Reversible airflow obstruction using spirometry, and
  — The exclusion of alternative diagnoses.

- **Establish patient-clinician partnership.**
  — Address patient's concerns.
  — Agree upon the goals of asthma therapy.
  — Agree upon a written action plan for patient self-management.

Reduce inflammation, symptoms, and exacerbations.

- **Prescribe anti-inflammatory medications to patients with mild, moderate, or severe persistent asthma** (i.e., inhaled steroids, cromolyn, or nedocromil).

- **Reduce exposures to precipitants of asthma symptoms.**
  — Assess patient's exposure and sensitivity to individual precipitants (e.g., allergens, irritants).
  — Provide written and verbal instructions on how to avoid or reduce factors that make the patient's asthma worse.

Monitor and manage asthma over time.

- **Train all patients to monitor their asthma.**
  — All patients should monitor symptoms.
  — Patients with moderate-to-severe persistent asthma should also monitor their peak flow.

- **See patients at least every 1 to 6 months**
  — Assess attainment of goals of asthma therapy and patient's concerns,
  — Adjust treatment, if needed,
  — Review the action plan with patient, and
  — Check patient's inhaler and peak flow technique.

Treat asthma episodes promptly.

- Prompt use of short-acting inhaled beta$_2$-agonists and, if episode is moderate to severe, a 3- to 10-day course of oral steroids.

- Prompt communication and followup with clinician.

1. Initial Assessment and Diagnosis of Asthma

Diagnosis of Asthma in Adults and Children Over 5 Years of Age

Recurrent episodes of coughing or wheezing are almost always due to asthma in both children and adults. Cough can be the sole symptom.

Findings that increase the probability of asthma include:

Medical history:

- Episodic wheeze, chest tightness, shortness of breath, or cough.

- Symptoms worsen in presence of aeroallergens, irritants, or exercise.

- Symptoms occur or worsen at night, awakening the patient.

- Patient has allergic rhinitis or atopic dermatitis.

- Close relatives have asthma, allergy, sinusitis, or rhinitis.

Physical examination of the upper respiratory tract, chest, and skin:

- Hyperexpansion of the thorax

- Sounds of wheezing during normal breathing or a prolonged phase of forced exhalation

- Increased nasal secretions, mucosal swelling, sinusitis, rhinitis, or nasal polyps

- Atopic dermatitis/eczema or other signs of allergic skin problems

▷ Assessment and monitoring

Pharmacologic therapy

Control of factors contributing to asthma severity

▷ Patient education for a partnership

To establish an asthma diagnosis, determine the following:

1. **History or presence of episodic symptoms of airflow obstruction** (i.e., wheeze, shortness of breath, tightness in the chest, or cough). Asthma symptoms vary throughout the day; absence of symptoms at the time of the examination does not exclude the diagnosis of asthma.

2. **Airflow obstruction is at least partially reversible.** Use spirometry to:

   Establish airflow obstruction: FEV_1 <80 percent predicted; FEV_1/FVC* <65 percent or below the lower limit of normal. (If obstruction is absent, see Additional Tests, page 16.)

   Establish reversibility: FEV_1 increases ≥12 percent and at least 200 mL after using a short-acting inhaled beta$_2$-agonist (e.g., albuterol, terbutaline).

   NOTE: Older adults may need to take oral steroids for 2 to 3 weeks and then take the spirometry test to measure the degree of reversibility achieved. Chronic bronchitis and emphysema may coexist with asthma in adults. The degree of reversibility indicates the degree to which asthma therapy may be beneficial.

3. **Alternative diagnoses are excluded** (e.g., vocal cord dysfunction, vascular rings, foreign bodies, or other pulmonary diseases). See page 16 for additional tests that may be needed.

   In general, FEV_1 predicted norms or reference values used for children should also be used for adolescents.

   ---

   *FEV_1, forced expiratory volume in 1 second
   FVC, forced vital capacity

Diagnosis in Infants and Children Younger Than 5 Years of Age

Because children with asthma are often mislabeled as having bronchiolitis, bronchitis, or pneumonia, many do not receive adequate therapy.

- The diagnostic steps listed previously are the same for this age group except that spirometry is not possible. A trial of asthma medications may aid in the eventual diagnosis.

- **Diagnosis is not needed to *begin* to treat wheezing associated with an upper respiratory viral infection, which is the most common precipitant of wheezing in this age group.** Patients should be monitored carefully.

- There are two general patterns of illness in infants and children who have wheezing with acute viral upper respiratory infections: a remission of symptoms in the preschool years and persistence of asthma throughout childhood.

Additional Tests for Adults and Children

Additional tests may be needed when asthma is suspected but spirometry is normal, when coexisting conditions are suspected, or for other reasons. These tests can aid diagnosis or confirm suspected contributors to asthma morbidity (e.g., allergens and irritants).

Reasons for Additional Tests	The Tests
• Patient has symptoms but spirometry is normal or near normal	• Assess diurnal variation of peak flow over 1 to 2 weeks. • Refer to a specialist for bronchoprovocation with methacholine, histamine, or exercise; negative test may help rule out asthma.
• Suspect infection, large airway lesions, heart disease, or obstruction by foreign object	• Chest x-ray
• Suspect coexisting chronic obstructive pulmonary disease, restrictive defect, or central airway obstruction	• Additional pulmonary function studies • Diffusing capacity test
• Suspect other factors contribute to asthma (These are not diagnostic tests for asthma.)	• Allergy tests—skin or in vitro • Nasal examination • Gastroesophageal reflux assessment

The factors associated with continuing asthma are allergies, a family history of asthma, and perinatal exposure to aeroallergens and passive smoke.

Patient Education After Diagnosis

Identify the concerns the patient has about being diagnosed with asthma by asking: "What worries you most about having asthma? What concerns do you have about your asthma?"

Address the patient's concerns and make at least these key points (see patient handout, "What Everyone Should Know About Asthma Control"):

- **Asthma can be managed and the patient can live a normal life.**

- **Asthma can be controlled when the patient works together with the medical staff.** The patient plays a big role in monitoring asthma, taking medications, and avoiding things that can cause asthma episodes.

- **Asthma is a chronic lung disease characterized by inflammation of the airways.** There may be periods when there are no symptoms, but the airways are swollen and sensitive to some degree all of the time. Long-term anti-inflammatory medications are important to control airway inflammation.

- **Many things in the home, school, work, or elsewhere can cause asthma attacks** (e.g., secondhand tobacco smoke, allergens, irritants). An asthma attack (also called episodes, flareups, or exacerbations) occurs when airways narrow, making it harder to breathe.

- **Asthma requires long-term care and monitoring.** Asthma cannot be cured, but it can be controlled. Asthma can get better or worse over time and requires treatment changes.

Patient education should begin at the time of diagnosis and continue at every visit.

Assessment of Asthma Severity

See figure 3 on page 23 to estimate the severity of chronic asthma in patients of all age groups. These levels of severity correspond to the "steps" of pharmacologic therapy discussed later.

General Guidelines for Referral to an Asthma Specialist

Based on the opinion of the Expert Panel, referral for consultation or care to a specialist in asthma care is recommended if assistance is needed for:

- **Diagnosis and assessment** (e.g., differential diagnosis is problematic, other conditions aggravate asthma, or confirmation is needed on the contribution of occupational or environmental exposures)

- **Specialized treatment and education** (e.g., considering patient for immunotherapy or providing additional education for allergen avoidance)

- **Other cases:**
  - Patient is not meeting the goals of asthma therapy (defined in next section) after 3 to 6 months. An earlier referral or consultation is appropriate if the physician concludes that the patient is unresponsive to therapy.
  - Life-threatening asthma exacerbation occurred.
  - Patient requires step 4 care (see figure 4 on page 24) or has used more than two bursts of oral steroids in 1 year. (Referral may be considered for patients requiring step 3 care.)
  - Patient is younger than age 3 and requires step 3 or 4 care. Referral should be considered for patients under age 3 who require step 2 care (see figure 5 on page 25).

An asthma specialist is usually a fellowship-trained allergist or pulmonologist or, occasionally, a physician with expertise in asthma management developed through additional training and experience.

Patients with significant psychiatric, psychosocial, or family problems that interfere with their asthma therapy should be referred to an appropriate mental health professional for counseling or treatment.

2. Pharmacologic Therapy: Managing Asthma Long Term

Assessment and monitoring

Pharmacologic therapy

Control of factors contributing to asthma severity

Patient education for a partnership

Establish the Goals of Asthma Therapy With the Patient

The goals of asthma therapy provide the criteria that the clinician and patient will use to evaluate the patient's response to therapy. The goals will provide the focus for all subsequent interactions with the patient.

First, determine the patient's personal goals of therapy by asking a few questions, such as: "What would you like to be able to do that you can't do now or can't do well because of your asthma?" "What would you like to accomplish with your asthma treatment?"

Then, share the general goals of asthma therapy with the patient and the family.

Finally, agree on the goals you and the patient will set as the foundation for the patient's treatment plan.

The Asthma Medications: Long-Term Control and Quick Relief

General Goals of Asthma Therapy

- **Prevent chronic asthma symptoms and asthma exacerbations during the day and night.** (Indicators: No sleep disruption by asthma. No missed school or work due to asthma. No or minimal need for emergency department visits or hospitalizations.)

- **Maintain normal activity levels**—including exercise and other physical activities.

- **Have normal or near-normal lung function.**

- **Be satisfied with the asthma care received.**

- **Have no or minimal side effects** while receiving optimal medications.

- **Long-term-control asthma medications are taken daily to achieve and maintain control of persistent asthma** (for dosage information, see pages 54–56). The most effective long-term-control medications for asthma are those that reduce inflammation. Inhaled steroids are the most potent inhaled anti-inflammatory medication currently available (see next page).

  Inhaled steroids are generally well tolerated and safe at recommended doses. To reduce the potential for adverse effects, **patients taking inhaled steroids should:**
  — Use a spacer/holding chamber.
  — Rinse and spit following inhalation.
  — Use the lowest possible dose to maintain control. Consider adding a long-acting inhaled beta$_2$-agonist to a low-to-medium dose of inhaled steroid rather than using a higher dose of inhaled steroid.[17,18]

Inhaled Steroids: The Most Effective Long-Term-Control Medication for Asthma

The daily use of inhaled steroids results in the following:[5,6,10-16]

- Asthma symptoms will diminish. Improvement will continue gradually (see study 1).

- Occurrence of severe exacerbations is greatly reduced.

- Use of quick-relief medication decreases (see study 2).

- Lung function improves significantly, as measured by peak flow, FEV_1, and airway hyperresponsiveness.

Problems due to asthma may return if patients stop taking inhaled steroids.

Frequency of dosing

Once-daily dosing with inhaled steroids for patients with mild asthma and twice-a-day dosing for many other patients, even with high doses of some preparations, have been effective.[7-9]

Study 1.

Daily Inhaled Steroids Control Moderate Persistent Asthma in Children 7 to 16 Years Old: Reduced Symptomatic Days*

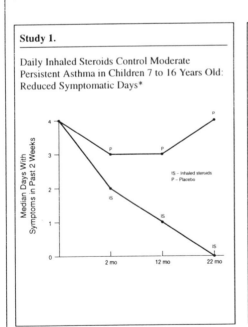

Study 2.

Inhaled Steroids Control Asthma in Adults: Significant Reduction in Need for Quick-Relief Medicine*

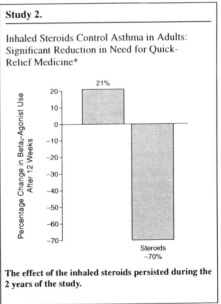

The effect of the inhaled steroids persisted during the 2 years of the study.

---

*Other endpoints—FEV_1, peak flow, airway hyperresponsiveness, and symptoms—significantly improved relative to the placebo group over 22 months of the children's study (N=116)[5] and over 2 years in the adult study (N=103).[6]

- **Quick-relief medications are used to provide prompt treatment of acute airflow obstruction and its accompanying symptoms** such as cough, chest tightness, shortness of breath, and wheezing. These medications include short-acting inhaled beta$_2$-agonists and oral steroids. Anticholinergics are included in special circumstances.

Stepwise Approach to Managing Asthma in Adults and in Children Over 5 Years of Age

All patients need to have a short-acting inhaled beta$_2$-agonist to take as needed for symptoms. Patients with mild, moderate, or severe persistent asthma require daily long-term-control medication to control their asthma.

See figure 4 for the recommended pharmacologic therapy at each level of asthma severity and pages 54–56 for dosage information. Also, see the glossary for the brand names of the medications mentioned in this guide.

Gaining Control of Asthma

The physician's judgment of an individual patient's needs and circumstances will determine at what step to initiate therapy. There are two appropriate approaches to gaining control of asthma:

- Start treatment at the step appropriate to the severity of the patient's asthma at the time of evaluation. If control is not achieved, gradually step up therapy until control is achieved and maintained.

OR

- At the onset, give therapy at a higher level to achieve rapid control and then step down to the minimum therapy needed to maintain control. A higher level of therapy can be accomplished by either adding a course of oral steroids to inhaled steroids, cromolyn, or nedocromil or using a higher dose of inhaled steroids.

- In the opinion of the Expert Panel, the **preferred approach is to start with more intensive therapy** in order to more rapidly suppress airway inflammation and thus gain prompt control.

If control is not achieved with initial therapy (e.g., within 1 month), the step selected, the therapy in the step, and possibly the diagnosis should be reevaluated.

Maintaining Control

Increases or decreases in medications may be needed as asthma severity and control vary over time. The Expert Panel's opinion is that **followup visits every 1 to 6 months are essential for monitoring asthma.** In addition, patients should be instructed to monitor their symptoms (and peak flow if used) and adjust therapy as described in the action plan (see Patient Handouts).

Step Down Therapy

Gradually reduce or "step down" long-term-control medications after several weeks or months of controlling persistent asthma (i.e., the goals of asthma therapy are achieved). In general, the last medication added to the medical regimen should be the first medication reduced.

Inhaled steroids may be reduced about 25 percent every 2 to 3 months until the lowest dose required to maintain control is reached. For patients with persistent asthma, anti-inflammatory medications should be continued.

For patients who are taking oral steroids daily on a long-term basis, referral for consultation or care by an asthma specialist is recommended. Patients should be closely monitored for adverse side effects. **Continuous attempts should be made to reduce daily use of oral steroids when asthma is controlled:**

- Maintain patients on the lowest possible dose of oral steroids (single dose daily or on alternate days).

- Use high doses of inhaled steroids to eliminate or reduce the need for oral steroids.

Step Up Therapy

The presence of one or more indicators of poor asthma control (see figure 6) **may suggest a need to increase or "step up" therapy.** Before increasing therapy, alternative reasons for poorly controlled asthma should be considered (see figure 7). Referral to a specialist for comanagement or consultation may be appropriate.

The addition of a 3- to 10-day course of oral steroids may be needed to reestablish control during a period of gradual deterioration or a moderate-to-severe exacerbation (see Managing Asthma Exacerbations, page 43). If symptoms do not recur after the course of steroids (and peak flow remains normal), the patient should continue in the same step. However, if the steroid course controls symptoms for less than 1 to 2 weeks, or if courses of steroids are repeated frequently, the patient should move to the next higher step in therapy.

Special Considerations for Infants, Children, and Adolescents

Infants and Preschool Children

Treatment of acute or chronic wheezing or cough should follow the stepwise approach presented in figure 5. In general, physicians should do the following when infants and young children consistently require treatment for symptoms more than two times per week:

- Prescribe daily inhaled anti-inflammatory medication (inhaled steroids, cromolyn, or nedocromil) as long-term-control asthma therapy. A trial of cromolyn or nedocromil is often given to patients with mild persistent asthma.

Figure 3.

Classification of Asthma Severity: Clinical Features Before Treatment

	Days With Symptoms	Nights With Symptoms	PEF or FEV_1*	PEF Variablity
Step 4 Severe Persistent	Continual	Frequent	≤60%	>30%
Step 3 Moderate Persistent	Daily	≥5/month	>60%- <80%	>30%
Step 2 Mild Persistent	3-6/week	3-4/month	≥80%	20-30%
Step 1 Mild Intermittent	≤2/week	≤2/month	≥80%	<20%

* Percent predicted values for forced expiratory volume in 1 second (FEV_1) and percent of personal best for peak expiratory flow (PEF) (relevant for children 6 years old or older who can use these devices).

NOTES:
• Patients should be assigned to the most severe step in which *any* feature occurs. Clinical features for individual patients may overlap across steps.
• An individual's classification may change over time.
• Patients at any level of severity of chronic asthma can have mild, moderate, or severe exacerbations of asthma. Some patients with intermittent asthma experience severe and life-threatening exacerbations separated by long periods of normal lung function and no symptoms.
• Patients with two or more asthma exacerbations per week (i.e., progressively worsening symptoms that may last hours or days) tend to have moderate-to-severe persistent asthma.

• Monitor the response to therapy carefully (e.g., frequency of symptoms over 2 to 4 weeks).

• If benefits are sustained for at least 3 months, a step down in therapy should be attempted.

• If clear benefit is not observed, treatment should be stopped. Alternative therapies or diagnoses should be considered.

• Consider oral steroids if an exacerbation caused by a viral respiratory infection is moderate to severe. If the patient has a history of severe exacerbations, consider steroids at the onset of the viral infection.

Medication delivery devices should be selected according to the child's ability to use them. Be aware that the dose received can vary considerably among delivery devices:

• **Children aged 2 or less**—nebulizer therapy is preferred for administering cromolyn or high doses of short-acting inhaled beta$_2$-agonists. A metered-dose inhaler (MDI) with a spacer/holding chamber that has a face mask may be used to take inhaled steroids.

Figure 4.

Stepwise Approach for Managing Asthma in Adults and Children Over 5 Years Old: Treatment

Long-Term Control

Preferred treatments are in bold print.

Step 4
Severe
Persistent

Daily medications:
- **Anti-inflammatory: inhaled steroid (high dose)*** AND
- Long-acting bronchodilator: either **long-acting inhaled beta$_2$-agonist** (adult: 2 puffs q 12 hours; child: 1–2 puffs q 12 hours), sustained-release theophylline, or long-acting beta$_2$-agonist tablets AND
- Steroid tablets or syrup long term; make repeated attempts to reduce systemic steroid and maintain control with high-dose inhaled steroid.

Step 3
Moderate
Persistent

Daily medication:
- Either
  —**Anti-inflammatory: inhaled steroid (medium dose)***
  OR
  —**Inhaled steroid (low-to-medium dose)*** and add a long-acting bronchodilator, especially for nighttime symptoms: either **long-acting inhaled beta$_2$-agonist** (adult: 2 puffs q 12 hours; child: 1-2 puffs q 12 hours), sustained-release theophylline, or long-acting beta$_2$-agonist tablets.
- If needed
  —Anti-inflammatory: **inhaled steroids (medium-to-high dose)***
  AND
  —Long-acting bronchodilator, especially for nighttime symptoms; either **long-acting inhaled beta$_2$-agonist**, sustained-release theophylline, or long-acting beta$_2$-agonist tablets.

Step 2
Mild
Persistent

Daily medication:
- **Anti-inflammatory: either inhaled steroid (low dose)* or cromolyn** (adult: 2–4 puffs tid-qid; child: 1–2 puffs tid-qid) or **nedocromil** (adult: 2–4 puffs bid-qid; child: 1–2 puffs bid-qid) (children usually begin with a trial of cromolyn or nedocromil).
- Sustained-release theophylline to serum concentration of 5–15 mcg/mL is an alternative, but not preferred, therapy. Zafirlukast or zileuton may also be considered for those ≥12 years old, although their position in therapy is not fully established.

Step 1
Mild
Intermittent

- No daily medication needed.

Quick-Relief

All Patients

Short-acting bronchodilator: **inhaled beta$_2$-agonist** (2–4 puffs) as needed for symptoms. Intensity of treatment will depend on severity of exacerbation.

*See Estimated Comparative Daily Dosages for Inhaled Steroids on page 56.

NOTES:
- *The stepwise approach presents general guidelines to assist clinical decisionmaking. Asthma is highly variable; clinicians should tailor medication plans to the needs of individual patients.*
- Gain control as quickly as possible. Either start with aggressive therapy (e.g., *add* a course of oral steroids or a higher dose of inhaled steroids to the therapy that corresponds to the patient's initial step of severity); or start at the step that corresponds to the patient's initial severity and step up treatment, if necessary.
- **Step down:** Review treatment every 1 to 6 months. Gradually decrease treatment to the least medication necessary to maintain control.
- **Step up:** If control is not maintained, consider step up. Inadequate control is indicated by increased use of short-acting beta$_2$-agonists and in: step 1 when patient uses a short-acting beta$_2$-agonist more than two times a week; steps 2 and 3 when patient uses short-acting beta$_2$-agonist on a daily basis or more than three to four times in 1 day. But before stepping up: Review patient inhaler technique, compliance, and environmental control (avoidance of allergens or other precipitant factors).
- A course of oral steroids may be needed at any time and at any step.
- Patients with exercise-induced bronchospasm should take two to four puffs of an inhaled beta$_2$-agonist 5 to 60 minutes before exercise.
- Referral to an asthma specialist for consultation or comanagement is *recommended* if there is difficulty maintaining control or if the patient requires step 4 care. Referral may be *considered* for step 3 care.
- For a list of brand names, see glossary.

Figure 5.

Stepwise Approach for Managing Infants and Young Children (5 Years of Age and Younger) With Acute or Chronic Asthma Symptoms

Long-Term Control

Step 4
Severe
Persistent

- Daily anti-inflammatory medication
  - High-dose inhaled steroid* with spacer and face mask
  - If needed, add oral steroids (2 mg/kg/day); reduce to lowest daily or alternate-day dose that stabilizes symptoms

Step 3
Moderate Persistent

- Daily anti-inflammatory medication. Either:
  - Medium-dose inhaled steroid* with spacer and face mask
  Once control is established, consider:
  - Lower medium-dose inhaled steroid* with spacer and face mask and nedocromil (1–2 puffs bid-qid)
  OR
  - Lower medium-dose inhaled steroid* with spacer and face mask and theophylline (10 mg/kg/day up to 16 mg/kg/day for children ≥1 year of age, to a serum concentration of 5–15 mcg/mL)**

Step 2
Mild
Persistent

- Daily anti-inflammatory medication.
  - Infants and young children usually begin with a trial of cromolyn (nebulizer is preferred—1 ampule tid-qid; or MDI—1–2 puffs tid-qid) or nedocromil (MDI only—1–2 puffs bid-qid)
  OR
  - Low-dose inhaled steroid* with spacer and face mask

Step 1
Mild
Intermittent

- No daily medication needed.

Quick-Relief

All Patients

Bronchodilator as needed for symptoms: Short-acting inhaled beta$_2$-agonist by nebulizer (0.05 mg/kg in 2–3 cc of saline) or inhaler with face mask and spacer (2–4 puffs; for exacerbations, repeat q 20 minutes for up to 1 hour) or oral beta$_2$-agonist.

With viral respiratory infection, use short-acting inhaled beta$_2$-agonist q 4 to 6 hours up to 24 hours (longer with physician consult) but, in general, if repeated more than once every 6 weeks, consider moving to next step up. Consider oral steroids if the exacerbation is moderate to severe or at the onset of the infection if the patient has a history of severe exacerbations.

* See Estimated Comparative Dosages for Inhaled Steroids on page 56
** For children <1 year of age: usual max mg/kg/day = 0.2 (age in weeks) + 5.

NOTES:
- *The stepwise approach presents general guidelines to assist clinical decisionmaking. Asthma is highly variable; clinicians should tailor medication plans to the needs of individual patients.*
- **Gain control** as quickly as possible. Either start with aggressive therapy (e.g., *add* a course of oral steroids or a higher dose of inhaled steroids to the therapy that corresponds to the patient's initial step of severity); or start at the step that corresponds to the patient's initial severity and step up treatment, if necessary.
- **Step down.** Review treatment every 1 to 6 months. If control is sustained for at least 3 months, a gradual stepwise reduction in treatment may be possible.
- **Step up.** If control is not achieved, consider step up. Inadequate control is indicated by increased use of short-acting beta$_2$-agonists and in: step 1 when patient uses a short-acting beta$_2$-agonist more than two times a week; steps 2 and 3 when patient uses short-acting beta$_2$-agonist on a daily basis OR more than three to four times a day. But before stepping up: review patient inhaler technique, compliance, and environmental control (avoidance of allergens or other precipitant factors).
- A course of oral steroids (prednisolone) may be needed at any time and step.
- Referral to an asthma specialist for consultation or comanagement is *recommended* for patients requiring step 3 or 4 care. Referral may be *considered* for step 2 care.
- For a list of brand names, see glossary.

- **Children 3 to 5 years of age**—MDI plus spacer/holding chamber may be used by many children of this age. If the desired therapeutic effects are not achieved, a nebulizer or an MDI plus spacer/holding chamber with a face mask may be required.

Spacers/holding chambers are devices that hold the aerosol medication so the patient can inhale it easily. This reduces the problem of coordinating the actuation of the MDI with the inhalation. Spacers/holding chambers come in many different shapes. These devices are not simply tubes that put space between the patient's mouth and the MDI. Examples of spacers/holding chambers are illustrated in the box on page 27.

Parents or caregivers need to be instructed in the proper use of appropriately sized face masks, spacers with face masks, and holding chamber devices. Acceptable use of the delivery device should be demonstrated in the office before the patient leaves. The ability of children to use the devices may vary widely.

School-Age Children and Adolescents

The pharmacologic management of school-age children and adolescents follows the same basic principles as those for adults, but with special consideration of growth, school, and social development.

- **Cromolyn or nedocromil is often tried first in children with mild or moderate persistent asthma.** This is because these medications are often effective anti-inflammatory therapies and have no known long-term systemic effects.

Figure 6.

Indicators of Poor Asthma Control—Consider Increasing Long-Term Medications*

- Awakened at night with symptoms
- An urgent care visit
- Patient has increased need for short-acting inhaled beta$_2$-agonists (excludes use for upper respiratory viral infections and exercise-induced bronchospasm) OR
  — At step 1: Used short-acting inhaled beta$_2$-agonists more than two times in a week
  — At steps 2–3: Used short-acting inhaled beta$_2$-agonists more than three to four times a day OR used this medication on a daily basis for a week or less
  — Patient used more than one canister of short-acting inhaled beta$_2$-agonist in one month

* This may mean a temporary increase in anti-inflammatory medication to regain control or a "step up" in long-term therapy. This will depend on the frequency of the above events, reasons for poor control (see figure 7), and the clinician's judgment.

Figure 7.

Assess Reasons for Poor Asthma Control Before Increasing Medications—ICE

• **Inhaler technique**	Check patient's technique.
• **Compliance**	Ask when and how much medication the patient is taking.
• **Environment**	Ask patient if something in his or her environment has changed.

Also consider:

• **Alternative diagnosis**	Assess patient for presence of concomitant upper respiratory disease or alternative diagnosis.

- **For children with severe persistent asthma, and for many with moderate persistent asthma, inhaled steroids are necessary for long-term-control therapy.** Cromolyn and nedocromil do not provide adequate control for these patients. See stepwise approach to pharmacotherapy (figure 4 on page 24) for treatment recommendations.

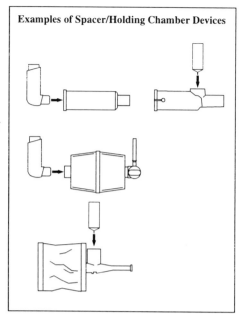

Examples of Spacer/Holding Chamber Devices

Inhaled Steroids and Growth

The potential but small risk of adverse effects on linear growth from the use of inhaled steroids is well balanced by their efficacy. Poor asthma control itself can result in retarded linear growth. Most studies do not demonstrate a negative effect on growth with dosages of 400 to 800 mcg a day of beclomethasone,[21-23] although a few short-term studies have.[24,25] Adverse effects on linear growth appear to be dose dependent. High doses of inhaled steroids have greater potential for growth suppression, but less potential than the alternative of oral steroids. Some caution (e.g., monitoring growth, stepping down therapy when possible) is suggested while this issue is studied further.

Action Plan for Schools

The clinician should prepare a written action plan for the student's school that explains when medications may be needed to treat episodes and to prevent exercise-induced bronchospasm. Recommendations to limit exposures to offending allergens or irritants and a written request for the child to carry quick-relief medications at school could be helpful. When possible, schedule daily medications so they do not need to be taken at school. (See patient handout, "School Self-Management Plan")

Managing Asthma in Older Adults

- Make adjustments or avoid asthma medications that can aggravate other conditions:
  - **Inhaled steroids.** Give supplements of calcium (1,000 to 1,500 mg per day), vitamin D (400 units a day), and, where appropriate, estrogen replacement therapy, especially for women using high doses of inhaled steroids.
  - **Oral steroids** may provoke confusion, agitation, and changes in glucose metabolism.

— **Theophylline and epinephrine** may exacerbate underlying heart conditions. Also, the risk of theophylline overdose may be higher because of reduced theophylline clearance in older patients.

- Inform patients about potential adverse effects on their asthma from medications used for other conditions, for example:
  — **Aspirin and other oral nonsteroidal anti-inflammatory medications** (arthritis, pain relief)
  — **Nonselective beta-blockers** (high blood pressure)
  — **Beta-blockers in some eye drops** (glaucoma)

- Chronic bronchitis and emphysema may coexist with asthma. A 2- to 3-week trial with oral steroids can help determine the presence of reversibility of airway obstruction and indicate the extent of potential benefit from asthma therapy.

Managing Special Situations

Managing Exercise-Induced Bronchospasm

Exercise-induced bronchospasm generally begins during exercise and reaches its peak 5 to 10 minutes after stopping. The symptoms often spontaneously resolve in another 20 to 30 minutes.

A diagnosis of exercise-induced bronchospasm is suggested by a history of cough, shortness of breath, chest pain or tightness, wheezing, or endurance problems during and after vigorous activity. The diagnosis can be confirmed by an objective measure of the problem (i.e., a 15 percent decrease in peak flow or FEV_1 between measurements taken before and after vigorous activity at 5-minute intervals for 20 to 30 minutes.)

For the vast majority of patients, exercise-induced bronchospasm should not limit either participation or success in vigorous activities. The following are the **recommended control measures:**

- **Two to four puffs of short-acting beta$_2$-agonist 5 to 60 minutes before exercise,** preferably as close to the start of exercise as possible. The effects of this pretreatment should last approximately 2 to 3 hours. A long-acting inhaled beta$_2$-agonist taken at least 30 minutes before exercise will last 10 to 12 hours.[26] Cromolyn or nedocromil can also be used before exercise with a duration of effect of 1 to 2 hours.[27–29]

- **A 6- to 10-minute warmup period before exercise** may benefit patients who can tolerate continuous exercise with minimal symptoms. The warmup may preclude a need for repeated medications.

- **Increase in long-term-control medications, if appropriate.** If symptoms occur with usual activities or exercise, a step up in long-term-control therapy may be warranted. Long-term control of asthma with anti-inflammatory medication (i.e., inhaled steroid, cromolyn, or nedocromil) can reduce the frequency and severity of exercise-induced bronchospasm.[30]

Teachers and coaches need to be notified that a child has exercise-induced bronchospasm. They should be told that the child is able to participate in activities but may need inhaled medication before activity. Athletes should disclose the medications they use and adhere to standards set by the U.S. Olympic Committee.[31] A complete, easy-to-use list of prohibited and approved medications can be obtained from the U.S. Olympic Committee's Drug Control Hotline (1-800-233-0393).

Managing Seasonal Asthma Symptoms

- **During the allergy season:** Use the stepwise approach to the long-term management of asthma to control symptoms.

- **Before the season:** If symptoms during a season are predictable, start daily anti-inflammatory therapy (inhaled steroids, cromolyn, or nedocromil) just before the anticipated onset of symptoms and continue this throughout the season.

Managing Asthma in Patients Undergoing Surgery

- Evaluate the patient's asthma over the past 6 months.

- Improve lung function to predicted values before surgery, possibly with a short course of oral steroids.

- Give patients who have received oral steroids for longer than 2 weeks during the past 6 months 100 mg of hydrocortisone every 8 hours intravenously during the surgical period. Reduce the dose rapidly within 24 hours following surgery.

Managing Asthma in Pregnant Women

Management of asthma in pregnant women is essential and is achieved with basically the same treatment as for nonpregnant women. Poorly controlled asthma during pregnancy can result in reduced oxygen supply to the fetus, increased perinatal mortality, increased prematurity, and low birth weight.[32] There is little to suggest an increased risk to the fetus for most drugs used to treat asthma.

Drugs or drug classes with potential risk to the fetus include brompheniramine, epinephrine, and alpha-adrenergic compounds (other than pseudoephedrine),[33-35] decongestants (other than pseudoephedrine), antibiotics (tetracycline, sulfona-mides, and ciprofloxacine), live virus vaccines, immunotherapy (initiation or increase in doses), and iodides.

3. Control of Factors Contributing to Asthma Severity

Avoiding or controlling factors that contribute to asthma severity will reduce symptoms and the need for medications. (See figure 8).

Assessment and monitoring

Pharmacologic therapy

▶ Control of factors contributing to asthma severity

▶ Patient education for a partnership

Patient Assessment and Education

Have each patient complete the "Patient Self-Assessment Form for Environmental and Other Factors That Can Make Asthma Worse" to assess exposures and identify factors that may contribute to asthma severity.

Educate patients in how to reduce their exposures to these factors (see patient handout, "How To Control Things That Make Your Asthma Worse," and box on page 33). Confirm suspected occupational exposures by having the patient record over 2 to 3 weeks symptoms, exposures, bronchodilator use, and peak flow at and away from work.

Inhaled Allergens and Persistent Asthma

To reduce the effects of specific allergens on a patient with persistent asthma (see figure 9):

- **Identify the specific allergens to which patient is exposed** (use "Patient Self-Assessment Form for Environmental and Other Factors That Can Make Asthma Worse").

Figure 8.

Allergen Control Significantly Improves Even Mild Asthma: An Illustrative Study with House-Dust Mites

Many studies support the effectiveness of allergen control in improving asthma and reducing the need for medication.[36-39] The controlled study of 20 children with mild asthma and house-dust mite allergy illustrates the effect control measures can have.[39]

- Major components of treatment used in the study:
  - Encased pillows, mattresses, and box springs in allergen-impermeable covers.
  - Washed blankets and mattress pads every 2 weeks in hot water.
  - Removed toys, upholstered furniture, and carpets from bedroom.

- After 1 month, the treatment group had:
  - Symptom days and days needing medicine significantly reduced to a minimal number
  - Airway hyperresponsiveness reduced significantly relative to the control group.

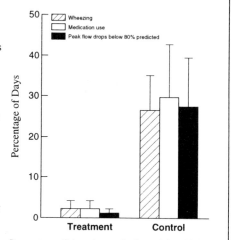

Percentage of days (± standard error) in which wheezing was noticed, medication was used, or peak flow dropped below 80% predicted.[39] Reproduced with permission.

Figure 9.

Determining the Need for Allergen Control in Patients With Persistent Asthma

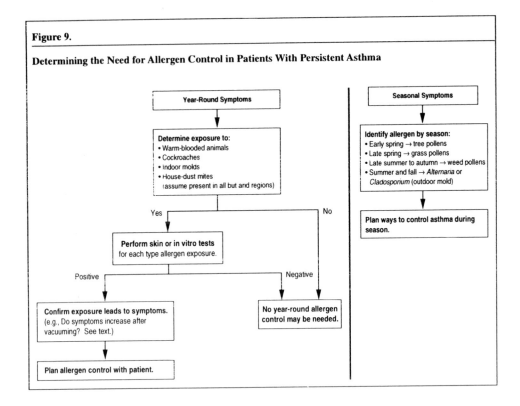

- **Determine and confirm sensitivity to the allergens** (skin or in vitro tests, medical history).

- **Obtain agreement with the patient to initiate one or two simple control measures** (see patient handout, "How To Control Things That Make Your Asthma Worse," and box on page 33).

- **Follow up with patient, adding control measures after first ones are implemented.**

Let the patient know that the benefits of many control measures will take some time to be felt. For dust-mite control it can take less than a month, whereas the benefits from removing an animal from the home may take 6 months or longer to become apparent. This is how long it may take before all the dander is out of the environment.

Allergy Testing

Skin or in vitro (e.g., RAST) tests are *alternative* methods to assess the sensitivity to the year-round allergens to which patients with persistent asthma are exposed (i.e., animal, house-dust mite, cockroach, or indoor mold allergens). Allergy testing is the only reliable way to determine sensitivity to year-round indoor allergens[40,41] and is important for justifying the expense and effort involved in implementing environmental controls. Allergy tests also reinforce

Control Measures for Factors Contributing to Asthma Severity

Factors Contributing to Asthma Severity	Control Measures: Instructions to Patients
Allergens	See patient handout, "How To Control Things That Make Your Asthma Worse."
Tobacco smoke	Strongly advise patient and others living in the home to *stop smoking*. Discuss ways to reduce exposure to other sources of tobacco smoke, such as from day care providers and the workplace.
Rhinitis	Intranasal steroids. Antihistamine/decongestant combinations may also be used.
Sinusitis	Medical measures to promote drainage. Antibiotic therapy is appropriate when complicating acute bacterial infection is present.
Gastroesophageal reflux	No eating within 3 hours of bedtime, head of bed elevated 6 to 8 inches, and appropriate medications (e.g., H_2-antagonist).
Sulfite sensitivity	No eating of shrimp, dried fruit, processed potatoes. No drinking of beer or wine.
Medication interactions	No beta-blockers (including ophthalmological preparations).
	Aspirin and other nonsteroidal anti-inflammatory medications. Inform adult patients with severe persistent asthma, nasal polyps, or a history of aspirin sensitivity about the risk of severe and even fatal episodes from using these drugs. Usually safe alternatives are acetaminophen or salsalate.
Occupational exposures	Discuss with asthma patients the importance of avoidance, ventilation, respiratory protection, and a tobacco smoke-free environment. If occupationally induced asthma, recommend complete cessation of exposure to initiating agent. Obtain permission from patient before contacting management or onsite health professionals about workplace exposure.
Viral respiratory infections	Annual influenza vaccinations should be given to patients with persistent asthma.

for the patients the need to take environmental control measures. Whether skin or in vitro tests are used will probably depend on whether the physician is knowledgeable about skin testing technique.

Order tests only for those substances to which you have determined the patient is exposed (i.e., do not order a panel of tests). **When allergy tests are positive, ask patients about the onset of symptoms when they are in contact with the allergen.** Positive answers to these questions confirm the likelihood that the allergy is contributing to asthma symptoms. However, lack of a positive response to these questions does not exclude the possibility that the allergen may be contributing to the patient's symptoms.

- **For animals and dust mites:** "Do nasal, eye, or chest symptoms occur in a room where carpets are being or have just been vacuumed?"

- **For indoor mold:** "Do nasal, eye, or chest symptoms appear when in damp or moldy rooms, such as basements?"

Immunotherapy

In the opinion of the Expert Panel and based on the evidence,[42-46] allergen immunotherapy may be considered for asthma patients when (1) there is clear evidence of a relationship between symptoms and exposure to an unavoidable allergen to which the patient is sensitive, (2) symptoms occur all year or during a major portion of the year, and (3) there is difficulty controlling symptoms with pharmacologic management because multiple medications are required or medications are ineffective or not accepted by the patient. The course of allergen immunotherapy is typically of 3 to 5 years' duration. If use of allergen immunotherapy is elected, it should be administered only in a medical office where facilities and trained personnel are available to treat any life-threatening reaction that can, but rarely does, occur.[47,48] In the Expert Panel's opinion, referral to an allergist should be made when patients are being considered for immunotherapy.

4. Periodic Assessment and Monitoring

▶ Assessment and monitoring

Pharmacologic therapy

Control of factors contributing to asthma severity

▶ Patient education for a partnership

Periodic clinical assessments every 1 to 6 months and patient self-monitoring are essential for asthma care because:

- Asthma symptoms and severity change, requiring changes in therapy.

- Patients' exposure to precipitants of asthma will change.

- Patients' memories and self-management practices fade with time. Reinforcement, review, and reminders are needed.

The frequency of patient visits depends on the severity of the asthma and the patient's ability to control and monitor symptoms. The first followup visit usually needs to be sooner than 1 month.

Working Within the Time Constraints of the Typical Office Visit

Each physician develops his or her own way of accomplishing the periodic assessment and patient education (see box on page 36 for an example). Here are ways some primary care physicians have been able to perform the recommended periodic assessment and patient education within the time constraints of routine office visits:

- **Give patients an assessment questionnaire to complete in the waiting room.** The answers to these questions determine the issues to be addressed during that visit. See "Patient Self-Assessment Form for Followup Visits" on page 70 for such an assessment questionnaire. This helps set priorities to be addressed.

- **Have patients come back to the office more often, especially at the beginning.** Break the assessment and education the patient needs into segments and perform these over a number of visits. For example, after the diagnosis of asthma, a patient could be given the "Patient Self-Assessment Form for Environmental and Other Factors That Can Make Asthma Worse" to be completed at home. A visit in a week or so could be set to review the form and your recommendations to the patient. Similarly, initial education on the use of a peak flow meter and action plan might be scheduled for a separate visit. An example of how the necessary patient education can be divided and conducted across visits is outlined in figure 10 on page 40. Review this and make adjustments, as needed, for your own practice.

- **Use nurses or office staff to do some of the tasks,** like checking MDI technique.

- Some managed care organizations have a home case manager to do followup assessments and education.

Patient Self-Monitoring

All patients should be taught to recognize symptoms and what to do when symptoms occur (see patient handout, "Asthma Action Plan"). Review the information in the Asthma Action Plan often, optimally at each office visit.

Long-term daily peak flow monitoring is recommended for those with moderate or severe persistent asthma or patients with a history of severe exacerbations. If long-term daily peak flow monitoring is not used by these patients, short-term monitoring (2 to 3 weeks) can be used to evaluate the severity of exacerbations to guide treatment decisions, evaluate response to changes in long-term treatment, and identify environmental or occupational exposures.

Educate patients on how to use the peak flow meter to help monitor and manage their asthma (see patient handout, "How To Use Your Peak Flow Meter," for details). Ask patients to demonstrate the use of their peak flow meter at every visit and use the reading as part of the clinical assessment. This will take less than a minute and should become a routine component of the clinic visit.

Specific recommendations regarding peak flow monitoring include:

- Use the patient's own personal best peak flow (see patient handout, "How To Use Your Peak Flow Meter") as the standard against which peak flow measurements should be compared.

- Use the same peak flow meter and, when needed, replace with same brand.

Spirometry and Peak Flow Measurement at Office Visits

The Expert Panel recommends that spirometry tests be done (1) at the initial assessment, (2) after treatment has stabilized symptoms and peak flow (to document a baseline of "normal" airway function), and (3) at least every 1 to 2 years when asthma is stable, more often when asthma is unstable, or at other times the clinician believes it is needed.

How I Organized My Visits To Accomplish the Periodic Assessment and Patient Education

- My staff gives asthma patients a self-assessment form to complete in the waiting room.
- My nurse evaluates the patients' inhaler technique and checks their peak flow before they see me.
- I am then able to direct my care to the patients' and families' concerns, problems in achieving the goals of therapy, medication issues, and other concerns I may identify with open-ended questions.

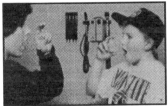

I feel my office has been very successful with this organized approach to the asthma office visit. It obviously required energy to organize the system and practice on the part of myself and my staff to make it work. But the routine periodic assessment and patient education needed for good asthma care are doable in the typical office visit.

Stuart Stoloff, MD
Private Family Practice
Carson City, Nevada

- Measure peak flow first thing in the morning before medications.

- A drop in peak flow below 80 percent of personal best indicates a need for added medications.

- A drop in peak flow below 50 percent of personal best indicates a severe exacerbation.

Clinician Assessment

At each visit, (1) identify patient's concerns about asthma and expectations for the visit, (2) assess achievement of the patient's goals and the general goals of asthma therapy, (3) review medications usage, and (4) teach and reinforce patient's self-management activities (the latter is addressed in the next chapter on "Education for a Partnership in Asthma Care"). These four activities can be achieved within the time constraints of routine medical visits, particularly when the patient completes the "Patient Self-Assessment Form for Followup Visits" in the waiting room.

Identify Patient Concerns and Expectations of the Visit

Review the self-assessment questionnaire and address the patient's concerns during the visit.

Assess Achievement of the Goals of Asthma Therapy

If the patient is not meeting the following goals of asthma therapy, assess the reasons (see figure 7 on page 26) and consider increasing the patient's medications.

Prevent chronic asthma symptoms and asthma exacerbations during the day and night.

- Perform physical examination (respiratory tract).

- Review patient's symptom history at each visit:
  — Daytime symptoms in the past 2 weeks
  — Nighttime symptoms in the past 2 weeks
  — Symptoms while exercising
  — Cause(s) of the symptoms
  — What the patient did to control the symptoms

- Use of quick-relief medications:
  — Number of times short-acting inhaled beta$_2$-agonists are used per week
  — Number of short-acting inhaled beta$_2$-agonist inhalers used in past month

- Emergency or hospital care.

- Missed any work or school due to asthma.

Maintain normal activity levels — including exercise and other physical activities.

- Reduction in usual activities or exercise.

- Disruption of caregivers' or parents' routine by their child's asthma.

Have normal or near-normal lung function.

- Objective measure of lung function—either spirometry or peak flow at each visit (see box on page 36).

- Number of times peak flow went below 80 percent personal best in past 2 weeks, if peak flow monitoring is performed.

Be satisfied with the asthma care received and the level of control—ask patient about this.

Have no or minimal side effects—shakiness, nervousness, bad taste, sore throat, cough, upset stomach—while receiving optimal medications.

Review Medications Usage and Skills

- Ask patients to review for you what medications they are taking, when they take them, and how often.

- Identify any problems patients have had taking medications as prescribed (e.g., missed doses). Note: Patients should bring all of their medications to each office visit.

- Ask patients to demonstrate their use of a placebo inhaler at each followup visit. Assess their performance using the checklist in the patient handout (see patient handout, "How To Use Your Metered-Dose Inhaler the Right Way"). Ask patients to demonstrate use of their peak flow meter, if used.

5. Education for a Partnership in Asthma Care

The goal of all patient education is to help patients take the actions needed to control their asthma.

Assessment and monitoring

Pharmacologic therapy

Control of factors contributing to asthma severity

▶ Patient education for a partnership

These actions are listed below and are described more fully in the patient hand-outs. See figure 10 on page 40 for an example of how to address these issues during routine office visits.

- Taking daily medications for long-term control as prescribed

- Using delivery devices effectively—metered-dose inhalers, spacers, nebulizers

- Identifying and controlling factors that make asthma worse

- Monitoring peak flow and/or symptoms

- Following the written action plan when symptoms or episodes occur

How To Increase the Likelihood of Compliance

Patients cannot be expected to perform a task they never agreed to do or one that is only mentioned once to them. Thus, two essential clinician activities for successful patient education are:

1. **Asking the patient for a verbal, sometimes written, agreement** to take specific action(s). You will need to explain the recommended action(s) and the benefits the patient can expect from doing them.

2. **Following up** and reinforcing the patient for the actions during subsequent visits or phone calls.

Other ways to increase compliance are:

- **Develop an Asthma Action Plan with the patient** (see patient handout). Involve adolescents and school-age children in developing their plan, as appropriate. Minimize the number of medications and daily doses to the fewest clinically possible. Give parents additional copies of the plan to give to day care providers and schools.

- **Fit the daily medication regimen into the patient's and family's routine.** Explain the difference between long-term-control and quick-relief medicines and how to use them. Ask patients (and parents) when would be the easiest times for them to take their daily medicines.

- **Identify and address obstacles and concerns. Ask patients about problems they think they might have doing the recommended action(s).** Ask questions that start with "what" or "how" to identify the obstacles (e.g., "What are things that might make it hard for you to take the action each day?"). Discuss ways to address the problems or provide alternative actions.

Figure 10.

Example of Delivery of Asthma Education by Clinicians During Patient Care Visits

Recommendations for Initial Visit

Assessment Questions Focus on: • Concerns • Goals of Therapy • Quality of Life • Expectations	Teach information in simple language	Teach and demonstrate skills
"What worries you most about your asthma?" "What do you want to accomplish at this visit?" "What do you want to be able to do that you can't do now because of your asthma?" "What do you expect from treatment?" "What medicines have you tried?" "What other questions do you have for me today?"	What is asthma? A chronic lung disease. The airways are very sensitive. They become inflamed and narrow; breathing becomes difficult. Two types of medicines are needed: • Long-term control: medications that prevent symptoms, often by reducing inflammation • Quick relief: short-acting bronchodilator relaxes muscles around airways Bring all medications to every appointment. When to seek medical advice. Provide appropriate telephone number.	Inhaler (see patient handout) and spacer/holding chamber use. Check performance. Self-monitoring skills tied to action plan: • Recognize intensity and frequency of asthma symptoms • Review the signs of deterioration and the need to reevaluate therapy: — Waking at night with asthma — Increased medication use — Decreased activity tolerance Use of an action plan (see patient handout)

Recommendations for First Followup Visit (2 to 4 weeks or sooner as needed)

Ask relevant questions from previous visit and also ask: "What medications are you taking?" "How and when are you taking them?" "What problems have you had using your medications?" "Please show me how you use your inhaled medications."	Use of two types of medications. Remind patient to bring all medications and the peak flow meter to every appointment for review. Self-evaluation of progress in asthma control using symptoms and peak flow as a guide.	Use of an action plan. Review and adjust as needed. Peak flow monitoring (see patient handout) and daily diary recording. Correct inhaler and spacer/holding chamber technique.

Recommendations for Second Followup Visit

Ask relevant questions from previous visits and also ask: "Have you noticed anything in your home, work, or school that makes your asthma worse?" "Describe for me how you know when to call your doctor or go to the hospital for asthma care." "What questions do you have about the action plan?" "Can we make it easier?" "Are your medications causing you any problems?"	Relevant environmental control/avoidance strategies (see patient handout). • How to identify and control home, work, or school exposures that can cause or worsen asthma • How to avoid cigarette smoke (active and passive) Review all medications and review and interpret peak flow and symptom scores from daily diary	Inhaler/spacer/holding chamber technique. Peak flow monitoring technique. Review use of action plan. Confirm that patient knows what to do if asthma gets worse.

Recommendations for All Subsequent Visits

Ask relevant questions from previous visits and also ask: "How have you tried to control things that make your asthma worse?" "Please show me how you use your inhaled medication."	Review and reinforce all: • Educational messages • Environmental control strategies at home, work, or school • Medications Review and interpret peak flow and symptom scores from daily diary.	Inhaler/spacer/holding chamber technique. Peak flow monitoring technique. Review use of action plan. Confirm that patient knows what to do if asthma gets worse. Periodically review and adjust written action plan.

- **Ask for agreement/plans to act.** Ask patients to summarize what recommended action(s) they plan to take, especially at the end of each visit.

- **Encourage or enlist family involvement.**

- **Follow up. At each visit, review the performance of the agreed-upon actions.** Praise appropriate actions and discuss how to improve other actions. Share evidence of the patient's improvement in lung function and symptoms. Remain encouraging when patients do not take the agreed-upon actions.

- **Assess the influence of the patient's cultural beliefs and practices that might affect asthma care.** Ask open-ended questions (e.g., "What will your friends and family think when you tell them you have asthma? What advice might they give to you?") If harmless or potentially beneficial folk remedies are mentioned by the patients, consider incorporating them into the treatment plan.

Teach Use of Inhaler and Peak Flow Meter

Most patients use their inhalers incorrectly, and this skill deteriorates over time. Patients' poor technique results in less medication getting to the airways. The initial inhaler training can be done in minutes with the simple skills-training method described below. Note that different inhalers may require different inhalation techniques. The necessary reviews at each visit are quick and easy and can be done by other staff members in the office.

Effective skills-training steps for teaching inhaler techniques are as follows:

1. **Tell** the patient the steps and give written instructions. (For written instructions, see patient handouts.)

2. **Demonstrate** how to use the inhaler following each of these steps.

3. Ask the patient to **demonstrate** how to use the inhaler. Let the patient refer to the handout on the first training. Subsequently, use the handout as a checklist to assess the patient's technique.

Figure 11.

How Often To Change Long-Term-Control Canisters

# Sprays	2 Sprays/ Day	4 Sprays/ Day	6 Sprays/ Day	8 Sprays/ Day	9 Sprays/ Day	12 Sprays/ Day	16 Sprays/ Day
60	30 days	15 days	n/a	n/a	n/a	n/a	n/a
100	n/a	25 days	16 days	12 days	n/a	n/a	n/a
104	n/a	26 days	17 days	13 days	n/a	n/a	n/a
112	n/a	28 days	18 days	14 days	n/a	n/a	n/a
120	60 days	30 days	20 days	15 days	n/a	n/a	n/a
200	n/a	50 days	33 days	25 days	22 days	16 days	12 days
240	n/a	60 days	40 days	30 days	26 days	20 days	15 days

* If the medication is taken as prescribed, the canister should be discarded as indicated above. Otherwise, the remaining puffs may not contain sufficient medication.

4. **Tell** patients what they did right and what they need to improve. Have them demonstrate their technique again, if needed. Focus the patient on improving one or two key steps (e.g., timing of actuation and inhalation) if the patient made multiple errors.

At each subsequent visit, perform the last two steps: patient demonstration and telling what they did right and what they need to improve. Train patients to use their peak flow meter using the same four skills-training steps above and the patient handout, "How To Use Your Peak Flow Meter."

Tips for Replacing Metered-Dose Inhalers

The *only* reliable way to determine whether a metered-dose inhaler is empty is to count the number of puffs used and subtract that number from the total number of sprays in the canister. Unfortunately, many patients believe they know when their inhalers are empty by floating the canister, spraying into the air, or tasting the medicine.

Clinicians and pharmacists can help patients determine the life of their long-term-control canisters by referring to the chart in figure 11 ("How Often To Change Long-Term-Control Canisters") or by dividing the number of sprays per canister (written on the canister and listed in the dosage chart on page 54) by the number of puffs prescribed per day. Determine the corresponding calendar date. Make an appointment before that date or make refills available after that date.

6. Managing Asthma Exacerbations at Home, in the Emergency Department, and in the Hospital

Assessment and monitoring

▶ Pharmacologic therapy

Control of factors contributing to asthma severity

▶ Patient education for a partnership

Home Management: Prompt Treatment Is Key

Educating patients to recognize and treat exacerbations early is the best strategy.

Education and preparation of patients to manage their exacerbations* are essential and should include:

- A written action plan and clear instructions on how to follow it. (See patient handout, "Asthma Action Plan," and figure 12).

- Instructions on how to recognize signs of worsening asthma and signs that indicate the need to call the doctor or seek emergency care.

- Prompt use of short-acting beta$_2$-agonists (two puffs every 20 minutes for 1 hour) and, for moderate-to-severe exacerbations, the addition of oral steroids. Increased therapy should be maintained for several days to stabilize symptoms and peak flow.

- Monitoring the response to the medications.

- Followup with patients to assess overall asthma control, the need to increase long-term-control medications, and the need to remove or withdraw from allergens or irritants that precipitated the exacerbation.

*Asthma exacerbations are episodes of progressively worsening shortness of breath, cough, wheezing, chest tightness, or some combination of these symptoms.

Risk Factors for Death From Asthma

History of Severe Exacerbations

- Past history of sudden severe exacerbations
- Prior intubation for asthma
- Prior admission for asthma to an intensive care unit

Asthma Hospitalizations and Emergency Visits

- ≥ 2 hospitalizations in the past year
- ≥ 3 emergency care visits in the past year
- Hospitalization or emergency visit in past month

Beta$_2$-Agonist and Oral Steroid Usage

- Use of >2 canisters per month of short-acting inhaled beta$_2$-agonist
- Current use of oral steroids or recent withdrawal from oral steroids

Complicating Health Problems

- Comorbidity (e.g., cardiovascular diseases or COPD)
- Serious psychiatric disease, including depression, or psychosocial problems
- Illicit drug use

Other Factors

- Poor perception of airflow obstruction or its severity
- Sensitivity to *Alternaria* (an outdoor mold)
- Low socioeconomic status and urban residence

Sources: See references 19, 49–52.

Figure 12.

Management of Asthma Exacerbations: Home Treatment
Give patients the Asthma Action Plan (page 63), which corresponds to this figure.

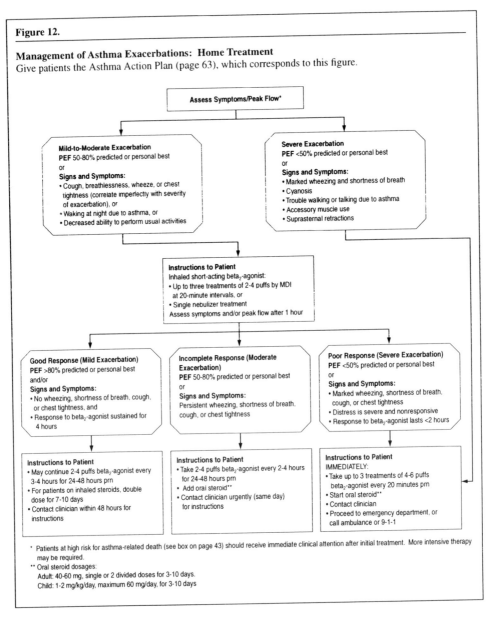

Assess Symptoms/Peak Flow*

Mild-to-Moderate Exacerbation
PEF 50-80% predicted or personal best
or
Signs and Symptoms:
• Cough, breathlessness, wheeze, or chest tightness (correlate imperfectly with severity of exacerbation), or
• Waking at night due to asthma, or
• Decreased ability to perform usual activities

Severe Exacerbation
PEF <50% predicted or personal best
or
Signs and Symptoms:
• Marked wheezing and shortness of breath
• Cyanosis
• Trouble walking or talking due to asthma
• Accessory muscle use
• Suprasternal retractions

Instructions to Patient
Inhaled short-acting beta₂-agonist:
• Up to three treatments of 2-4 puffs by MDI at 20-minute intervals, or
• Single nebulizer treatment
Assess symptoms and/or peak flow after 1 hour

Good Response (Mild Exacerbation)
PEF >80% predicted or personal best and/or
Signs and Symptoms:
• No wheezing, shortness of breath, cough, or chest tightness, and
• Response to beta₂-agonist sustained for 4 hours

Incomplete Response (Moderate Exacerbation)
PEF 50-80% predicted or personal best
or
Signs and Symptoms:
Persistent wheezing, shortness of breath, cough, or chest tightness

Poor Response (Severe Exacerbation)
PEF <50% predicted or personal best
or
Signs and Symptoms:
• Marked wheezing, shortness of breath, cough, or chest tightness
• Distress is severe and nonresponsive
• Response to beta₂-agonist lasts <2 hours

Instructions to Patient
• May continue 2-4 puffs beta₂-agonist every 3-4 hours for 24-48 hours prn
• For patients on inhaled steroids, double dose for 7-10 days
• Contact clinician within 48 hours for instructions

Instructions to Patient
• Take 2-4 puffs beta₂-agonist every 2-4 hours for 24-48 hours prn
• Add oral steroid**
• Contact clinician urgently (same day) for instructions

Instructions to Patient
IMMEDIATELY:
• Take up to 3 treatments of 4-6 puffs beta₂-agonist every 20 minutes prn
• Start oral steroid**
• Contact clinician
• Proceed to emergency department, or call ambulance or 9-1-1

* Patients at high risk for asthma-related death (see box on page 43) should receive immediate clinical attention after initial treatment. More intensive therapy may be required.
** Oral steroid dosages:
  Adult: 40-60 mg, single or 2 divided doses for 3-10 days.
  Child: 1-2 mg/kg/day, maximum 60 mg/day, for 3-10 days

Patients at high risk of asthma-related death (see box on page 43) **require special attention** — intensive education, monitoring, and care. They should be counseled to seek medical care early during an exacerbation and instructed about when and how to call for an ambulance. Patients with moderate-to-severe persistent asthma or a history of severe exacerbations should have the medication (e.g., steroid tablets or liquid) and equipment (e.g., peak flow meter, compressor-driven nebulizer for young children) for assessing and treating exacerbations at home.

Prehospital Emergency Medicine/Ambulance Management

It is recommended that emergency workers administer short-acting inhaled beta$_2$-agonists and supplemental oxygen to patients who have signs or symptoms of asthma.[53] Subcutaneous epinephrine or terbutaline are NOT recommended but can be used if inhaled medication is not available (see dosage information on page 57).

Emergency Department and Hospital Management of Exacerbations

Treat Without Delay

Assess patient's peak flow or FEV$_1$ and administer medication(s) upon patient's arrival without delay. After therapy is initiated, obtain a brief, focused history and physical examination pertinent to the exacerbation. Perform a more detailed history, physical, and lab studies only after therapy has started.

The goals for treating asthma exacerbations are rapid reversal of airflow obstruction, reduction in the likelihood of recurrence, and correction of significant hypoxemia. To achieve these goals, the management of asthma exacerbations in the emergency department and hospital (see figure 13 and dosage chart on page 57) includes:

- **Oxygen for most patients** to maintain SaO$_2$ ≥90 percent (>95 percent in pregnant women, infants, and patients with coexistent heart disease). Monitor oxygen saturation until a significant clinical improvement has occurred.

- **Short-acting inhaled beta$_2$-agonists every 20 to 30 minutes for three treatments for all patients** (see box on page 48). The onset of action is about 5 minutes. Subsequent therapy depends on response (see figure 13). Subcutaneous beta$_2$-agonists provide no proven advantage over inhaled medication.

- **Oral steroids should be given to most patients** — those with moderate-to-severe exacerbations, patients who fail to respond promptly and completely to an inhaled beta$_2$-agonist, and patients admitted into the hospital. Oral steroids speed recovery and reduce the likelihood of recurrence. Onset of action is greater than 4 hours.[57-59] Often, a 3- to 10-day course of oral steroids at discharge is useful.

NOTE: Anticholinergics added to albuterol may be considered. Adding high doses of ipratropium bromide (0.5 mg in adults, 0.25 mg in children) to albuterol in a nebulizer has been shown to cause additional bronchodilation in some but not all studies,[54-56] particularly in patients with severe airflow obstruction.

> **Effectiveness of MDI Plus Spacer/Holding Chamber vs. Nebulizer**
>
> Equivalent bronchodilation can be achieved by a beta$_2$-agonist given by MDI with a spacer/holding chamber under the supervision of trained personnel or by nebulizer therapy.[62-64] Continuous administration with a nebulizer may be more effective in children and severely obstructed adults[65-68] and patients who have difficulty with an MDI plus spacer/holding chamber.

Figure 13.

Management of Asthma Exacerbations: Emergency Department and Hospital-Based Care

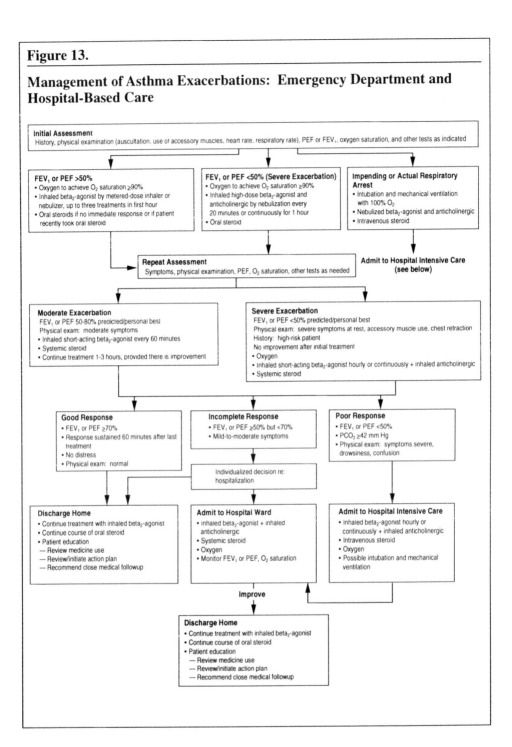

— For patients who take oral steroids long term, give supplemental doses, even if the exacerbation is mild.
— In infants and children, give oral steroids early in the course of an asthma exacerbation.
— Oral administration of prednisone is usually preferred to intravenous methylprednisolone because it is less invasive and the effects are equivalent.[60,61]

Repeat Assessment

The Expert Panel recommends repeat assessments of patients with severe exacerbations after the first dose and the third dose (about 60 to 90 minutes after initiating treatment) of short-acting inhaled beta$_2$-agonists. Evaluate the patient's subjective response, physical findings, and lung function. Consider arterial blood gas measurement for evaluating arterial carbon dioxide (PCO_2) in patients with suspected hypoventilation, severe distress, or with FEV_1 or peak flow ≤ 30 percent of predicted after treatment.

Special Considerations for Infants

Infants require special attention due to their greater risk for respiratory failure.

• Use oral steroids early in the episode.

• Monitor oxygen saturation by pulse oximetry. SaO_2 should be >95 percent at sea level.

• Assess infants for signs of serious distress, including use of accessory muscles, paradoxical breathing, cyanosis, a respiratory rate >60, or oxygen saturation <91 percent.

• Assess response to therapy. A lack of response to beta$_2$-agonist therapy noted by physical exam or oxygen saturation is an indication for hospitalization.

Therapies Not Recommended for Treating Exacerbations

Theophylline/aminophylline is NOT recommended therapy in the emergency department because it appears to provide no additional benefit to short-acting inhaled beta$_2$-agonists and may produce adverse effects.[69-73] In hospitalized patients, intravenous methylxanthines are not beneficial in children with severe asthma[74-76] and their addition remains controversial for adults.[77,78]

Chest physical therapy and mucolytics are not recommended. Anxiolytic and hypnotic drugs are contraindicated. Antibiotics are NOT recommended for asthma treatment but may be needed for comorbid conditions (e.g., patients with fever and purulent sputum or with evidence of bacterial pneumonia). Aggressive hydration is NOT recommended for older children and adults. Assess fluid status and make appropriate corrections for infants and young children to reduce their risk of dehydration.

Hospital Asthma Care

In general, the principles of care in the hospital are similar to those for care in the emergency department and involve treatment with aerosolized bronchodilators, systemic steroids, oxygen, and frequent assessments (see figure 13). Clinical assessment of respiratory distress and fatigue and objective measurement of airflow (peak flow or FEV_1) and oxygen saturation with pulse oximetry should be performed. Most patients respond well to therapy; however, a small minority will show signs of worsening ventilation.

Signs of impending respiratory failure include declining mental clarity, worsening fatigue, and a PCO_2 of ≥ 42 mm Hg. Respiratory failure tends to progress rapidly and is hard to reverse. The decision to intubate is based on clinical judgment; however, intubation is best done semi-electively, before the crisis of respiratory arrest. Therefore, the Expert Panel recommends that intubation should not be delayed once it is deemed necessary. Intubation should be performed by physicians with extensive experience in intubation and airway management. Consultation or comanagement by a physician expert in ventilator management is appropriate.

Patient Discharge From the Emergency Department or Hospital

Patients can be discharged from the emergency department and hospital when peak flow or FEV_1 is ≥ 70 percent of predicted or personal best and symptoms are minimal. Patients should be assessed for discharge on an individual basis if they have a peak flow or FEV_1 of ≥ 50 but <70 percent of predicted or personal best and mild symptoms. Take into consideration the risk factors

Before Discharge, Provide Patients With the Following:

- **Sufficient short-acting inhaled beta$_2$-agonist and oral steroids** to complete the course of therapy or to continue therapy until the followup appointment. Patients given oral steroids should continue taking them for 3 to 10 days. **Patients may be asked to start taking or to increase inhaled steroids** in an attempt to improve the patient's long-term-control regimen.

- **Written and verbal instructions** on when to increase medications or return for care should asthma worsen. The plan provided in the emergency department can be quite simple. Before discharge from the hospital, patients should receive a more complete written action plan (see patient handout, page 63) on when to take their medicines.

- **Training on how to monitor peak flow** should be *provided* in the hospital and *considered* for patients in the emergency department. Also, consider issuing peak flow meters. Patients in both settings should receive instruction on monitoring their symptoms.

- **Training on necessary environmental control measures and inhaler technique, whenever possible.**

- **Referral for a followup medical appointment.** Tell patients from the emergency department to go to a followup appointment within 3 to 5 days or set up an appointment for them. When possible, phone or fax a notice to the patient's physician that the patient came to the emergency department. For both emergency department and hospital patients, emphasize the need for continual, regular care in an outpatient setting. If patients do not have a physician, refer them or arrange a followup visit with a primary care physician, a clinic, or an asthma specialist.

for asthma-related death (see box on page 43). Hospitalized patients should have their medications changed to an oral or inhaled regimen and then be observed for 24 hours before discharge.

References

1. National Heart, Lung, and Blood Institute, National Asthma Education and Prevention Program. *Expert Panel Report 2: Guidelines for the Diagnosis and Management of Asthma.* National Institutes of Health pub no 97-4051. Bethesda, MD, 1997.

2. Pappas G, Hadden WC, Kozak LJ, Fisher GF. Potentially avoidable hospitalizations: inequalities in rates between US socioeconomic groups. *Am J Public Health* 1997;87:811-16.

3. Friday GA Jr, Khine H, Lin MS, Caliguiri LA. Profile of children requiring emergency treatment for asthma. *Ann Allergy Asthma Immunol* 1997; 78:221-224.

4. Hartert TV, Windom HH, Peebles RS Jr, Freidhoff LR, Togias A. Inadequate outpatient medical therapy for patients with asthma admitted to two urban hospitals. *Am J Med* 1996;100:386-394.

5. van Essen-Zandvliet EE, Hughes MD, Waalkens HJ. Duiverman EJ, Pocock SJ, Kerrebijn KF. Effects of 22 months of treatment with inhaled steroids and/or beta$_2$-agonists on lung function, airway responsiveness, and symptoms in children with asthma. *Am Rev Respir Dis* 1992;146:547-54.

6. Haahtela T, Jarvinen M, Kava T, et al. Comparison of a beta$_2$-agonist, terbutaline, with an inhaled corticosteroid, budesonide, in newly detected asthma. *N Engl J Med* 1991;325:388-92.

7. Jones AH, Langdon CG, Lee PS, et al. Pulmicort Turbuhaler once daily as initial prophylactic therapy for asthma. *Respir Med* 1994;88:293-9.

8. Pincus DJ, Szefler SJ, Ackerson LM, Martin RJ. Chronotherapy of asthma with inhaled steroids: the effect of dosage timing on drug efficacy. *J Allergy Clin Immunol* 1995;95:1172-8.

9. Noonan M, Chervinsky P, Busse WW, et al. Fluticasone propionate reduces oral prednisone use while it improves asthma control and quality of life. *Am J Respir Crit Care Med* 1995;152:1467-73.

10. Haahtela T, Jarvinen M, Kava T, et al. Effects of reducing or discontinuing inhaled budesonide in patients with mild asthma. *N Engl J Med* 1994; 331:700-5.

11. Waalkens HJ, Van Essen-Zandvliet EE, Hughes MD, et al. Cessation of long-term treatment with inhaled corticosteroid (budesonide) in children with asthma results in deterioration. *Am Rev Respir Dis* 1993;148:1252-7.

12. Dahl R, Lundback E, Malo JL, et al. A dose-ranging study of fluticasone propionate in adult patients with moderate asthma. *Chest* 1993;104:1352-8.

13. Fabbri L, Burge PS, Croonenborgh L, et al. on behalf of an International Study Group. Comparison of fluticasone propionate with beclomethasone dipropionate in moderate to severe asthma treated for one year. *Thorax* 1993;48:817-23.

14. Gustafsson P, Tsanakas J, Gold M, Primhak R. Radford M, Gillies E. Comparison of the efficacy and safety of inhaled fluticasone 200 mcg/day with inhaled beclomethasone dipropionate 400 mcg/day in mild and moderate asthma. *Arch Dis Child* 1993;69:206-11.

15. Jeffery PK, Godfrey RW, Adelroth E, Nelson F, Rogers A, Johansson SA. Effects of treatment on airway inflammation and thickening of basement membrane reticular collagen in asthma. *Am Rev Respir Dis* 1992;145:890-9.

16. Rafferty P, Tucker LG, Frame MH, Fergusson RJ, Biggs BA, Crompton GK. Comparison of budesonide and beclomethasone dipropionate in patients with severe chronic asthma: assessment of relative prednisolone-sparing effects. *Br J Dis Chest* 1985;79:244-50.

17. Greening AP, Wind P, Northfield M, Shaw G. Added salmeterol versus higher-dose steroid in asthma patients with symptoms on existing inhaled steroid. *Lancet* 1994;344:219-24.

18. Woolcock A, Lundback B, Ringdal N, Jacques LA. Comparison of addition of salmeterol to inhaled steroids with doubling of the dose of inhaled steroid. *Am J Respir Crit Care Med* 1996;153:1481-8.

19. Suissa S, Ernst P, Bolvin JF, et al. A cohort analysis of excess mortality in asthma and the use of inhaled beta$_2$-agonists. *Am J Respir Crit Care Med* 1994;149(3 Pt 1):604-10.

20. Drazen JM, Israel E. Boushey HA, et al. Comparison of regularly scheduled with as-needed use of albuterol in mild asthma. *N Engl J Med* 1996;335:841-7.

21. Wolthers OD. Long-, intermediate- and short-term growth studies in asthmatic children treated with inhaled glucosteroids. *Eur Respir J* 1996;9:821-7.

22. Kamada AK, Szefler SJ, Martin RJ, et al. and the Asthma Clinical Research Network. Issues in the use of inhaled glucocorticoids. *Am J Respir Crit Care Med* 1996;153:1739-48.

23. Barnes PJ, Pedersen S. Efficacy and safety of inhaled steroids in asthma. *Am Rev Respir Dis* 1993;148:S1-S26.

24. Tinkelman DG, Reed CE, Nelson HS, Offord KP. Aerosol beclomethasone dipropionate compared with theophylline as primary treatment of chronic, mild to moderately severe asthma in children. *Pediatrics* 1993;92:64-77.

25. Doull IJM, Freezer NJ. Holgate ST. Growth of pre-pubertal children with mild asthma treated with inhaled beclomethasone dipropionate. *Am J Respir Crit Care Med* 1995;151:1715-9.

26. Kemp JP, Dockhorn RJ, Busse WW, Bleecker ER, Van As A. Prolonged effect of inhaled salmeterol against exercise-induced bronchospasm. *Am J Respir Crit Care Med* 1994;150:1612-5.

27. Albazzaz MK, Neale MG, Patel KR. Dose-response study of nebulized nedocromil sodium in exercise induced asthma. *Thorax* 1989;44:816-9.

28. de Benedictis FM, Tuteri G, Pazzelli P, Bertotto A, Bruni L, Vaccaro R. Cromolyn versus nedocromil: duration of action in exercise-induced asthma in children. *J Allergy Clin Immunol* 1995;96:510-4.

29. Woolley M, Anderson SD, Quigley BM. Duration of terbutaline sulfate and cromolyn sodium alone and in combination on exercise-induced asthma. *Chest* 1990;97:39-45.

30. Vathenen AS, Knox AJ, Wisniewski A, Tattersfield AE. Effect of inhaled budesonide on bronchial reactivity to histamine, exercise, and eucapnic dry air hyperventilation in patients with asthma. *Thorax* 1991;46:811-6.

31. Nastasi KJ, Heinly TL, Blaiss MS. Exercise-induced asthma and the athlete. *J Asthma* 1995;32:249-57.

32. Nelson HS, Weber RW. Endocrine aspects of allergic diseases. In: Bierman CW, Pearlman DS, eds. *Allergic Diseases From Infancy to Adulthood.* Philadelphia: WB Saunders, 1988. ch. 15.

33. Schatz M, Zeiger RS, Harden KM, et al. The safety of inhaled beta-agonist bronchodilators during pregnancy. *J Allergy Clin Immunol* 1988;82:686-95.

34. *Federal Register.* 21 CFR Parts 201, 202. 1979;44(124):37434-37467.

35. Briggs GG, Freeman RK, Yaffe SJ. *Drugs in Pregnancy and Lactation: A Reference Guide to Fetal and Neonatal Risk,* 2nd ed. Baltimore, MD: Williams & Wilkins, 1986.

36. Peroni DG, Boner AL, Vallone G, Antolini I, Warner JO. Effective allergen avoidance at high altitude reduces allergen-induced bronchial hyperresponsiveness. *Am J Respir Crit Care Med* 1994;149(6):1442-6.

37. Piacentini GL, Martinati L, Fornari A, et al. Antigen avoidance in a mountain environment: influence on basophil releasability in children with allergic asthma. *J Allergy Clin Immunol* 1993;92(5):644-50.

38. Simon HU, Grotzer M, Nikolaizik WH, Blaser K, Schoni MH. High altitude climate therapy reduces peripheral blood T lymphocyte activation, eosinophilia, and bronchial obstruction in children with house-dust mite allergic asthma. *Pediatr Pulmonol* 1994;17(5):304-11.

39. Murray AB, Ferguson AC. Dust-free bedrooms in the treatment of asthmatic children with house dust or house dust mite allergy: a controlled trial. *Pediatrics* 1983;71:418-22.

40. Murray AB, Milner RA. The accuracy of features in the clinical history for predicting atopic sensitization to airborne allergens in children. *J Allergy Clinical Immunol* 1995;96:588-96.

41. Adinoff AD, Rosloniec DM, McCall LL, Nelson HS. Immediate skin test reactivity to Food and Drug Administration-approved standardized extracts. *J Allergy Clin Immunol* 1990;86:766-74.

42. Abramson MJ, Puy RM, Weiner JM. Is allergen immunotherapy effective in asthma? A meta-analysis of randomized controlled trials. *Am J Respir Crit Care Med* 1995;151:969-74.

43. Reid MJ, Moss RB, Hsu YP, Kwasnicki JM, Commerford TM, Nelson BL. Seasonal asthma in northern California: allergic causes and efficacy of immunotherapy. *J Allergy Clin Immunol* 1986;78:590-600.

44. Malling HJ, Dreborg S, Weeke B. Diagnosis and immunotherapy of mould allergy. V. Clinical efficacy and side effects of immunotherapy with *Cladosporium herbarum*. *Allergy* 1986;41:507-19.

45. Creticos PS, Reed CE, Norman PS, et al. Ragweed immunotherapy in adult asthma. *N Engl J Med* 1996;334(8):501-6.

46. Horst M, Hejjaoui A, Horst V, Michel FB, Bousquet J. Double-blind, placebo-controlled rush immunotherapy with a standardized *Alternaria* extract. *J Allergy Clin Immunol* 1990;85:460-72.

47. American Academy of Allergy and Immunology Board of Directors. Guidelines to minimize the risk from systemic reactions caused by immunotherapy with allergenic extracts. *J Allergy Clin Immunol* 1994;93:811-2.

48. Frew AJ. Injection immunotherapy. British Society for Allergy and Clinical Immunology Working Party. *BMJ* 1993;307:919-23.

49. Kallenbach JM, Frankel AH, Lapinsky SE, et al. Determinants of near fatality in acute severe asthma. *Am J Med* 1993;95:265-72.

50. Rodrigo C, Rodrigo G. Assessment of the patient with acute asthma in the emergency department. A factor analytic study. *Chest* 1993;104:1325-8.

51. Greenberger PA, Miller TP, Lifschultz B. Circumstances surrounding deaths from asthma in Cook County (Chicago) Illinois. *Allergy Proc* 1993;14:321-6.

52. O'Hollaren MT, Yuninger JW, Offord KP, et al. Exposure to an aeroallergen as a possible precipitating factor in respiratory arrest in young patients with asthma. *N Engl J Med* 1991;324:359-63.

53. Fergusson RJ, Stewart CM, Wathen CG, Moffat R, Crompton GK. Effectiveness of nebulised salbutamol administered in ambulances to patients with acute severe asthma. *Thorax* 1995;50:81-2.

54. Schuh S, Johnson DW, Callahan S, Canny G, Levison H. Efficacy of frequent nebulized ipratropium bromide added to frequent high-dose albuterol therapy in severe childhood asthma. *J Pediatr* 1995;126:639-45.

55. Kelly HW, Murphy S. Corticosteroids for acute, severe asthma. *DICP* 1991;25:72-9.

56. Karpel JP, Schacter EN, Fanta C, et al. A comparison of ipratropium and albuterol vs. albuterol alone for the treatment of acute asthma. *Chest* 1996;110:611-6.

57. Rowe BH, Keller JL, Oxman AD. Effectiveness of steroid therapy in acute exacerbations of asthma: a meta-analysis. *Am J Emerg Med* 1992;10:301-10.

58. Scarfone RJ, Fuchs SM, Nager AL, Shane SA. Controlled trial of oral prednisone in the emergency department treatment of children with acute asthma. *Pediatrics* 1993;2:513-8.

59. Connett GJ, Warde C, Wooler E, Lenney W. Prednisolone and salbutamol in the hospital treatment of acute asthma. *Arch Dis Child* 1994;70:170-3.

60. Harrison BD, Stokes TC, Hart GJ, Vaughan DA, Ali NJ, Robinson AA. Need for intravenous hydrocortisone in addition to oral prednisolone in patients admitted to hospital with severe asthma without ventilatory failure. *Lancet* 1986;1(8474):181-4.

61. Ratto D, Alfaro C, Sipsey J, Glovsky MM, Sharma OP. Are intravenous corticosteroids required in status asthmaticus? *JAMA* 1988;260:527-9.

62. Idris AH, McDermott MF, Raucci JC, Morrabel A, McGorray S, Hendeles L. Emergency department treatment of severe asthma. Metered-dose inhaler plus holding chamber is equivalent in effectiveness to nebulizer. *Chest* 1993;103:665-72.

63. Colacone A, Afilalo M, Wolkove N, Kreisman H. A comparison of albuterol administered by metered dose inhaler (and holding chamber) or wet nebulizer in acute asthma. *Chest* 1993;104:835-41.

64. Kerem E, Levison H, Schuh S, et al. Efficacy of albuterol administered by nebulizer versus spacer device in children with acute asthma. *J Pediatr* 1993;123:313-7.

65. Lin RY, Sauter D, Newman T, Sirleaf J, Walters J, Tavakol M. Continuous versus intermittent albuterol nebulization in the treatment of acute asthma. *Ann Emerg Med* 1993;22:1847-53.

66. Rudnitsky GS, Eberlein RS, Schoffstall JM, Mazur JE, Spivey WH. Comparison of intermittent and continuously nebulized albuterol for treatment of asthma in an urban emergency department. *Ann Emerg Med* 1993;22:1842-6.

67. Papo MC, Frank J, Thompson AE. A prospective, randomized study of continuous versus intermittent nebulized albuterol for severe status asthmaticus in children. *Crit Care Med* 1993;21:1479-86.

68. Kelly HW, Murphy S. Beta-adrenergic agonists for acute, severe asthma. *Ann Pharmacother* 1992;26:81-91.

69. Fanta CH, Rossing TH, McFadden ER Jr. Treatment of acute asthma: is combination therapy with sympathomimetics and methylxanthines indicated? *Am J Med* 1986;80:5-10.

70. Rossing TH, Fanta CH, Goldstein DH, Snapper JR, McFadden ER Jr. Emergency therapy of asthma: comparison of the acute effects of parenteral and inhaled sympathomimetics and infused aminophylline. *Am Rev Respir Dis* 1980;122:365-71.

71. Murphy DG, McDermott MF, Rydman RJ, Sloan EP, Zalenski RJ. Aminophylline in the treatment of acute asthma when beta$_2$-adrenergics and steroids are provided. *Arch Intern Med* 1993;153:1784-88.

72. Rodrigo C, Rodrigo G. Treatment of acute asthma. Lack of therapeutic benefit and increase of the toxicity from aminophylline given in addition to high doses of salbutamol delivered by metered-dose inhaler with a spacer. *Chest* 1994;106:1071-6.

73. Coleridge J, Cameron P, Epstein J, Teichtahl H. Intravenous aminophylline confers no benefit in acute asthma treated with intravenous steroids and inhaled bronchodilators. *Aust N Z J Med* 1993;23:348-54.

74. Strauss RE, Wertheim DL, Bonagura VR, Valacer DJ. Aminophylline therapy does not improve outcome and increases adverse effects in children hospitalized with acute asthmatic exacerbations. *Pediatrics* 1994;93:205-10.

75. Carter E, Cruz M, Chesrown S, Shieh G, Reilly K, Hendeles L. Efficacy of intravenously administered theophylline in children hospitalized with severe asthma. *J Pediatr* 1993;122:470-6.

76. DiGiulio GA, Kercsmar CM, Krug SE, Alpert SE, Marx CM. Hospital treatment of asthma: lack of benefit from theophylline given in addition to nebulized albuterol and intravenously administered corticosteroid. *J Pediatr* 1993;122:464-9.

77. Huang D, O'Brien RG, Harman E, et al. Does aminophylline benefit adults admitted to the hospital for an acute exacerbation of asthma? *Ann Intern Med* 1993;119:1155-60.

78. Self TH, Abou-Shala N, Burns R, et al. Inhaled albuterol and oral prednisone therapy in hospitalized adult asthmatics. Does aminophylline add any benefit? *Chest* 1990;98:1317-21.

Appendices

Dosages for Medications

Glossary

Patient Handouts

Patient Self-Assessment Forms

*These questions are examples and do not represent a standardized assessment or diagnostic
instrument. The validity and reliability of these questions have not been assessed.

Usual Dosages for Long-Term-Control Medications*

Medication	Dosage Form	Adult Dose	Child Dose	Comments
Inhaled Steroids (see Estimated Comparative Daily Dosages for Inhaled Steroids, page 56)				• Most effective anti-inflammatory currently available
Oral Steroids				
Methylprednisolone	2, 4, 8, 16, 32 mg tablets	• 7.5–60 mg daily in a single dose or qod as needed for control	• 0.25–2 mg/kg daily in single dose or qod as needed for control	• For long-term treatment of severe persistent asthma, administer single dose in a.m. either daily or on alternate days (which may lessen adrenal suppression). One study suggests improved efficacy and no increase in adrenal suppression when administered at 3:00 p.m.
Prednisolone	5 mg tabs, 5 mg/5 cc, 15 mg/5 cc	• Short-course "burst": 40–60 mg per day as single or 2 divided doses for 3–10 days	• Short course "burst": 1–2 mg/kg/day, maximum 60 mg/day, for 3–10 days	• Short courses or "bursts" are effective for establishing control when initiating therapy or during a period of gradual deterioration.
Prednisone	1, 2.5, 5, 10, 20, 25 mg tabs; 5 mg/cc, 5 mg/5 cc			• The burst should be continued until patient achieves 80% of peak flow personal best or symptoms resolve. This usually requires 3–10 days but may require longer. There is no evidence that tapering the dose following improvement prevents relapse.
Cromolyn and Nedocromil				
Cromolyn	MDI 1 mg/puff (200 sprays/canister) Nebulizer solution 20 mg/ampule	2–4 puffs tid-qid 1 ampule tid-qid	1–2 puffs tid-qid 1 ampule tid-qid	• An initial trial in children with mild-to-moderate persistent asthma is often given due to strong safety profile.
				• Can usually see therapeutic effect of cromolyn within 2 weeks: takes 4 to 6 weeks to determine maximum effect
Nedocromil	MDI 1.75 mg/puff (104 sprays/canister)	2–4 puffs bid-qid	1–2 puffs bid-qid	• Dose of cromolyn by MDI may be inadequate, so nebulizer may be preferred
Long-Acting Bronchodilators				
Salmeterol	*Inhaled* MDI 21 mcg/puff, 60 or 120 puffs (120 sprays/canister) DPI 50 mcg/blister	2 puffs q 12 hours 1 blister q 12 hours	1–2 puffs q 12 hours 1 blister q 12 hours	• Should not be used in place of anti-inflammatory therapy. • Use with inhaled steroids in step 3. • May use one dose nightly for symptoms. • Duration of bronchodilation is 12 hours.
Sustained-release albuterol	*Tablet* 4 mg tablet	4 mg q 12 hours	0.3–0.6 mg/kg/day, not to exceed 8 mg/day	• **Should not be used for symptom relief or for exacerbations.**

Usual Dosages for Long-Term-Control Medications* *continued*

Medication	Dosage Form	Adult Dose	Child Dose	Comments
Theophylline	Liquids Sustained-release tablets and capsules	Starting dose 10 mg/kg/day up to 300 mg max; usual max 800 mg/day	Starting dose 10 mg/kg/day; usual max: • ≥1 year of age: 16 mg/kg/day • <1 year: 0.2 (age in weeks) + 5 = mg/kg/day	• Adjuvant to inhaled steroids for nocturnal symptoms • Alternative, but not preferred, long-term therapy at step 2. • Adjust dosage to achieve peak serum concentration of 5-15 mcg/mL at steady-state (at least 48 hours on same dosage) • Due to wide interpatient variability in theophylline metabolic clearance, **routine serum theophylline level monitoring is important.**
Leukotriene Modifiers				
Zafirlukast	20 mg tablet	40 mg daily (1 tablet bid)		• May be considered at step 2 for patients ≥12 years of age, although their position in therapy is not fully established • For zafirlukast, administration with meals decreases bioavailability; take at least 1 hour before or 2 hours after meals • For patients taking zafirlukast and warfarin, closely monitor prothrombin and adjust warfarin dosage • For zileuton, monitor hepatic enzymes (ALT)
Zileuton	300 mg tablet 600 mg tablet	2,400 mg daily (two 300-mg tablets or one 600-mg tablet, qid)		

NOTE: All chlorofluorocarbon (CFC)-propelled inhalers are being phased out. The new non-CFC products should have similar effectiveness and safety levels as the original product.

* For a list of brand names, see glossary, page 58.

Estimated Comparative Daily Dosages for Inhaled Steroids

Adults

Inhaled Steroid	Low Dose	Medium Dose	High Dose
Beclomethasone dipropionate	168–504 mcg	504–840 mcg	>840 mcg
42 mcg/puff	4–12 puffs—42 mcg	12–20 puffs—42 mcg	>20 puffs—42 mcg
84 mcg/puff	2–6 puffs—84 mcg	6–10 puffs—84 mcg	>10 puffs—84 mcg
Budesonide DPI	200–400 mcg	400–600 mcg	>600 mcg
200 mcg/dose	1–2 inhalations	2–3 inhalations	>3 inhalations
Flunisolide	500–1,000 mcg	1,000–2,000 mcg	>2,000 mcg
250 mcg/puff	2–4 puffs	4–8 puffs	>8 puffs
Fluticasone	88–264 mcg	264–660 mcg	>660 mcg
MDI:			
44, 110, 220 mcg/puff	2–6 puffs—44 mcg or 2 puffs—110 mcg	2–6 puffs—110 mcg	>6 puffs—110 mcg or >3 puffs—220 mcg
DPI:			
50, 100, 250 mcg/dose	2–6 inhalations—50 mcg	3–6 inhalations—100 mcg	>6 inhalations—100 mcg or >2 inhalations—250 mcg
Triamcinolone acetonide	400–1,000 mcg	1,000–2,000 mcg	>2,000 mcg
100 mcg/puff	4–10 puffs	10–20 puffs	>20 puffs

Children ≤12 years

Inhaled Steroid	Low Dose	Medium Dose	High Dose
Beclomethasone dipropionate	84–336 mcg	336–672 mcg	>672 mcg
42 mcg/puff	2–8 puffs—42 mcg	8–16 puffs—42 mcg	>16 puffs—42 mcg
84 mcg/puff	1–4 puffs—84 mcg	4–8 puffs—84 mcg	>8 puffs—84 mcg
Budesonide DPI	100–200 mcg	200–400 mcg	>400 mcg
200 mcg/dose		1–2 inhalations—200 mcg	>2 inhalations—200 mcg
Flunisolide	500–750 mcg	1,000–1,250 mcg	>1,250 mcg
250 mcg/puff	2–3 puffs	4–5 puffs	>5 puffs
Fluticasone	88–176 mcg	176–440 mcg	>440 mcg
MDI:			
44, 110, 220 mcg/puff	2–3 puffs—44 mcg	4–10 puffs—44 mcg or 2–4 puffs—110 mcg	>4 puffs—110 mcg or >2 puffs—220 mcg
DPI:			
50, 100, 250 mcg/dose	2–4 inhalations—50 mcg	2–4 inhalations—100 mcg	>4 inhalations—100 mcg or >2 inhalations—250 mcg
Triamcinolone acetonide	400–800 mcg	800–1,200 mcg	>1,200 mcg
100 mcg/puff	4–8 puffs	8–12 puffs	>12 puffs

- *Clinician judgment of patient response is essential to appropriate dosing.* Once asthma is controlled, medication doses should be carefully titrated to the minimum dose required to maintain control, thus reducing the potential for adverse effect.
- Data from *in vitro* and clinical trials suggest that different inhaled corticosteroid preparations are not equivalent on a per puff or microgram basis. However, few data directly compare the preparations. *The Expert Panel developed recommended dose ranges for different preparations based on available data.*
- Inhaled corticosteroid safety data suggest dose ranges for children equivalent to beclomethasone dipropionate 200–400 mcg/day (low dose), 400–800 mcg/day (medium dose), and >800 mcg/day (high dose).

Dosages of Drugs for Asthma Exacerbations in Emergency Medical Care or Hospital*

Medication	Dosages		Comments
	Adults	Children	
Inhaled short-acting beta₂-agonists			
Albuterol Nebulizer solution (5 mg/mL)	2.5–5 mg every 20 min for 3 doses, then 2.5–10 mg every 1–4 hours as needed, or 10–15 mg/hour continuously.	0.15 mg/kg (minimum dose 2.5 mg) every 20 min for 3 doses, then 0.15–0.3 mg/kg up to 10 mg every 1–4 hours as needed, or 0.5 mg/kg/hour by continuous nebulization.	Only selective beta₂-agonists are recommended. For optimal delivery, dilute aerosols to minimum of 4 mL at gas flow of 6–8 L/min
Metered-dose inhaler (90 mcg/puff)	4–8 puffs every 20 min up to 4 hours, then every 1–4 hours as needed.	4–8 puffs every 20 min for 3 doses, then every 1–4 hours as needed	As effective as nebulized therapy if patient is able to coordinate inhalation maneuver. Use spacer/holding chamber.
Bitolterol and pirbuterol			Have not been studied in severe asthma exacerbations.
Systemic (injected) beta₂-agonists			
Epinephrine 1:1000 (1 mg/mL)	0.3–0.5 mg every 20 min for 3 doses SQ	0.01 mg/kg up to 0.3–0.5 mg every 20 min for 3 doses SQ	No proven advantage of systemic therapy over aerosol
Terbutaline (1 mg/mL)	0.25 mg every 20 min for 3 doses SQ.	0.01 mg/kg every 20 min for 3 doses then every 2–6 hours as needed SQ.	No proven advantage of systemic therapy over aerosol.
Anticholinergics			
Ipratropium bromide Nebulizer solution (0.25 mg/mL)	0.5 mg every 30 min for 3 doses then every 2–4 hours as needed	0.25 mg every 20 min for 3 doses, then every 2 to 4 hours	May mix in same nebulizer with albuterol. Should not be used as first-line therapy; should be added to beta₂-agonist therapy. Dose delivered from MDI is low and has not been studied in asthma exacerbations.
Metered-dose inhaler (18 mcg/puff)	4–8 puffs as needed	4–8 puffs as needed.	
Steroids			
Prednisone Methylprednisolone Prednisolone	120–180 mg/day in 3 or 4 divided doses for 48 hours, then 60–80 mg/day until PEF reaches 70% of predicted or personal best.	1 mg/kg every 6 hours for 48 hours then 1–2 mg/kg/day (maximum = 60 mg/day) in 2 divided doses until PEF 70% of predicted or personal best.	Adult "burst" at discharge: 40–60 mg in single or 2 divided doses for 3–10 days. Child "burst" at discharge: 1–2 mg/kg/day, maximum 60 mg/day for 3–10 days.

* For a list of brand names, see glossary page 58.

Glossary*

Asthma Long-Term-Control Medications

Generic name	Brand name
Corticosteroids: Inhaled	
beclomethasone	Beclovent®
	Vanceril®, Vanceril®—Double Strength
budesonide	Pulmicort Turbuhaler®
flunisolide	AeroBid®. AeroBid-M®
fluticasone	Flovent®
triamcinolone	Azmacort®
Cromolyn and Nedocromil: Inhaled	
cromolyn sodium	Intal®
nedocromil sodium	Tilade®
Leukotriene Modifiers: Oral	
zafirlukast	Accolate®
zileuton	Zyflo®
Long-Acting Beta2-Agonists	
salmeterol (inhaled)	Serevent®
albuterol (extended release)	Volmax®
	Proventil Repetabs®
Theophylline: Oral	
	Aerolate® III
	Aerolate® JR
	Aerolate® SR
	Choledyl® SA
	Elixophyllin®
	Quibron®-T
	Quibron®-T/SR
	Slo-bid®
	Slo-Phyllin®
	Theo-24®
	Theochron®
	Theo-Dur®
	Theolair®
	Theolair®-SR
	T-Phyl®
	Uni-Dur®
	Uniphyl®

Asthma Quick-Relief Medications

Generic name	Brand name
Short-Acting Beta2-Agonists: Inhaled	
albuterol	Airet®
	Proventil®
	Proventil HFA®
	Ventolin®
	Ventolin® Rotacaps
bitolterol	Tornalate®
pirbuterol	Maxair®
terbutaline	Brethaire®
	Brethine® (tablet only)
	Bricanyl® (tablet only)

**This list does not include metaproterenol, which is not recommended for relief of acute broncho-spasm due to its potential for excessive cardiac stimulation, especially in high doses.

Generic name	Brand name
Anticholinergics: Inhaled	
ipratropium bromide	Atrovent®
Corticosteroids: Oral	
methylprednisolone	Medrol®
prednisone	Prednisone
	Deltasone®
	Orasone®
	Liquid Pred®
	Prednisone Intensol®
prednisolone	Prelone®
	Pediapred®

* This glossary is a complete list of brand names associated with the appropriate generic names of asthma medications, as listed in the United States Pharmacopeial Convention, Inc., *Approved Drug Products and Legal Requirements*, Volume III, 17th edition, 1997, and the USP DI *Drug Information for Health Care Professionals,* Volume I, 17th edition, 1997. This list does not constitute an endorsement of these products by the National Heart, Lung, and Blood Institute.

What Everyone Should Know About Asthma Control

You will learn to take care of your asthma over time. For now, you will be off to a good start if you know just five key things. These five things should guide your efforts to take care of your asthma.

Asthma can be managed so that you can live a normal life.

Your asthma should not keep you from doing what you want. It should not keep you from going to work or school. If it does, talk to your doctor about your treatment.

Asthma is a disease that makes the airways in your lungs inflamed.

This means your airways are swollen and sensitive. The swelling is there all of the time, even when you feel just fine. The swelling can be controlled with medicine and by staying away from things that bother your airways.

Many things in your home, school, work, and other places can cause asthma attacks.

An asthma attack occurs when your airways narrow, making it harder to breathe. Asthma attacks are some-times called flareups, exacerbations, or episodes.

Things in the air that you are allergic to (like pollen) can cause an asthma attack. So can things that bother your airways like tobacco smoke. You can learn to stay away from the things that cause you to have asthma attacks.

Asthma needs to be watched and cared for over a very long time.

Asthma cannot be cured, but it can be treated. You can become free of symp-toms all or most of the time. But your asthma does NOT go away when your symptoms go away. You will need to keep taking care of your asthma.

Also, over the years your asthma may change. Your asthma could get worse so you need more medicine. That's why you need to keep in touch with your doctor.

Asthma can be controlled when you manage your asthma and work with your doctor.

You play a big role in taking care of your asthma with your doctor's help. Your job is to:

- Take your medicines as your doctor suggests,

- Watch for signs that your asthma is getting worse and act quickly to stop the attack,

- Stay away from things that can bother your asthma,

- Ask your doctor about any concerns you have about your asthma, and

- See your doctor at least every 6 months.

When you do these things, you will gain—and keep—control of your asthma.

You can help prevent asthma attacks by staying away from things that make your asthma worse. This guide suggests many ways to help you do this.

You need to find out what makes your asthma worse. Some things that make asthma worse for some people are not a problem for others. You do not need to do all of the things listed in this guide.

Look at the things listed in dark print below. Put a check next to the ones that you know make your asthma worse. Ask your doctor to help you find out what else makes your asthma worse. Then, decide with your doctor what steps you will take. Start with the things in your bedroom that bother your asthma. Try something simple first.

☐ Tobacco Smoke

- ☐ If you smoke, ask your doctor for ways to help you quit. Ask family members to quit smoking, too.
- ☐ Do not allow smoking in your home or around you.
- ☐ Be sure no one smokes at a child's day care center.

☐ Dust Mites

Many people with asthma are allergic to dust mites. Dust mites are like tiny "bugs" you cannot see that live in cloth or carpet.

Things that will help the most:

- ☐ Encase your mattress in a special dust-proof cover.*
- ☐ Encase your pillow in a special dust-proof cover* or wash the pillow each week in hot water. Water must be hotter than 130°F to kill the mites.
- ☐ Wash the sheets and blankets on your bed each week in hot water.

Other things that can help:

- ☐ Reduce indoor humidity to less than 50 percent. Dehumidifiers or central air conditioners can do this.
- ☐ Try not to sleep or lie on cloth-covered cushions or furniture.
- ☐ Remove carpets from your bedroom and those laid on concrete, if you can.
- ☐ Keep stuffed toys out of the bed or wash the toys weekly in hot water.

☐ Animal Dander

Some people are allergic to the flakes of skin or dried saliva from animals with fur or feathers.

The best thing to do:

- ☐ Keep furred or feathered pets out of your home.

If you can't keep the pet outdoors, then:

- ☐ Keep the pet out of your bedroom and keep the bedroom door closed.
- ☐ Cover the air vents in your bedroom with heavy material to filter the air.*
- ☐ Remove carpets and furniture covered with cloth from your home. If that is not possible, keep the pet out of the rooms where these are.

☐ Cockroach

Many people with asthma are allergic to the dried droppings and remains of cockroaches.

- ☐ Keep all food out of your bedroom.
- ☐ Keep food and garbage in closed containers (never leave food out).

- [ ] Use poison baits, powders, gels, or paste (for example, boric acid). You can also use traps.
- [ ] If a spray is used to kill roaches, stay out of the room until the odor goes away.

Vacuum Cleaning

- [ ] Try to get someone else to vacuum for you once or twice a week, if you can. Stay out of rooms while they are being vacuumed and for a short while afterward.
- [ ] If you vacuum, use a dust mask (from a hardware store), a double-layered or microfilter vacuum cleaner bag,* or a vacuum cleaner with a HEPA filter.*

Indoor Mold

- [ ] Fix leaky faucets, pipes, or other sources of water.
- [ ] Clean moldy surfaces with a cleaner that has bleach in it.

Pollen and Outdoor Mold

What to do during your allergy season (when pollen or mold spore counts are high):

- [ ] Try to keep your windows closed.
- [ ] Stay indoors with windows closed during the midday and afternoon, if you can. Pollen and some mold spore counts are highest at that time.
- [ ] Ask your doctor whether you need to take or increase anti-inflammatory medicine before your allergy season starts.

Smoke, Strong Odors, and Sprays

- [ ] If possible, do not use a wood-burning stove, kerosene heater, or fireplace.
- [ ] Try to stay away from strong odors and sprays, such as perfume, talcum powder, hair spray, and paints.

Exercise, Sports, Work, or Play

- [ ] You should be able to be active without symptoms. See your doctor if you have asthma symptoms when you are active—like when you exercise, do sports, play, or work hard.
- [ ] Ask your doctor about taking medicine before you exercise to prevent symptoms.
- [ ] Warm up for about 6 to 10 minutes before you exercise.
- [ ] Try not to work or play hard outside when the air pollution or pollen levels (if you are allergic to the pollen) are high.

Other Things That Can Make Asthma Worse

- [ ] **Flu:** Get a flu shot.
- [ ] **Sulfites in foods:** Do not drink beer or wine or eat shrimp, dried fruit, or processed potatoes if they cause asthma symptoms.
- [ ] **Cold air:** Cover your nose and mouth with a scarf on cold or windy days.
- [ ] **Other medicines:** Tell your doctor about all the medicines you may take. Include cold medicines, aspirin, and even eye drops.

---

*To find out where to get products mentioned in this guide, call:

Asthma and Allergy Foundation of America (800-727-8462)

Allergy and Asthma Network/Mothers of Asthmatics, Inc. (800-878-4403)

American Academy of Allergy, Asthma, and Immunology (800-822-2762)

National Jewish Medical and Research Center (Lung Line) (800-222-5864)

How To Use Your Metered-Dose Inhaler the Right Way

Using an inhaler seems simple, but most patients do not use it the right way. When you use your inhaler the wrong way, less medicine gets to your lungs. (Your doctor may give you other types of inhalers.)

For the next 2 weeks, read these steps aloud as you do them or ask someone to read them to you. Ask your doctor or nurse to check how well you are using your inhaler.

Use your inhaler in one of the three ways pictured below (A or B are best, but C can be used if you have trouble with A and B).

Steps for Using Your Inhaler

Getting ready	1. Take off the cap and shake the inhaler.
	2. Breathe out all the way.
	3. Hold your inhaler the way your doctor said (A, B, or C below).
Breathe in slowly	4. As you start breathing in **slowly** through your mouth, press down on the inhaler **one** time. (If you use a holding chamber, first press down on the inhaler. Within 5 seconds, begin to breathe in slowly.)
	5. Keep breathing in **slowly**, as deeply as you can.
Hold your breath	6. Hold your breath as you count to 10 slowly, if you can.
	7. For inhaled quick-relief medicine (beta$_2$-agonists), wait about 1 minute between puffs. There is no need to wait between puffs for other medicines.

A. Hold inhaler 1 to 2 inches in front of your mouth (about the width of two fingers).

B. Use a spacer/holding chamber. These come in many shapes and can be useful to any patient.

C. Put the inhaler in your mouth. Do not use for steroids.

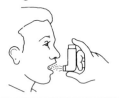
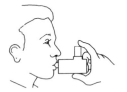
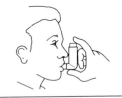

Clean Your Inhaler as Needed

Look at the hole where the medicine sprays out from your inhaler. If you see "powder" in or around the hole, clean the inhaler. Remove the metal canister from the L-shaped plastic mouthpiece. Rinse only the mouthpiece and cap in warm water. Let them dry over-night. In the morning, put the canister back inside. Put the cap on.

Know When To Replace Your Inhaler

For medicines you take each day (an example):
Say your new canister has 200 puffs (number of puffs is listed on canister) and you are told to take 8 puffs per day.

$$8 \text{ puffs per day} \overline{)\,200 \text{ puffs in canister}}^{\,25 \text{ days}}$$

So this canister will last 25 days.

If you started using this inhaler on May 1, replace it on or before May 25.

You can write the date on your canister.

For quick-relief medicine take as needed and count each puff.

Do not put your canister in water to see if it is empty. This does not work.

ASTHMA ACTION PLAN FOR _____ Doctor's Name _____ Date _____

Doctor's Phone Number _____ Hospital/Emergency Room Phone Number _____

GREEN ZONE: Doing Well

- No cough, wheeze, chest tightness, or shortness of breath during the day or night
- Can do usual activities

And, if a peak flow meter is used,
Peak flow: more than _____
(80% or more of my best peak flow)

My best peak flow is: _____

Take These Long-Term-Control Medicines Each Day (include an anti-inflammatory)

Medicine	How much to take	When to take it

Before exercise ☐ _____ ☐ 2 or ☐ 4 puffs 5 to 60 minutes before exercise

---

YELLOW ZONE: Asthma Is Getting Worse

- Cough, wheeze, chest tightness, or shortness of breath, or
- Waking at night due to asthma, or
- Can do some, but not all, usual activities

-Or-

Peak flow: _____ to _____
(50% - 80% of my best peak flow)

FIRST ➡ **Add: Quick-Relief Medicine – and keep taking your GREEN ZONE medicine**

_____ (short-acting beta₂-agonist)   ☐ 2 or ☐ 4 puffs, every 20 minutes for up to 1 hour
                                        ☐ Nebulizer, once

SECOND ➡ **If your symptoms (and peak flow, if used) return to GREEN ZONE after 1 hour of above treatment:**
☐ Take the quick-relief medicine every 4 hours for 1 to 2 days.
☐ Double the dose of your inhaled steroid for _____ (7-10) days.

-Or-

If your symptoms (and peak flow, if used) do not return to GREEN ZONE after 1 hour of above treatment:

☐ Take: _____ (short-acting beta₂-agonist) ☐ 2 or ☐ 4 puffs or ☐ Nebulizer

☐ Add: _____ (oral steroid) _____ mg. per day For _____ (3-10) days

☐ Call the doctor ☐ before/ ☐ within _____ hours after taking the oral steroid.

RED ZONE: Medical Alert!

- Very short of breath, or
- Quick-relief medicines have not helped, or
- Cannot do usual activities, or
- Symptoms are same or get worse after 24 hours in Yellow Zone

-Or-

Peak flow: less than_____
(50% of my best peak flow)

Take this medicine:

☐ _____ (short-acting beta₂-agonist) ☐ 4 or ☐ 6 puffs or ☐ Nebulizer

☐ _____ (oral steroid) _____ mg.

Then call your doctor NOW. Go to the hospital or call for an ambulance if:
- You are still in the red zone after 15 minutes AND
- You have not reached your doctor.

DANGER SIGNS

- Trouble walking and talking due to shortness of breath
- Lips or fingernails are blue

➡ ■ Take ☐ 4 or ☐ 6 puffs of your quick-relief medicine AND
■ Go to the hospital or call for an ambulance (_____) NOW!

– 63 –

School Self-Management Plan

Asthma and Allergy
Foundation of America
1125 15th St., N.W., Suite 502
Washington, DC 20005

STUDENT ASTHMA
ACTION CARD

Endorsed by

National Asthma
Education Program

Name: _____ Grade: _____ Age: _____

Teacher: _____ Room: _____

Parent/Guardian Name: _____ Ph: (H) _____

Address:_____ Ph: (W) _____

Parent/Guardian Name: _____ Ph: (H) _____

Address:_____ Ph: (W) _____

| ID Photo |

Emergency Phone Contact #1 _____ _____ _____

Name Relationship Phone

Emergency Phone Contact #2 _____ _____ _____

Name Relationship Phone

Physician Student Sees for Asthma: _____ Ph: _____

Other Physician: _____ Ph: _____

DAILY ASTHMA MANAGEMENT PLAN

- Identify the things which start an asthma episode (Check each that applies to the student.)

☐ Exercise ☐ Strong odors or fumes ☐ Other _____

☐ Respiratory infections ☐ Chalk dust _____

☐ Change in temperature ☐ Carpets in the room

☐ Animals ☐ Pollens

☐ Food _____ ☐ Molds

Comments _____

- Control of School Environment

(List any environmental control measures, pre-medications, and/or dietary restrictions that the student needs to prevent an asthma episode.)

_____

_____

_____

- Peak Flow Monitoring

Personal Best Peak Flow number: _____

Monitoring Times: _____ _____ _____

- Daily Medication Plan

	Name	Amount	When to Use
1.	_____	_____	_____
2.	_____	_____	_____
3.	_____	_____	_____
4.	_____	_____	_____

School Self-Management Plan (continued)

EMERGENCY PLAN

Emergency action is necessary when the student has symptoms such as _____, _____, _____, _____ or has a peak flow reading of _____.

- **Steps to take during an asthma episode:**

  1. Give medications as listed below.

  2. Have student return to classroom if _____ _____

  3. Contact parent if _____

  4. Seek emergency medical care if the student has any of the following:

     ✔ No improvement 15-20 minutes after initial treatment with medication and a relative cannot be reached.

     ✔ Peak flow of _____

     ✔ Hard time breathing with:

        • Chest and neck pulled in with breathing
        • Child is hunched over
        • Child is struggling to breathe

     ✔ Trouble walking or talking

     ✔ Stops playing and can't start activity again

     ✔ Lips or fingernails are gray or blue

     } **IF THIS HAPPENS, GET EMERGENCY HELP NOW!**

- **Emergency Asthma Medications**

	Name	Amount	When to Use
1.			
2.			
3.			
4.			

COMMENTS / SPECIAL INSTRUCTIONS

_____
_____
_____
_____

FOR INHALED MEDICATIONS

☐ I have instructed _____ in the proper way to use his/her medications. It is my professional opinion that _____ should be allowed to carry and use that medication by him/herself.

☐ It is my professional opinion that _____ should not carry his/her inhaled medication by him/herself.

_____   _____
Physician Signature   Date

_____   _____
Parent Signature   Date

How To Use Your Peak Flow Meter

A peak flow meter helps you check how well your asthma is controlled. Peak flow meters are most helpful for people with moderate or severe asthma.

This guide will tell you (1) how to find your personal best peak flow number, (2) how to use your personal best number to set your peak flow zones, (3) how to take your peak flow, and (4) when to take your peak flow to check your asthma each day.

Starting Out: Find Your Personal Best Peak Flow Number

To find your personal best peak flow number, take your peak flow each day for 2 to 3 weeks. Your asthma should be under good control during this time. Take your peak flow as close to the times listed below as you can. (These times for taking your peak flow are only for finding your personal best peak flow. To check your asthma each day, you will take your peak flow in the morning. This is discussed on the next page.)

- Between noon and 2:00 p.m. each day.

- Each time you take your quick-relief medicine to relieve symptoms. (Measure your peak flow <u>after</u> you take your medicine.)

- Any other time your doctor suggests.

Write down the number you get for each peak flow reading. The highest peak flow number you had during the 2 to 3 weeks is your personal best.

Your personal best can change over time. Ask your doctor when to check for a new personal best.

Your Peak Flow Zones

Your peak flow zones are based on your personal best peak flow number. The zones will help you check your asthma and take the right actions to keep it controlled. The colors used with each zone come from the traffic light.

 Green Zone (80 to 100 percent of your personal best) signals **good control.** Take your usual daily long-term-control medicines, if you take any. Keep taking these medicines even when you are in the yellow or red zones.

 Yellow Zone (50 to 79 percent of your personal best) signals **caution: your asthma is getting worse.** Add quick-relief medicines. You might need to increase other asthma medicines as directed by your doctor.

 Red Zone (below 50 percent of your personal best) signals **medical alert!** Add or increase quick-relief medicines and call your doctor <u>now</u>.

Ask your doctor to write an action plan for you that tells you:

- The peak flow numbers for <u>your</u> green, yellow, and red zones. Mark the zones on your peak flow meter with colored tape or a marker.

- The medicines you should take while in each peak flow zone.

How To Take Your Peak Flow

1. Move the marker to the bottom of the numbered scale.

2. Stand up or sit up straight.

3. Take a deep breath. Fill your lungs all the way.

4. Hold your breath while you place the mouthpiece in your mouth, between your teeth. Close your lips around it. Do **not** put your tongue inside the hole.

5. Blow out as hard and fast as you can. Your peak flow meter will measure how fast you can blow out air.

6. Write down the number you get. But if you cough or make a mistake, do not write down the number. Do it over again.

7. Repeat steps 1 through 6 two more times. Write down the highest of the three numbers. This is your peak flow number.

8. Check to see which peak flow <u>zone</u> your peak flow number is in. Do the actions your doctor told you to do while in that zone.

Your doctor may ask you to write down your peak flow numbers each day. You can do this on a calendar or other paper. This will help you and your doctor see how your asthma is doing over time.

Checking Your Asthma: When To Use Your Peak Flow Meter

- **Every morning** when you wake up, *before* you take medicine. Make this part of your daily routine.

- **When you are having asthma symptoms or an attack.** And after taking medicine for the attack. This can tell you how bad your asthma attack is and whether your medicine is working.

- Any other time your doctor suggests.

If you use more than one peak flow meter (such as at home and at school), be sure that both meters are the same brand.

Bring to Each of Your Doctor's Visits:

- Your peak flow meter.

- Your peak flow numbers if you have written them down each day.

Also, ask your doctor or nurse to check how you use your peak flow meter—just to be sure you are doing it right.

Patient Self-Assessment Form for Environmental and Other Factors That Can Make Asthma Worse

Patient Name: _____ Date: _____

Do you cough, wheeze, have chest tightness, or feel short of breath year-round? (If no, go to next question) If yes:	No _____	Yes _____
• Are there **pets** or animals in your home, school, or day care?	No _____	Yes _____
• Is there moisture or **dampness** in any room of your home?	No _____	Yes _____
• Have you seen **mold** or smelled musty odors any place in your home?	No _____	Yes _____
• Have you seen **cockroaches** in your home?	No _____	Yes _____
• Do you use a **humidifier** or swamp cooler in your home?	No _____	Yes _____

Does your coughing, wheezing, chest tightness, or shortness of breath get worse at certain times of the year? (If no, go to next question) If yes: Do your symptoms get worse in the:	No _____	Yes _____
• Early spring? (Trees)	No _____	Yes _____
• Late spring? (Grasses)	No _____	Yes _____
• Late summer to autumn? (Weeds)	No _____	Yes _____
• Summer and fall? (*Alternaria, Cladosporium*)	No _____	Yes _____

Do you **smoke**?	No _____	Yes _____
Does anyone smoke at home, work, or day care?	No _____	Yes _____

Is a **wood-burning stove or fireplace** used in your home?	No _____	Yes _____
Are **kerosene, oil, or gas stoves or heaters** used without vents in your home?	No _____	Yes _____
Are you exposed to **fumes or odors** from cleaning agents, sprays, or other chemicals?	No _____	Yes _____

Do you cough or wheeze during the week, but not on weekends when away from **work or school**?	No _____	Yes _____
Do your eyes and nose get irritated soon after you get to work or school?	No _____	Yes _____
Do your coworkers or classmates have symptoms like yours?	No _____	Yes _____
Are isocyanates, plant or animal products, smoke, gases, or fumes used where you work?	No _____	Yes _____
Is it cold, hot, dusty, or humid where you work?	No _____	Yes _____

Do you have a **stuffy nose** or postnasal drip, either at certain times of the year or year-round?	No _____	Yes _____
Do you sneeze often or have itchy, watery eyes?	No _____	Yes _____

Do you have **heartburn?**	No _____	Yes _____
Does food sometimes come up into your throat?	No _____	Yes _____
Have you had coughing, wheezing, or shortness of breath at night in the past 4 weeks?	No _____	Yes _____
Does your infant vomit then cough or have wheezy cough at night?	No _____	Yes _____
Are these symptoms worse after feeding?	No _____	Yes _____

Have you had wheezing, coughing, or shortness of breath **after eating** shrimp, dried fruit, or canned or processed potatoes?	No _____	Yes _____
After drinking beer or wine?	No _____	Yes _____

Are you taking any prescription medicines or over-the-counter **medicines**?	No _____	Yes _____
If yes, which ones? _____	No _____	Yes _____

Do you use eye drops?	No _____	Yes _____
Do you use any medicines that contain beta-blockers (e.g., blood pressure medicine)?	No _____	Yes _____
Do you ever take aspirin or other nonsteroidal anti-inflammatory drugs (like ibuprofen)?	No _____	Yes _____
Have you ever had coughing, wheezing, chest tightness, or shortness of breath after taking any medication?	No _____	Yes _____

Do you cough, wheeze, have chest tightness, or feel short of breath during or after **exercising**?	No _____	Yes _____

Patient Self-Assessment Form for Followup Visits

Patient Name: _____ Date: _____

Please answer the questions below in the space provided on the right.

Since your last visit:

1. Has your asthma been any worse?   No _____ Yes _____
2. Have there been any changes in your home, work, or school environment (such as a new pet, someone smoking)?   No _____ Yes _____
3. Have you had any times when your symptoms were a lot worse than usual?   No _____ Yes _____
4. Has your asthma caused you to miss work or school or reduce or change your activities?   No _____ Yes _____
5. Have you missed any regular doses of your medicines for any reason?   No _____ Yes _____
6. Have your medications caused you any problems? (shakiness, nervousness, bad taste, sore throat, cough, upset stomach)   No _____ Yes _____
7. Have you had any emergency room visits or hospital stays for asthma?   No _____ Yes _____
8. Has the cost of your asthma treatment kept you from getting the medicine or care you need for your asthma?   No _____ Yes _____

In the past 2 weeks,

9. Have you had a cough, wheezing, shortness of breath or chest tightness during:
   - the day   No _____ Yes _____
   - night   No _____ Yes _____
   - exercise or play?   No _____ Yes _____
10. (If you use a peak flow meter) Did your peak flow go below 80 percent of your personal best?   No _____ Yes _____
11. How many days have you used your inhaled quick-relief medicine?   Number of days _____
12. Have you been satisfied with the way your asthma has been?   No _____ Yes _____

13. What are some concerns or questions you would like us to address at this visit?

_____

_____

_____

For staff use.
- ☐ Peak Flow Technique
- ☐ MDI Technique
- ☐ Reviewed Action Plan: ☐ Daily meds   ☐ Emergency meds

Diagnosis and Evaluation of the Child With Attention-Deficit/ Hyperactivity Disorder

- *Clinical Practice Guideline*
- *Technical Report Summary*

Clinical Practice Guideline:
Diagnosis and Evaluation of the Child With Attention-Deficit/Hyperactivity Disorder

Author:

Subcommittee on Attention-Deficit/Hyperactivity Disorder
Committee on Quality Improvement

American Academy of Pediatrics
PO Box 927, 141 Northwest Point Blvd
Elk Grove Village, IL 60009-0927

Subcommittee on Attention-Deficit/ Hyperactivity Disorder

James M. Perrin, MD, Co-Chairperson
Martin T. Stein, MD, Co-Chairperson

Robert W. Amler, MD
Thomas A. Blondis, MD
Heidi M. Feldman, MD, PhD

Bruce P. Meyer, MD
Bennett A. Shaywitz, MD
Mark L. Wolraich, MD

Consultants:

Anthony DeSpirito, MD
Charles J. Homer, MD, MPH

Sydney Zentall, PhD

Liaison Representatives:

Karen Pierce, MD, American Academy of Child and Adolescent Psychiatry
Theodore G. Ganiats, MD, American Academy of Family Physicians

Brian Grabert, MD, Child Neurology Society
Ronald T. Brown, PhD, Society for Pediatric Psychology

Committee on Quality Improvement 1999–2000

Charles J. Homer, MD, MPH, Chairperson

Richard D. Baltz, MD
Gerald B. Hickson, MD
Paul V. Miles, MD

Thomas B. Newman, MD, MPH
Joan E. Shook, MD
William M. Zurhellen, MD

Liaison Representatives:

Betty A. Lowe, MD, National Association of Children's Hospitals and Related Institutions
Ellen Schwalenstocker, MBA, National Association of Children's Hospitals and Related Institutions
Michael J. Goldberg, MD, Council on Sections

Richard Shiffman, MD, Section on Computers and Other Technologies
Jan Ellen Berger, MD, Committee on Medical Liability
F. Lane France, MD, Committee on Practice and Ambulatory Medicine

Abstract

This clinical practice guideline provides recommendations for the assessment and diagnosis of school-aged children with attention-deficit/hyperactivity disorder (ADHD). This guideline, the first of 2 sets of guidelines to provide recommendations on this condition, is intended for use by primary care clinicians working in primary care settings. The second set of guidelines will address the issue of treatment of children with ADHD.

The Committee on Quality Improvement of the American Academy of Pediatrics selected a committee composed of pediatricians and other experts in the fields of neurology, psychology, child psychiatry, development, and education, as well as experts from epidemiology and pediatric practice. In addition, this panel consists of experts in education and family practice. The panel worked with Technical Resources International, Washington, DC, under the auspices of the Agency for Healthcare Research and Quality, to develop the evidence base of literature on this topic. The resulting evidence report was used to formulate recommendations for evaluation of the child with ADHD. Major issues contained within the guideline address child and family assessment; school assessment, including the use of various rating scales; and conditions seen frequently among children with ADHD. Information is also included on the use of current diagnostic coding strategies. The deliberations of the committee were informed by a systematic review of evidence about prevalence, coexisting conditions, and diagnostic tests. Committee decisions were made by consensus where definitive evidence was not available. The committee report underwent review by sections of the American Academy of Pediatrics and external organizations before approval by the Board of Directors.

The guideline contains the following recommendations for diagnosis of ADHD: 1) in a child 6 to 12 years old who presents with inattention, hyperactivity, impulsivity, academic underachievement, or behavior problems, primary care clinicians should initiate an evaluation for ADHD; 2) the diagnosis of ADHD requires that a child meet *Diagnostic and Statistical Manual of Mental Disorders, Fourth Edition* criteria; 3) the assessment of ADHD requires evidence directly obtained from parents or caregivers regarding the core symptoms of ADHD in various settings, the age of onset, duration of symptoms, and degree of functional impairment; 4) the assessment of ADHD requires evidence directly obtained from the classroom teacher (or other school professional) regarding the core symptoms of ADHD, duration of symptoms, degree of functional impairment, and associated conditions; 5) evaluation of the child with ADHD should include assessment for associated (coexisting) conditions; and 6) other diagnostic tests are not routinely indicated to establish the diagnosis of ADHD but may be used for the assessment of other coexisting conditions (eg, learning disabilities and mental retardation).

This clinical practice guideline is not intended as a sole source of guidance in the evaluation of children with ADHD. Rather, it is designed to assist primary care clinicians by providing a framework for diagnostic decisionmaking. It is not intended to replace clinical judgment or to establish a protocol for all children with this condition and may not provide the only appropriate approach to this problem.

Attention-deficit/hyperactivity disorder (ADHD) is the most common neurobehavioral disorder of childhood. ADHD is also among the most prevalent chronic health conditions affecting school-aged children. The core symptoms of ADHD include inattention, hyperactivity, and impulsivity.[1,2] Children with ADHD may experience significant functional problems, such as school difficulties, academic underachievement,[3] troublesome interpersonal relationships with family members[4,5] and peers, and low self-esteem. Individuals with ADHD present in childhood and may continue to show symptoms as they enter adolescence[6] and adult life.[7] Pediatricians and other primary care clinicians frequently are asked by parents and teachers to evaluate a child for ADHD. Early recognition, assessment, and management of this condition can redirect the educational and psychosocial development of most children with ADHD.[8,9]

Recorded prevalence rates for ADHD vary substantially, partly because of changing diagnostic criteria over time,[10-13] and partly because of variations in ascertainment in different settings and the frequent use of referred samples to estimate rates. Practitioners of all types (primary care, subspecialty, psychiatry, and nonphysician mental health providers) vary greatly in the degree to which they use *Diagnostic and Statistical Manual of Mental Health Disorders, Fourth Edition (DSM-IV)* criteria to diagnose ADHD. Reported rates also vary substantially in different geographic areas and across countries.[14]

With increasing epidemiologic and clinical research, diagnostic criteria have been revised on multiple occasions over the past 20 years.[10-13] A recent review of prevalence rates in school-aged community samples (rather than referred samples) indicates rates varying from 4% to 12%, with estimated prevalence based on combining these studies of ~8% to 10%. In the general population,[15-23,24] 9.2% (5.8%–13.6%) of males and 2.9% (1.9%–4.5%) of females are found to have behaviors consistent with ADHD. With the *DSM-IV* criteria (compared with earlier versions), more females have been diagnosed with the predominantly inattentive type.[25,26] Prevalence rates also vary significantly depending on whether they reflect school samples 6.9% (5.5%–8.5%) versus community samples 10.3% (8.2%–12.7%).

Public interest in ADHD has increased along with debate in the media concerning the diagnostic process and treatment strategies.[27] Concern has been expressed about the over-diagnosis of ADHD by pointing to the several-fold increase in prescriptions for stimulant medication among children during the past decade.[28] In addition, there are significant regional variations in the amount of stimulants prescribed by physicians.[29] Practice surveys among primary care pediatricians and family physicians reveal wide variations in practice patterns about diagnostic criteria and methods.[30]

ADHD commonly occurs in association with oppositional defiant disorder, conduct disorder, depression, anxiety disorder,[16] and with many developmental disorders, such as speech and language delays and learning disabilities.

This diagnostic guideline is intended for use by primary care clinicians to evaluate children between 6 and 12 years of age for ADHD, consistent with best available empirical studies. Special attention is given to assessing school performance and behavior, family functioning, and adaptation. In light of the high prevalence of ADHD in pediatric practice, the guideline should assist primary care clinicians in these assessments. The diagnosis usually requires several steps. Clinicians will generally need to carry out the evaluation in more than 1 visit, often indeed 2 to 3 visits. The guideline is not intended for children with mental retardation, pervasive developmental disorder, moderate to severe sensory deficits such as visual and hearing impairment, chronic disorders associated with medications that may affect behavior, and those who have experienced child abuse and sexual abuse. These children too may have ADHD, and this guideline may help clinicians in considering this diagnosis; nonetheless, this guideline primarily reviews evidence relating to the diagnosis of ADHD in relatively uncomplicated cases in primary care settings.

Methodology

To initiate the development of a practice guideline for the diagnosis and evaluation of children with ADHD directed toward primary care physicians, the American Academy of Pediatrics (AAP) worked with several colleague organizations to organize a working panel representing a wide range of primary care and subspecialty groups. The committee, chaired by 2 general pediatricians (1 with substantial additional experience and training in developmental and behavioral pediatrics), included representatives from the American Academy of Family Physicians, the American Academy of Child and Adolescent Psychiatry, the Child Neurology Society, and the Society for Pediatric Psychology, as well as developmental and behavioral pediatricians and epidemiologists.

This group met over a period of 2 years, during which it reviewed basic literature on current practices in the diagnosis of ADHD and developed a series of questions to direct an evidence-based review of the prevalence of ADHD in community and primary care practice settings, the rates of coexisting conditions, and the utility of several diagnostic methods and devices. The AAP committee collaborated with the Agency for Healthcare Research and Quality in its support of an evidence-based review of several of these key items in the diagnosis of ADHD. David Atkins, MD, provided liaison from the Agency for Healthcare Research and Quality, and Technical Resources International conducted the evidence review.

The Technical Resources International report focused on 4 specific areas for the literature review: the prevalence of ADHD among children 6 to 12 years of age in the general population and the coexisting conditions that may occur with ADHD; the prevalence of ADHD among children in primary care settings and the coexisting conditions that may occur; the accuracy of various screening methods for diagnosis; and the prevalence of abnormal findings on commonly used medical screening tests. The literature search was conducted using Medline and PsycINFO databases, references from review articles, rating scale manuals, and articles identified by the subcommittee. Only articles published in English between 1980 and 1997 were included. The study population was limited to children 6 to 12 years of age, and only studies using general, unselected populations in communities, schools, or the primary clinical setting were used. Data on screening tests were taken from studies conducted in any setting. Articles accepted for analysis were abstracted twice by trained personnel and a clinical specialist. Both abstracts for each article were compared and differences between them resolved. A multiple logistic regression model with random effects was used to analyze simultaneously for age, gender, diagnostic tool, and setting using EGRET software. Results were presented in evidence tables and published in the final evidence report.[24]

The draft practice guideline underwent extensive peer review by committees and sections within the AAP, by numerous outside organizations, and by other individuals identified by the subcommittee. Liaisons to the subcommittee also were invited to distribute the draft to entities within their organizations. The resulting comments were compiled and reviewed by the subcommittee co-chairpersons, and relevant changes were incorporated into the draft based on recommendations from peer reviewers.

The recommendations contained in the practice guideline are based on the best available data (Fig 1). Where data were lacking, a combination of evidence and expert consensus was used. Strong recommendations were based on high-quality scientific evidence, or, in the absence of high-quality data, strong expert consensus. Fair and weak recommendations were based on lesser quality or limited data and expert consensus. Clinical options were identified as interventions because the subcommittee could not find compelling evidence for or against. These clinical options are interventions that a reasonable health care provider might or might not wish to implement in his or her practice.

RECOMMENDATION 1: In a child 6 to 12 years old who presents with inattention, hyperactivity, impulsivity, academic underachievement, or behavior problems, primary care clinicians should initiate an evaluation for ADHD (strength of evidence: good; strength of recommendation: strong).

The major justification for this recommendation is the high prevalence of ADHD in school-aged populations. School-aged children with a variety of developmental and behavioral concerns present to primary care clinicians.[31] Primary care pediatricians and family physicians recognize behavior problems that may impact academic achievement in 18% of school-aged children seen in their offices and clinics. Hyperactivity or inattention is diagnosed in 9% of children.[32]

Presentations of ADHD in clinical practice vary. In many cases, concerns derive from parents, teachers, other professionals, or nonparental caregivers.

Fig 1. Diagnosis and Evaluation of the Child with Attention-Deficit/Hyperactivity Disorder Clinical Algorithm

A

1

Child 6 to 12 years of age presents with parent (or other caregiver) or teacher concerns about academic under-achievement and/or specific behaviors OR clinician assesses these conditions during health supervision screening

Primary care clinician should consider ADHD in a child presenting with any of the following concerns:
- can't sit still/hyperactive
- lack of attention/poor concentration/doesn't seem to listen/daydreams
- acts without thinking/impulsive
- behavior problems
- academic underachievement

School assessment includes:
- Documentation of specific elements:
  – inattention
  – hyperactivity
  – impulsivity
- Use of teacher ADHD-specific behavior checklist (short-form)
- Teacher narrative including:
  – classroom behavior
  – learning patterns
  – classroom interventions
  – degree of functional impairment
- Evidence of school work
  – report card
  – samples of school work

Family assessment includes:
- Documentation of specific elements by interview or use of ADHD-specific checklist of:
  – inattention
  – hyperactivity
  – impulsivity
- Documentation should include
  – multiple settings
  – age of onset
  – duration of symptoms
  – degree of functional impairment

2

Assessment of the child by the primary care clinician includes:
- standard history and physical examination
- neurological examination
- family assessment
- school assessment

3

Does child meet *DSM-IV* criteria for ADHD?

4

Yes → Go to Box 8

No → (Go to Box 5)

Meeting ADHD criteria using the *DSM-IV* must include whether symptoms interfere with functioning and performance in more than one setting and last longer than 6 months

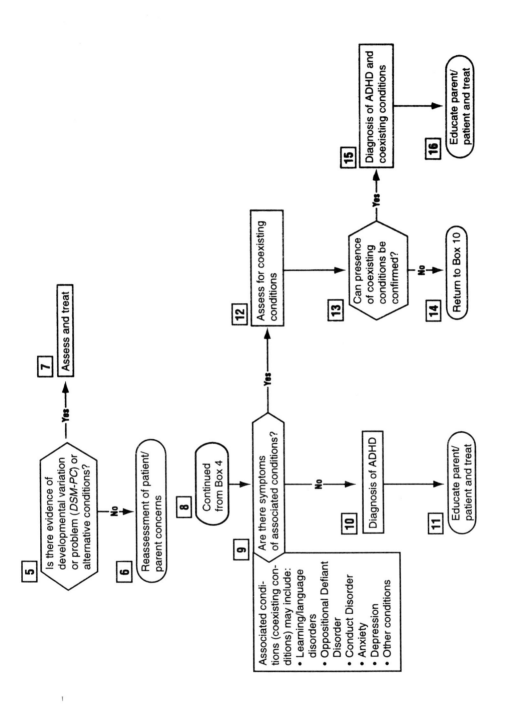

B

5 Is there evidence of developmental variation or problem (*DSM-PC*) or alternative conditions? — **Yes** → **7** Assess and treat

No ↓

6 Reassessment of patient/parent concerns

8 Continued from Box 4

9 Are there symptoms of associated conditions?

Associated conditions (coexisting conditions) may include:
• Learning/language disorders
• Oppositional Defiant Disorder
• Conduct Disorder
• Anxiety
• Depression
• Other conditions

No → **10** Diagnosis of ADHD → **11** Educate parent/patient and treat

Yes ↓

12 Assess for coexisting conditions

13 Can presence of coexisting conditions be confirmed?

No → **14** Return to Box 10

Yes ↓

15 Diagnosis of ADHD and coexisting conditions → **16** Educate parent/patient and treat

- 83 -

Common presentations include referral from school for academic under-achievement and failure, disruptive classroom behavior, inattentiveness, problems with social relationships, parental concerns regarding similar phenomena, poor self-esteem, or problems with establishing or maintaining social relationships. Children with core ADHD symptoms of hyperactivity and impulsivity are identified by teachers, because they often disrupt the classroom. Even mild distractibility and motor symptoms, such as fidgetiness, will be apparent to most teachers. In contrast, children with the inattentive subtype of ADHD, where hyperactive and impulsive symptoms are absent or minimal, may not come to the attention of teachers. These children may present with school underachievement.

Symptoms may not be apparent in a structured clinical setting that is free from the demands and distraction of the home and school.[33] Thus, if parents do not bring concerns to the primary clinician, then early detection of ADHD in primary care may not occur. Clinical practices during routine health supervision may assist in early recognition of ADHD.[34,35] Options include direct history from parents and children. The following general questions may be useful at all visits for school-aged children to heighten attention about ADHD and as an initial screening for school performance.

1. How is your child doing in school?
2. Are there any problems with learning that you or the teacher has seen?
3. Is your child happy in school?
4. Are you concerned with any behavioral problems in school, at home, or when your child is playing with friends?
5. Is your child having problems completing classwork or homework?

Alternatively, a previsit questionnaire may be sent to parents or given while the family is waiting in the reception area.[36] When making an appointment for a health supervision visit for a school-aged child, 1 or 2 of these questions may be asked routinely to sensitize parents to the concerns of their child's clinician. For example, "Your child's clinician is interested in how your child is doing in school. You might check with her teacher and discuss any concerns with your child's physician." Wall posters, pamphlets, and books in the waiting area that focus on educational achievements and school-aged behaviors send a message that this is an office or clinic that considers these issues important to a child's development.[37]

RECOMMENDATION 2: The diagnosis of ADHD requires that a child meet DSM-IV criteria (strength of evidence: good; strength of recommendation: strong).

Establishing a diagnosis of ADHD requires a strategy that minimizes over-identification and under-identification. Pediatricians and other primary care health professionals should apply *DSM-IV* criteria in the context of their clinical assessment of a child. The use of specific criteria will help to ensure a more accurate diagnosis and decrease variation in how the diagnosis is made.

The *DSM-IV* criteria, developed through several iterations by the American Psychiatric Association, are based on clinical experience and an expanding research foundation.[13] These criteria have more support in the literature than other available diagnostic criteria. The *DSM-IV* specification of behavior items, required numbers of items, and levels of impairment reflect the current consensus among clinicians, particularly psychiatry. The consensus includes increasing research evidence, particularly in the distinctions that the *DSM-IV* makes for the dimensions of attention and hyperactivity-impulsivity.[38]

The *DSM-IV* criteria define 3 subtypes of ADHD (see Table 1 for specific inattention and hyperactive-impulsive items).

• ADHD primarily of the inattentive type (ADHD/I, meeting at least 6 of 9 inattention behaviors)
• ADHD primarily of the hyperactive-impulsive type (ADHD/HI, meeting at least 6 of 9 hyperactive-impulsive behaviors)
• ADHD combined type (ADHD/C, meeting at least 6 of 9 behaviors in both the inattention and hyperactive-impulsive lists)

Children who meet diagnostic criteria for the behavioral symptoms of ADHD but who demonstrate no functional impairment do not meet the diagnostic criteria for ADHD.[13] The symptoms of ADHD should be present in 2 or more settings (eg, at home and in school), and the behaviors must adversely affect functioning in school or in a social situation. Reliable and clinically valid measures of dysfunction applicable to the primary care setting have been difficult to develop. The diagnosis comes from a synthesis of information obtained from parents; school reports; mental health care professionals, if they have been involved; and an interview/examination of the child. Current *DSM-IV* criteria require evidence of symptoms before 7 years of age. In some cases, the symptoms of ADHD may not be recognized by parents or teachers until the child is older than 7 years of age, when school tasks become more challenging. Age of onset and duration of symptoms may be obtained from parents in the course of a comprehensive history.

Teachers, parents, and child health professionals typically encounter children with behaviors relating to activity, impulsivity, and attention who may not fully meet *DSM-IV* criteria. *The Diagnostic and Statistical Manual for Primary Care (DSM-PC), Child and Adolescent Version,*[39] provides a guide to the more common behaviors seen in pediatrics. The manual describes common variations in behavior, as well as more problematic behaviors, at levels less than those specified in the *DSM-IV* (and with less impairment). The behavioral descriptions of the *DSM-PC* have not yet been tested in community studies to determine the prevalence or severity of developmental variations and moderate problems in the areas of inattention and hyperactivity or impulsivity. They do, however, provide guidance to clinicians in the evaluation of children with these symptoms and help to direct clinicians to many elements of treatment for children with problems with attention, hyperactivity, or impulsivity (Tables 2 and 3). The *DSM-PC* also considers environmental influ-

Table 1. Diagnostic Criteria for ADHD

A. Either 1 or 2:
1) Six (or more) of the following symptoms of **inattention** have persisted for at least 6 months to a degree that is maladaptive and inconsistent with developmental level:

Inattention
   a) Often fails to give close attention to details or makes careless mistakes in schoolwork, work, or other activities
   b) Often has difficulty sustaining attention in tasks or play activities
   c) Often does not seem to listen when spoken to directly
   d) Often does not follow through on instructions and fails to finish schoolwork, chores, or duties in the workplace (not due to oppositional behavior or failure to understand instructions)
   e) Often has difficulty organizing tasks and activities
   f) Often avoids, dislikes, or is reluctant to engage in tasks that require sustained mental effort (such as schoolwork or homework)
   g) Often loses things necessary for tasks or activities (eg, toys, school assignments, pencils, books, or tools)
   h) Is often easily distracted by extraneous stimuli
   i) Is often forgetful in daily activities

(2) Six (or more) of the following symptoms of **hyperactivity-impulsivity** have persisted for at least 6 months to a degree that is maladaptive and inconsistent with developmental level:

Hyperactivity
   a) Often fidgets with hands or feet or squirms in seat
   b) Often leaves seat in classroom or in other situations in which remaining seated is expected
   c) Often runs about or climbs excessively in situations in which it is inappropriate (in adolescents or adults, may be limited to subjective feelings of restlessness)
   d) Often has difficulty playing or engaging in leisure activities quietly
   e) Is often "on the go" or often acts as if "driven by a motor"
   f) Often talks excessively

Impulsivity
   g) Often blurts out answers before questions have been completed
   h) Often has difficulty awaiting turn
   i) Often interrupts or intrudes on other (eg, butts into conversations or games)

B. Some hyperactive-impulsive or inattentive symptoms that caused impairment were present before 7 years of age.

C. Some impairment from the symptoms is present in 2 or more settings (eg, at school [or work] or at home).

D. There must be clear evidence of clinically significant impairment in social, academic, or occupational functioning.

E. The symptoms do not occur exclusively during the course of a pervasive developmental disorder, schizophrenia, or other psychotic disorder and are not better accounted for by another mental disorder (eg, mood disorder, anxiety disorder, dissociative disorder, or personality disorder).

Code based on type:
314.01 **Attention-Deficit/Hyperactivity Disorder, Combined Type:**
   if both Criteria A1 and A2 are met for the past 6 months
314.00 **Attention-Deficit/Hyperactivity Disorder, Predominantly Inattentive Type:**
   if criterion A1 is met but criterion A2 is not met for the past 6 months
314.01 **Attention-Deficit/Hyperactivity Disorder, Predominantly Hyperactive, Impulsive Type:**
   if criterion A2 is met but criterion A1 is not met for the past 6 months
314.9 **Attention-Deficit/Hyperactivity Disorder Not Otherwise Specified**

Reprinted with permission from the *Diagnostic and Statistical Manual of Mental Disorders, 4th Ed. (DSM-IV)*. Copyright 1994. American Psychiatric Association.

Table 2. Developmental Variation: Impulsive/Hyperactive Behaviors

DEVELOPMENTAL VARIATION	COMMON DEVELOPMENTAL PRESENTATIONS
V65.49 Hyperactive/Impulsive variation	*Early childhood*
Young children in infancy and in the preschool years are normally very active and impulsive and may need constant supervision to avoid injury. Their constant activity may be stressful to adults who do not have the energy or patience to tolerate the behavior.	The child runs in circles, doesn't stop to rest, may bang into objects or people, and asks questions constantly.
During school years and adolescence, activity may be high in play situations and impulsive behaviors may normally occur, especially in peer pressure situations.	*Middle childhood* The child plays active games for long periods. The child may occasionally do things impulsively, particularly when excited.
High levels of hyperactive/impulsive behavior do not indicate a problem or disorder if the behavior does not impair function.	*Adolescence* The adolescent engages in active social activities (eg, dancing) for long periods, may engage in risky behaviors with peers.

SPECIAL INFORMATION

Activity should be thought of not only in terms of actual movement, but also in terms of variations in responding to touch, pressure, sound, light, and other sensations. Also, for the infant and young child, activity and attention are related to the interactions between the child and caregiver, eg, when sharing attention and playing together.

Activity and impulsivity often normally increase when the child is tired or hungry and decrease when sources of fatigue or hunger are addressed.

Activity normally may increase in new situations or when the child may be anxious. Familiarity then reduces activity.

Both activity and impulsivity must be judged in the context of the caregiver's expectations and the level of stress experienced by the caregiver. When expectations are unreasonable, the stress level is high, and/or the parent has an emotional disorder (especially depression), the adult may exaggerate the child's level of activity/impulsivity.

Activity level is a variable of temperature. The activity level of some children is on the high end of normal from birth and continues to be high throughout their development.

Taken from: American Academy of Pediatrics. *The Classification of Child and Adolescent Mental Diagnoses in Primary Care. Diagnostic and Statistical Manual for Primary Care (DSM-PC). Child and Adolescent Version.* Elk Grove Village, IL:American Academy of Pediatrics;1996.

Table 3. *DSM-PC:* Developmental Variation: Inattentive Behaviors

DEVELOPMENTAL VARIATION

V65.49 Inattention variation
A young child will have a short attention span that will increase as the child matures. The inattention should be appropriate for the child's level of development and not cause any impairment.

COMMON DEVELOPMENTAL PRESENTATIONS

Early childhood
The preschooler has difficulty attending, except briefly, to a storybook or a quiet task such as coloring or drawing.

Middle childhood
The child may not persist very long with a task the child does not want to do such as read an assigned book, homework, or a task that requires concentration such as cleaning something.

Adolescence
The adolescent is easily distracted from tasks he or she does not desire to perform.

SPECIAL INFORMATION

Infants and preschoolers usually have very short attention spans and normally do not persist with activities for long, so that diagnosing this problem in younger children may be difficult. Some parents may have a low tolerance for developmentally appropriate inattention.

Although watching television cartoons for long periods of time appears to reflect a long attention span, it does not reflect longer attention spans because most television segments require short (2- to 3-minute) attention spans and they are very stimulating.

Normally, attention span varies greatly depending upon the child's or adolescent's interest and skill in the activity, so much so that a short attention span for a particular task may reflect the child's skill or interest in that task.

Taken from: American Academy of Pediatrics. *The Classification of Child and Adolescent Mental Diagnoses in Primary Care. Diagnostic and Statistical Manual for Primary Care (DSM-PC). Child and Adolescent Version.* Elk Grove Village, IL: American Academy of Pediatrics; 1996.

ences on a child's behavior and provides information on differential diagnosis with a developmental perspective.

Given the lack of methods to confirm the diagnosis of ADHD through other means, it is important to recognize the limitations of the *DSM-IV* definition. Most of the development and testing of the *DSM-IV* has occurred through studies of children seen in psychiatric settings. Much less is known about its use in other populations, such as those seen in general pediatric or family practice settings. Despite the agreement of many professionals working in this field, the *DSM-IV* criteria remain a consensus without clear empirical data supporting the number of items required for the diagnosis. Current criteria do not take into account gender differences or developmental variations in behavior. Furthermore, the behavioral characteristics specified in the *DSM-IV*, despite efforts to standardize them, remain subjective and may be interpreted differently by different observers. Continuing research will likely clarify the validity of the *DSM-IV* criteria (and subsequent modifications) in the diagnosis. These complexities in the diagnosis mean that clinicians using *DSM-IV* criteria must apply them in the context of their clinical judgment.

No instruments used in primary care practice reliably assess the nature or degree of functional impairment of children with ADHD. With information obtained from the parent and school, the clinician can make a clinical judgment about the effect of the core and associated symptoms of ADHD on academic achievement, classroom performance, family and social relationships, independent functioning, self-esteem, leisure activities, and self-care (such as bathing, toileting, dressing, and eating).

The following 2 recommendations establish the presence of core behavior symptoms in multiple settings.

RECOMMENDATION 3: The assessment of ADHD requires evidence directly obtained from parents or caregivers regarding the core symptoms of ADHD in various settings, the age of onset, duration of symptoms, and degree of functional impairment (strength of evidence: good; strength of recommendation: strong).

Behavior symptoms may be obtained from parents or guardians using 1 or more methods, including open-ended questions (eg, "What are your concerns about your child's behavior in school?"), focused questions about specific behaviors, semi-structured interview schedules, questionnaires, and rating scales. Clinicians who obtain information from open-ended or focused questions must obtain and record the relevant behaviors of inattention, hyperactivity, and impulsivity from the *DSM-IV*. The use of global clinical impressions or general descriptions within the domains of attention and activity is insufficient to diagnose ADHD. As data are gathered about the child's behavior, an opportunity becomes available to evaluate the family environment and parenting style. In this way, behavioral symptoms may be evaluated in the context of the environment that may have important characteristics for a particular child.

Specific questionnaires and rating scales have been developed to review and quantify the behavioral characteristics of ADHD (Table 4). The ADHD-specific questionnaires and rating scales have been shown to have an odds ratio greater than 3.0 (equivalent to sensitivity and specificity greater than 94%) in studies differentiating children with ADHD from normal, age-matched, community controls.[24] Thus, ADHD-specific rating scales accurately distinguish between children with and without the diagnosis of ADHD. Almost all studies of these scales and checklists have taken place under ideal condi-

Table 4. Total ADHD-Specific Checklists: Ability to Detect ADHD vs Normal Controls

Study	Behavior Rating Scale	Age	Gender	Effect Size	95% Confidence Limits
Conners (1997)	CPRS-R:L-ADHD Index (Conners Parent Rating Scale—1997 Revised Version: Long Form, ADHD Index Scale)	6–17	MF	3.1	2.5, 3.7
Conners (1997)	CTRS-R:L-ADHD Index (Conners Teacher Rating Scale—1997 Revised Version: Long Form, ADHD Index Scale)	6–17	MF	3.3	2.8, 3.8
Conners (1997)	CPRS-R:L-*DSM-IV* Symptoms (Conners Parent Rating Scale—1997 Revised Version: Long Form, *DSM-IV* Symptoms Scale)	6–17	MF	3.4	2.8, 4.0
Conners (1997)	CTRS-R:L-*DSM-IV* Symptoms (Conners Teacher Rating Scale—1997 Revised Version: Long Form, *DSM-IV* Symptoms Scale)	6–17	MF	3.7	3.2, 4.2
Breen (1989)	SSQ-O-I (Barkley's School Situations Questionnaire—Original Version, Number of Problem Settings Scale)	6–11	F	1.3	0.5, 2.2
Breen (1989)	SSQ-O-II (Barkley's School Situations Questionnaire—Original Version, Mean Severity Scale)	6–11	F	2.0	1.0, 2.9
Combined				2.9	2.2, 3.5

Taken from: Green M, Wong M, Atkins D, et al. *Diagnosis of Attention Deficit/Hyperactivity Disorder. Technical Review 3.* Rockville, MD: US Department of Health and Human Services, Agency for Health Care Policy and Research; 1999. AHCPR publication 99-0050.

tions, ie, comparing children in referral sites with apparently healthy children. These instruments may function less well in primary care clinicians' offices than indicated in the tables. In addition, questions on which these rating scales are based are subjective and subject to bias. Thus, their results may convey a false sense of validity and must be interpreted in the context of the overall evaluation of the child. Whether these scales provide additional benefit beyond careful clinical assessment informed by *DSM-IV* criteria is not known. *RECOMMENDATION 3A: Use of these scales is a clinical option when evaluating children for ADHD (strength of evidence: strong; strength of recommendation: strong).*

Global, nonspecific questionnaires and rating scales that assess a variety of behavioral conditions, in contrast with the ADHD-specific measures, generally have an odds ratio <2.0 (equivalent to sensitivity and specificity <86%) in studies differentiating children referred to psychiatric practices from children who were not referred to psychiatric practices (Table 5). Thus, these

Table 5. Total Scales of Broadband Checklists: Ability to Detect Referred vs Nonreferred

Study	Behavior Rating Scale	Age	Gender	Effect Size	95% Confidence Limits
Achenbach (1991b)	CBCL/4-18-R, Total Problem Scale (Child Behavior Checklist for Ages 4–18, Parent Form)	4–11	M	1.4	1.3, 1.5
Achenbach (1991b)	Same as above	4–11	F	1.3	1.2, 1.4
Achenbach (1991c)	CBCL/TRF-R, Total Problem Scale (Child Behavior Checklist, Teacher Form)	5–11	M	1.2	1.0, 1.4
Achenbach (1991c)	Same as above	5–11	F	1.1	1.0, 1.3
Naglieri, LeBuffe, Pfeiffer (1994)	DSMD-Total Scale (Devereaux Scales of Mental Disorders)	5–12	MF	1.0	0.8, 1.3
Conners (1997)	CPRS-R:L-Global Problem Index (1997 Revision of Conners Parent Rating Scale, Long Version)	—	MF	2.3	1.9, 2.6
Conners (1997)	CTRS-R:L-Global Problem Index (1997 Revision of Conners Teacher Rating Scale, Long Version)	—	MF	2.0	1.7, 2.3
Combined				1.5	1.2, 1.8

Taken from: Green M, Wong M, Atkins D, et al. *Diagnosis of Attention Deficit/Hyperactivity Disorder. Technical Review 3.* Rockville, MD: US Department of Health and Human Services, Agency for Health Care Policy and Research; 1999. AHCPR publication 99-0050.

broadband scales do not distinguish well between children with and without ADHD. *RECOMMENDATION 3B: Use of broadband scales is not recommended in the diagnosis of children for ADHD, although they may be useful for other purposes (strength of evidence: strong; strength of recommendation: strong).*

More research is needed on the use of the ADHD-specific and global rating scales in pediatric practices for the purposes of differentiating children with ADHD from other children with different behavior or school problems.

RECOMMENDATION 4: The assessment of ADHD requires evidence directly obtained from the classroom teacher (or other school professional) regarding the core symptoms of ADHD, the duration of symptoms, the degree of functional impairment, and coexisting conditions. A physician should review any reports from a school-based multidisciplinary evaluation where they exist, which will include assessments from the teacher or other school-based professional (strength of evidence: good; strength of recommendation: strong).

The evaluation of ADHD must establish whether core behavior symptoms of inattention, hyperactivity, and impulsivity are present in >1 setting to meet *DSM-IV* criteria for the condition. Children 6 to 12 years of age generally are students in an elementary school setting, where they spend a substantial proportion of waking hours. Therefore, a description of their behavioral characteristics in the school setting is highly important to the evaluation. With permission from the legal guardian, the clinician should review a report from the child's school. The classroom teacher typically has more information about the child's behavior than do other professionals at the school and, when possible, should provide the report. Alternatively, a school counselor or principal often is helpful in coordinating the teacher's reporting and may be able to provide the required information.

Behavior symptoms may be obtained using 1 or more methods such as verbal narratives, written narratives, questionnaires, or rating scales. Clinicians who obtain information from narratives or interviews must obtain and record the relevant behaviors of inattention, hyperactivity, and impulsivity from the *DSM-IV*. The use of global clinical impressions or general descriptions within the domains of attention and activity is insufficient to diagnose ADHD.

The ADHD-specific questionnaires and rating scales also are available for teachers (Table 4). Teacher ADHD-specific questionnaires and rating scales have been shown to have an odds ratio >3.0 (equivalent to sensitivity and specificity greater than 94%) in studies differentiating children with ADHD from normal peers in the community.[24] Thus, teacher ADHD-specific rating scales accurately distinguish between children with and without the diagnosis of ADHD. Whether these scales provide additional benefit beyond narratives or descriptive interviews informed by *DSM-IV* criteria is not known. *RECOMMENDATION 4A: Use of these scales is a clinical option when diagnosing children for ADHD (strength of evidence: strong; strength of recommendation: strong).*

Teacher global questionnaires and rating scales that assess a variety of behavioral conditions, in contrast with the ADHD-specific measures, generally have an odds ratio <2.0 (equivalent to sensitivity and specificity <86%) in studies differentiating children referred to psychiatric practices from children who were not referred to psychiatric practices (Table 5). Thus, these broadband scales do not distinguish between children with and without ADHD. *RECOMMENDATION 4B: Use of teacher global questionnaires and rating scales is not recommended in the diagnosing of children for ADHD, although they may be useful for other purposes (strength of evidence: strong; strength of recommendation: strong).*

If a child 6 to 12 years of age routinely spends considerable time in other structured environments such as after-school care centers, additional information about core symptoms can be sought from professionals in those settings, contingent on parental permission. The ADHD-specific questionnaires may be used to evaluate the child's behavior in these settings. For children who are educated in their homes by parents, evidence of the presence of core behavior symptoms in settings other than the home should be obtained as an essential part of the evaluation.

Frequently there are significant discrepancies between parent and teacher ratings.[40] These discrepancies may be in either direction; symptoms may be reported by teachers and not parents or vice versa. These discrepancies may be attributable to differences between the home and school in terms of expectations, levels of structure, behavioral management strategies, and/or environmental circumstances. The finding of a discrepancy between the parents and teachers does not preclude the diagnosis of ADHD. A helpful clinical approach for understanding the sources of the discrepancies and whether the child meets *DSM-IV* criteria is to obtain additional information from other informants, such as former teachers, religious leaders, or coaches.

RECOMMENDATION 5: Evaluation of the child with ADHD should include assessment for coexisting conditions (strength of evidence: strong; strength of recommendation: strong).

A variety of other psychological and developmental disorders frequently coexist in children who are being evaluated for ADHD. As many as one third of children with ADHD have 1 or more coexisting conditions (Table 6). Although the primary care clinician may not always be in a position to make a precise diagnosis of coexisting conditions, consideration and examination for such a coexisting condition should be an integral part of the evaluation. A review of all coexisting conditions (such as motor disabilities, problems with parent-child interaction, or family violence) is not possible within the scope of this review. More common psychological disorders include conduct and oppositional defiant disorder, mood disorders, anxiety disorders, and learning disabilities. The pediatrician should also consider ADHD as a coexisting condition when considering these other conditions. Evidence for most of these coexisting disorders may be readily detected by the primary care clinician. For example, frequent sadness and preference for isolated activities may alert the physician to the presence of depressive symptoms, whereas a family history of anxiety disorders coupled with a patient history characterized by frequent fears and difficulties with separation from caregivers may be suggestive of symptoms associated with an anxiety disorder. Several screening tests are available that can detect areas of concern for many of the mental health disorders that coexist with ADHD. Although these scales have not been tested for use in primary care settings and are not diagnostic tests for either ADHD or associated mental health conditions, some clinicians may find them useful to establish high risk for coexisting psychological conditions. Similarly, poor school performance may indicate a learning disability. Testing may be required to determine whether a discrepancy exists between the child's learning potential (intelligence quotient) and his actual academic progress (achievement test scores), indicating the presence of a learning disability. Most studies of rates of coexisting conditions have come from referral pop-

Table 6. Summary of Prevalence of Selected Coexisting Conditions in Children With ADHD

Comorbid Disorder	Estimated Prevalence (%)	Confidence Limits for Estimated Prevalence (%)
Oppositional defiant disorder	35.2	27.2, 43.8
Conduct disorder	25.7	12.8, 41.3
Anxiety disorder	25.8	17.6, 35.3
Depressive disorder	18.2	11.1, 26.6

Taken from: Green M, Wong M, Atkins D, et al. *Diagnosis of Attention Deficit/Hyperactivity Disorder. Technical Review 3.* Rockville, MD: US Dept of Health and Human Services. Agency for Health Care Policy and Research; 1999. AHCPR publication 99-0050.

ulations. The following data generally reflect the relatively small number of studies from community or primary care settings.

Conduct Disorder and Oppositional Defiant Disorder

Oppositional defiant or conduct disorders coexist with ADHD in ~35% of children.[24] The diagnostic features of conduct disorder include "a repetitive and persistent pattern of behavior in which the basic rights of others or major age-appropriate social norms or rules are violated."[13] Oppositional defiant disorder (a less severe condition) includes persistent symptoms of "negativistic, defiant, disobedient, and hostile behaviors toward authority figures."[13] Frequently, children and adolescents with persisting oppositional defiant disorder later develop symptoms of sufficient severity to qualify for a diagnosis of conduct disorder. Longitudinal follow-up for children with conduct disorders that coexist with ADHD indicates that these children fare more poorly in adulthood relative to their peers diagnosed with ADHD alone.[41] For example, 1 study has reported the highest rates of police contacts and self-reported delinquency in children with ADHD and coexisting conduct disorder (30.8%) relative to their peers diagnosed with ADHD alone (3.4%) or conduct disorder alone (20.7%). Preliminary studies suggest that these coexisting conditions are more frequent in children with the predominantly hyperactive-impulsive and combined subtypes.[25,26]

Mood Disorders/Depression

The coexistence of ADHD and mood disorders (eg, major depressive disorder and dysthymia) is ~18%.[39] Frequently, the family history of children with ADHD includes other family members with a history of major depressive disorder.[42] In addition, children who have coexisting ADHD and mood disorders also may have a poorer outcome during adolescence relative to their peers who do not have this pattern of co-occurrence.[43] For example, adolescents with coexisting mood disorders and ADHD are at increased risk for suicide attempts.[44] Preliminary studies suggest that these coexisting conditions are more frequent in children with the predominantly inattentive and combined subtypes.[25,26]

Anxiety

The coexisting association between ADHD and anxiety disorders has been estimated to be ~25%.[24] In addition, the risk for anxiety disorders among relatives of children and adolescents diagnosed with ADHD is higher than for typically developing children, although some research suggests that ADHD and anxiety disorders transmit independently from families.[45] In either case, it is important to obtain a careful family history. Preliminary studies suggest that these coexisting conditions are more frequent in children with the predominantly inattentive and combined subtypes.[25,26]

Learning Disabilities

Only 1 published study examined the coexistence of ADHD and learning disabilities in children evaluated in general pediatric settings using *DSM-IV* criteria for the diagnosis of ADHD.[46] The prevalence of learning disabilities as a coexisting condition cannot be determined in the same manner as other psychological disorders because studies have employed dimensional (looking at the condition on a spectrum) rather than categorical diagnoses. Rates of learning disabilities that coexist with ADHD in settings other than primary care have been reported to range from 12% to 60%.[24]

To date, no definitive data describe the differences among groups of children with different learning disabilities coexisting with ADHD in the areas of sociodemographic characteristics, behavioral and emotional functioning, and response to various interventions. Nonetheless, the subgroup of children with learning disabilities, compared with their ADHD peers who do not have a learning disability, is most in need of special education services. Preliminary studies suggest that these coexisting conditions are more frequent in children with the predominantly inattentive and combined subtypes.[25,26]

RECOMMENDATION 6: *Other diagnostic tests are not routinely indicated to establish the diagnosis of ADHD (strength of evidence: strong; strength of recommendation: strong).*

Other diagnostic tests contribute little to establishing the diagnosis of ADHD. A few older studies have indicated associations between blood lead levels and child behavior symptoms, although most studies have not.[47-49] Although lead encephalopathy in younger children may predispose to later behavior and developmental problems, very few of these children will have elevated lead levels at school age. Thus, regular screening of children for high lead levels does not aid in the diagnosis of ADHD.

Studies have shown no significant associations between abnormal thyroid hormone levels and the presence of ADHD.[50-52] Children with the rare disorder of generalized resistance to thyroid hormone have higher rates of ADHD than other populations, but these children demonstrate other characteristics of that condition. This association does not argue for routine screening of thyroid function as part of the effort to diagnose ADHD.

Brain imaging studies and electroencephalography do not show reliable differences between children with ADHD and controls. Although some studies have demonstrated variation in brain morphology comparing children with and without ADHD, these findings do not discriminate reliably between children with and without this condition. In other words, although group means may differ significantly, the overlap in findings among children with and without ADHD creates high rates of false-positives and false-negatives.[53-55] Similarly, some studies have indicated higher rates of certain electroencephalogram abnormalities among children with ADHD,[56-58] but again the overlap between children with and without ADHD and the lack of consistent findings among multiple reports indicate that current literature do not support the routine use of electroencephalograms in the diagnosis of ADHD.

Continuous performance tests have been designed to obtain samples of a child's behavior (generally measuring vigilance or distractibility), which may correlate with behaviors associated with ADHD. Several such tests have been developed and tested, but all of these have low odds ratios (all <1.2, equivalent to a sensitivity and specificity <70%) in studies differentiating children with ADHD from normal comparison controls.[24,45,59,60] Therefore, current data do not support the use of any available continuous performance tests in the diagnosis of ADHD.

Areas for Future Research

The research issues pertaining to the diagnosis of ADHD relate to the diagnostic criteria themselves as well as the methods used to establish the diagnosis. The *DSM-IV* has helped to define behavioral criteria for ADHD more specifically. Although research has established the dimensional concepts of inattention and hyperactivity-impulsivity, further research is required to validate these subtypes. Because most of the existing research has been conducted with referred convenience samples, primarily in psychiatric settings, further research is required to determine whether the findings of previous research are generalizable to the type of children currently diagnosed and treated by primary care clinicians. Although the current *DSM-IV* criteria are appropriate for the age range included in this guideline, there is, as yet, inadequate information about its applicability to individuals younger or older than the age range for this guideline. Further research should clarify the developmental course of ADHD symptomatology. An additional difficulty for primary care is that existing evidence indicates that the behaviors used in making a *DSM-IV* diagnosis of ADHD fall on a spectrum. Currently, decisions about the inappropriateness of the behaviors in children depend on subjective judgments of observers/reporters. There are no data to offer precise estimates of when diagnostic behaviors become inappropriate. This is particularly problematic to primary care clinicians, who care for a number of patients who fit into borderline or gray areas. The inadequacy of research on this aspect is central to the issue of which children should be diagnosed with ADHD and treated with stimulant medication. Further research using normative or community-based samples to develop more valid and precise diagnostic criteria is essential.

The diagnostic process is also an area requiring further research. Because no pathognomonic findings currently establish the diagnosis, further research should examine the utility of existing methods, with the goal of developing a more definitive process. Specific examples include the need for additional information about the reliability and validity of teacher and parent rating scales and the reliability and validity of different interviewing methods. Further, given the prominence of impairment in the current diagnostic requirements, it is imperative to develop and assess better measurements of impairment that can be applied practically in the primary care setting. The research into diagnostic methods also should include those methods helpful in identifying clinically relevant coexisting conditions.

Lastly, research is required to identify more clearly the current practices of primary care physicians beyond using self-report. Such research is critical in determining the practicality of guideline recommendations as a method to determine changes in practice and to determine whether changes have an actual impact on the treatment and outcome of children with the diagnosis of ADHD.

Conclusion

This guideline offers recommendations for the diagnosis and evaluation of school-aged children with ADHD in primary care practice. The guideline emphasizes: 1) the use of explicit criteria for the diagnosis using *DSM-IV* criteria; 2) the importance of obtaining information regarding the child's symptoms in more than 1 setting and especially from schools; and 3) the search for coexisting conditions that may make the diagnosis more difficult or complicate treatment planning. The guideline further provides current evidence regarding various diagnostic tests for ADHD. It should help primary care providers in their assessment of a common child health problem.

Acknowledgments

The Practice Guideline, "Diagnosis and Evaluation of the Child With Attention-Deficit/Hyperactivity Disorder," was reviewed by appropriate committees and sections of the AAP, including the Chapter Review Group, a focus group of office-based pediatricians representing each AAP District: Gene R. Adams, MD; Robert M. Corwin, MD; Diane Fuquay, MD; Barbara M. Harley, MD; Thomas J. Herr, MD, Chair Person; Kenneth E. Mathews, MD; Robert D. Mines, MD; Lawrence C. Pakula, MD; Howard B. Weinblatt, MD; and Delosa A. Young, MD. The Practice Guideline was also reviewed by relevant outside medical organizations as part of the peer review process as well as by several patient advocacy organizations.

References

1. Reiff MI, Banez GA, Culbert TP. Children who have attentional disorders: diagnosis and evaluation. *Pediatr Rev.* 1993;14:455–465
2. Barkley RA. *Attention Deficit Hyperactivity Disorder: A Handbook for Diagnosis and Treatment.* 2nd ed. New York, NY: Guilford Press; 1996
3. Zentall SS. Research on the educational implications of attention deficit hyperactivity disorder. *Exceptional Child.* 1993;60:143–153
4. Schachar R, Taylor E, Wieselberg MB, Ghorley G, Rutter M. Changes in family functioning and relationships in children who respond to methylphenidate. *J Am Acad Child Adolesc Psychiatry.* 1987;26:728–732
5. Almond BW Jr, Tanner JL, Goffman HF. *The Family Is the Patient: Using Family Interviews in Children's Medical Care.* 2nd ed. Baltimore, MD: Williams & Wilkins; 1999:307–313
6. Biederman J, Faraone SV, Milberger S, et al. Predictors of persistence and remissions of ADHD into adolescence: results from a four-year prospective follow-up study. *J Am Acad Child Adolesc Psychiatry.* 1996;35:343–351
7. Biederman J, Faraone SV, Spencer T, et al. Patterns of psychiatric comorbidity, cognition, and psychosocial functioning in adults with attention deficit hyperactivity disorder. *Am J Psychiatry.* 1993;150:1792–1798
8. Baumgaertel A, Copeland L, Wolraich ML. Attention deficit-hyperactivity disorder. In: *Disorders of Development and Learning: A Practical Guide to Assessment and Management.* 2nd ed. St Louis, MO: Mosby Yearbook, Inc; 1996:424–456
9. Cantwell DP. Attention deficit disorder: a review of the past 10 years. *J Am Acad Child Adolesc Psychiatry.* 1996;35:978–987
10. American Psychiatric Association. *Diagnostic and Statistical Manual for Mental Disorders.* 2nd ed. Washington, DC: American Psychiatric Association; 1967
11. American Psychiatric Association. *Diagnostic and Statistical Manual for Mental Disorders.* 3rd ed. Washington, DC: American Psychiatric Association; 1980
12. American Psychiatric Association. *Diagnostic and Statistical Manual for Mental Disorders-Revised.* 3rd ed. Washington, DC: American Psychiatric Association; 1987
13. American Psychiatric Association. *Diagnostic and Statistical Manual for Mental Disorders.* 4th ed. Washington, DC: American Psychiatric Association; 1994
14. Drug Enforcement Agency. Washington, DC (personal communication)
15. August GJ, Garfinkel BD. Behavioral and cognitive subtypes of ADHD. *J Am Acad Child Adolesc Psychiatry.* 1989;28:739–748
16. August GJ, Realmuto GM, MacDonald AW III, Nugent SM, Crosby R. Prevalence of ADHD and comorbid disorders among elementary school children screened for disruptive behavior. *J Abnorm Child Psychol.* 1996;24:571–595
17. Bird H, Canino G, Rubio-Stipec M, et al. Estimates of the prevalence of childhood maladjustment in a community survey in Puerto Rico. *Arch Gen Psychiatry.* 1988;45:1120–1126
18. Cohen P, Cohen J, Kasen S, Velez CN. An epidemiological study of disorders in late childhood and adolescence I: age and gender-specific prevalence. *J Child Psychol Psychiatry.* 1993;34:851–867
19. King C, Young RD. Attentional deficits with and without hyperactivity: teacher and peer perceptions. *J Abnorm Child Psychol.* 1982;10:483–495

20. Kuperman S, Johnson B, Arndt S, Lingren S, Wolraich M. Quantitative EEG differences in a nonclinical sample of children with ADHD and undifferentiated ADD. *J Am Acad Child Adolesc Psychiatry.* 1996;35:1009–1017

21. Newcorn J, Halperin JM, Schwartz S, et al. Parent and teacher ratings of attention-deficit hyperactivity disorder symptoms: implications for case identification. *J Dev Behav Pediatr.* 1994;15:86–91

22. Shaffer D, Fisher P, Dulcan MK, et al. The NIMH Diagnostic Interview Schedule for Children Version 2.3 (DISC-2.3): description, acceptability, prevalence rates, and performance in the MECA study. Methods for the Epidemiology of Child and Adolescent Mental Disorders Study. *J Am Acad Child Adolesc Psychiatry.* 1996;35:865–877

23. Shekim WO, Kashani J, Beck N, et al. The prevalence of attention deficit disorders in a rural midwestern community sample of nine-year-old children. *J Am Acad Child Adolesc Psychiatry.* 1985;24:765–770

24. Green M, Wong M, Atkins D, et al. *Diagnosis of Attention Deficit/Hyperactivity Disorder: Technical Review 3.* Rockville, MD: US Department of Health and Human Services, Agency for Health Care Policy and Research; 1999. Agency for Health Care Policy and Research publication 99-0050

25. Wolraich ML, Hannah JN, Pinnock TY, Baumgaertel A, Brown J. Comparison of diagnostic criteria for attention deficit/hyperactivity disorder in a county-wide sample. *J Am Acad Child Adolesc Psychiatry.* 1996;35:319–324

26. Wolraich M, Hannah JN, Baumgaertel A, Pinnock TY, Feurer I. Examination of *DSM-IV* criteria for attention deficit/hyperactivity disorder in a county-wide sample. *J Dev Behav Pediatr.* 1998;19:162–168

27. Gibbs N. Latest on Ritalin. *Time.* 1998;152:86–96

28. Safer DJ, Zito JM, Fine EM. Increased methylphenidate usage for attention deficit disorder in the 1990s. *Pediatrics.* 1996;98:1084–1088

29. Rappley MD, Gardiner JC, Jetton JR, Houang RT. The use of methylphenidate in Michigan. *Arch Pediatr Adolesc Med.* 1995;149:675–679

30. Wolraich ML, Lindgren S, Stromquist A, et al. Stimulant medication use by primary care physicians in the treatment of attention deficit hyperactivity disorder. *Pediatrics.* 1990;86:95–101

31. Mulhern S, Dworkin PH, Bernstein B. Do parental encounters predict a diagnosis of attention deficit hyperactivity disorder? *J Dev Behav Pediatr.* 1994;15:348–352

32. Wasserman R, Kelleher KJ, Bocian A, et al. Identification of attentional and hyperactivity problems in primary care: a report from Pediatric Research in Office Settings and the Ambulatory Sentinel Practice Network. *Pediatrics.* 1999;103(3). URL: http://www.pediatrics.org/cgi/content/full/103/3/e38

33. Sleator EK, Ullmann RK. Can the physician diagnose hyperactivity in the office? *Pediatrics.* 1981;67:13–17

34. American Academy of Pediatrics. *Guidelines for Health Supervision III.* 3rd ed. Elk Grove Village, IL: American Academy of Pediatrics; 1997

35. Green M, ed. National Center for Education in Maternal and Child Health. *Bright Futures: Guidelines for Health Supervision of Infants, Children, and Adolescents.* Arlington, VA: National Center for Education in Maternal and Child Health; 1994

36. Stein MT. Preparing families for the toddler and preschool years. *Contemp Pediatr.* 1998;15:88

37. Dixon S, Stein M. *Encounters With Children: Pediatric Behavior and Development.* 3rd ed. St Louis, MO: Mosby; 1999

38. McBurnett K, Pfiffner LJ, Willcutt E, et al. Experimental cross-validation of *DSM-IV* types of attention-deficit/hyperactivity disorder. *J Am Acad Child Adolesc Psychiatry.* 1999;38:17–24

39. American Academy of Pediatrics. *The Classification of Child and Adolescent Mental Diagnoses in Primary Care: Diagnostic and Statistical Manual for Primary Care (DSM-PC) Child and Adolescent Version.* Elk Grove Village, IL: American Academy of Pediatrics; 1996

40. Lahey BB, McBurnett K, Piacentini, JC, et al. Agreement of parent and teacher rating scales with comprehensive clinical assessments of attention deficit disorder with hyperactivity. *J Psychopathol Behav Assess.* 1987;9:429–439

41. Ingrams S, Hechtman L, Morganstern G. Outcome issues in ADHD: adolescent and adult long term outcome. In: *Mental Retardation and Developmental Disabilities.* In press

42. Biederman J, Milberger S, Farone SV, Guite J, Warburton R. Associations between childhood asthma and ADHD: issues of psychiatric comorbidity and familiarity. *J Am Acad Child Adolesc Psychiatry.* 1994;33:842–848

43. Biederman J, Newcorn PJ, Sprich S. Comorbidity of attention deficit hyperactivity disorder with conduct, depressive, anxiety, and other disorders. *Am J Psychiatry.* 1991;148: 564–577

44. Brent DA, Perper JA, Goldstein CE, Kolko DJ, Zelenak JP. Risk factors for adolescent suicide: a comparison of adolescent suicide victims with suicidal inpatients. *Arch Gen Psychiatry.* 1988;45:581–588

45. Faraone SV, Biederman J, Mennin D, Gershon J, Tsuang MT. A prospective four-year follow-up study of children at risk for ADHD: psychiatric, neuropsychological, and psychosocial outcome. *J Am Acad Child Adolesc Psychiatry.* 1996;35:1449–1459

46. August GJ, Garfinkel BD. Behavioral and cognitive subtypes of ADHD. *J Am Acad Child Adolesc Psychiatry.* 1989;28:739–748

47. Kahn CA, Kelly PC, Walker WO Jr. Lead screening in children with attention deficit hyperactivity disorder and developmental delay. *Clin Pediatr (Phila).* 1995;34:498–501

48. Tuthill RW. Hair lead levels related to children's classroom attention-deficit behavior. *Arch Environ Health.* 1996;51:214–220

49. Gittelman R, Eskenazi B. Lead and hyperactivity revisited: an investigation of non-disadvantaged children. *Arch Gen Psychiatry.* 1983;40:827–833

50. Elia J, Gulotta C, Rose SR, Marin G, Rapoport JL. Thyroid function and attention-deficit hyperactivity disorder. *J Am Acad Child Adolesc Psychiatry.* 1994;33:169–172

51. Spencer T, Biederman J, Wilens T, Guite J, Harding M. ADHD and thyroid abnormalities: a research note. *J Child Psychol Psychiatry.* 1995;36:879–885

52. Weiss RE, Stein MA, Trommer B, Refetoff S. Attention-deficit hyperactivity disorder and thyroid function. *J Pediatr.* 1993;123:539–545

53. Shaywitz BA, Shaywitz SE, Byrne T, Cohen DJ, Rothman S. Attention deficit disorder: quantitative analysis of CT. *Neurology.* 1983;33:1500–1503

54. Castellanos FX, Giedd JN, Marsh WL, et al. Quantitative brain magnetic resonance imaging in attention-deficit hyperactivity disorder. *Arch Gen Psychiatry.* 1996;53:607–616

55. Lyoo IK, Noam GG, Lee CK, et al. The corpus callosum and lateral ventricles in children with attention-deficit hyperactivity disorder: a brain magnetic resonance imaging study. *Biol Psychiatry.* 1996;40:1060–1063

56. Matsuura M, Okubo Y, Toru M, et al. A cross-national EEG study of children with emotional and behavioral problems: a WHO collaborative study in the Western Pacific Region. *Biol Psychiatry.* 1993;34:59–65

57. Lahat E, Avital E, Barr J, et al. BAEP studies in children with attention deficit disorder. *Dev Med Child Neurol.* 1995;37:119–123

58. Kuperman S, Johnson B, Arndt S, et al. Quantitative EEG differences in a nonclinical sample of children with ADHD and undifferentiated ADD. *J Am Acad Child Adolesc Psychiatry.* 1996;35:1009–1017

59. Seidel WT, Joschko M. Assessment of attention in children. *Clin Neuropsychology.* 1991; 5:53–66

60. Dykman RA, Ackerman PT. Attention deficit disorder and specific reading disability: separate but often overlapping disorders. *J Learn Disabil.* 1991;24:96–103

Technical Report Summary:
Diagnosis of Attention-Deficit/
Hyperactivity Disorder

Author:

Agency for Health Care Policy and Research

Summary

The Agency for Health Care Policy and Research (AHCPR) is developing scientific information for other agencies and organizations on which to base clinical guidelines, performance measures, and other quality improvement tools, under the Agency's Evidence-Based Practice Initiative, which was launched in the fall of 1996. This technical review summarizes current scientific evidence on the prevalence of attention-deficit/hyperactivity disorder and on the value of various evaluation methods.

Overview

Attention-deficit/hyperactivity disorder (ADHD) is one of the most common childhood-onset psychiatric disorders. It is distinguished by symptoms of inattention, hyperactivity, and impulsivity. ADHD may be accompanied by learning disabilities, depression, anxiety, conduct disorder, and oppositional defiant disorder. The etiology of ADHD is unknown, and the disorder may have several different causes. Investigators have studied, for example, the relation of ADHD to elevated lead levels, abnormal thyroid function, morphologic brain differences, and electroencephalograph (EEG) patterns.

With current public awareness of ADHD, pediatricians and health care providers are reporting increases in referral rates of children with suspected ADHD. Numerous rating scales and medical tests for evaluation and diagnosis of ADHD are available, with mixed expert opinion on their usefulness.

The Agency for Health Care Policy and Research (AHCPR) sponsored the development of this technical review to summarize current scientific evidence from the literature on the prevalence of ADHD and on the value of various evaluation methods. The following questions provided a framework for the analysis:

1. What percentage of the U.S. general population ages 6 to 12 years has ADHD? Of those with ADHD, what percentage has one or more of the following comorbidities: learning disabilities, depression, anxiety, conduct disorder, and oppositional defiant disorder?
2. What percentage of children ages 6 to 12 years presenting at pediatricians' or family physicians' offices in the United States meets diagnostic criteria for ADHD? Of those with ADHD, what percentage has one or more of the following comorbidities: learning disabilities, depression, anxiety, conduct disorder, and oppositional defiant disorder?
3. What is the accuracy (i.e., sensitivity, specificity, positive predictive value) and reliability (i.e., inter/intra-rater agreement) of behavioral rating screening tests for ADHD compared with a reference standard?
4. What is the prevalence of abnormal findings on selected medical screening tests commonly recommended as standard components of an evaluation of a child with suspected ADHD?

Diagnostic screening tests, as analyzed under questions 3 and 4, were of two types: behavioral rating scales and medical screening tests. The behavior rating scales selected for consideration consisted of both ADHD-specific scales and "broad-band" scales designed to screen for various symptoms (including ADHD symptoms). The medical screening tests considered included commonly recommended tests that are standard components of an evaluation of a child with suspected ADHD: electroencephalography, lead concentration level testing, thyroid hormone level testing, hearing and vision screening, imaging tests, neurological screening, and continuous performance tests (CPTs).

Reporting the Evidence

The evidence on ADHD prevalence and diagnosis reported here was gathered from 87 published articles and 10 behavioral scale manuals. Studies must have been peer reviewed and published in the English language between 1980 and 1997. These 97 sources were identified during searches of the databases MEDLINE and PsycINFO and from reference lists in review articles, research study articles, and a draft guideline on ADHD obtained from the American Academy of Child and Adolescent Psychiatry (currently in development), recent journal publications, citations suggested by members of the American Academy of Pediatricians, and a database of bibliographies on studies that used or evaluated the Child Behavior Checklists (CBCL). Abstracts of more than 4,000 identified citations were reviewed, from which 507 articles and 10 manuals were retrieved and subjected to further consideration. The published studies had to be soundly designed and conform to specified inclusion and exclusion criteria to qualify for consideration.

Methodology

Data from the 97 accepted articles/manuals were abstracted, tabulated systematically, and subjected to statistical analysis. A multiple logistic regression model with random effects was used to analyze simultaneously for the effect of age, gender, diagnostic tool, and setting. This model accommodates the fact that each study estimated ADHD rates under slightly different conditions. The analysis was done using the EGRET software.

Findings

The significant findings derived from the analysis are summarized below.

Prevalence of ADHD in General Population

- Gender, diagnostic tool (DSM-III or DSM-III-R), and setting (community or school setting) are significant contributors to the ADHD rate, but age (5 to 9 years versus 10 to 12 years) is not a significant factor.

- ADHD prevalence is much higher when academic and behavioral functioning impairment criteria are not considered (16.1 percent without impairment criteria versus 6.8 percent with). Boys have higher rates of ADHD than do girls.

Prevalence of Comorbid ADHD in General Population

- One-third of children diagnosed with ADHD also qualify for a diagnosis of oppositional defiant disorder (ODD).
- One-fourth of children diagnosed with ADHD also qualify for a diagnosis of conduct disorder (CD).
- Less than one-fifth of children with ADHD also have a depressive disorder.
- More than one-fourth of children with ADHD qualify for a diagnosis of anxiety disorder.
- Almost one-third of children with ADHD also have more than one comorbid condition.
- Overall, the prevalence rates of comorbid ADHD are high. Estimates of the prevalence rates of various comorbid conditions in children with ADHD range from 12.36 percent (learning disorders) to 35.15 percent (conduct disorder).

Prevalence of ADHD in Pediatric Clinic Setting

- Results on prevalence of ADHD in a pediatric clinic setting are varied. A 1997 study finds prevalence conforms to that of the general population; a 1988 study shows much smaller prevalence.

Prevalence of Comorbid ADHD in Pediatric Clinic Setting

- Results on prevalence of comorbid ADHD in a pediatric clinic setting are varied. A 1997 study finds a high prevalence, similar to that in the general population; a 1988 study gives much lower rates.

Behavior Rating Scales, ADHD Specific

- The Conners Rating Scales, 1997 Revision, contain two highly effective indices for discriminating between ADHD children and normal controls. The Barkley School Situations Questionnaire is less effective. These results are based on studies conducted under ideal conditions; actual performance of the scales in physicians' offices is expected to be poorer.
- Hyperactivity subscales that effectively discriminate between ADHD children and normal controls include DSM-III-R SNAP and Conners Abbreviated Teacher Questionnaire (CATQ, HI). The ACTeRS scale performed poorly. These results are based on studies conducted under ideal conditions; actual performance of the scales in physicians' offices is expected to be poorer.

- An inattention subscale that effectively discriminates between ADHD children and normal controls is the DSM-III-R SNAP checklist. The ACTeRS scale performed poorly. These results are based on studies conducted under ideal conditions; actual performance of the scales in physicians' offices is expected to be poorer.
- An impulsivity subscale that effectively discriminates between ADHD children and normal controls is the DSM-III-R SNAP checklist.

Broad-Band Behavioral Rating Scales

- None of the broad-band scales analyzed—the CPCL/4-18-R Total Problem Scale, DSMD Total Problem Scale, CPRS-R:L Global Problem Index, and CTRS-R:L Global Problem Index—effectively discriminate between referred and nonreferred children. Thus, they are not useful as tools to detect clinical-level problems in children presenting at a pediatrician's office.
- Externalizing, internalizing, and adaptive functioning scales did not effectively detect referred versus nonreferred children.

Medical Screening Tests

- Analysis of six studies on the relation between elevated lead levels and ADHD showed that lead levels are not useful as a general diagnostic tool for ADHD. This is strengthened by the fact that ADHD prevalence appears to be increasing even as lead levels in the population appear to be decreasing.
- Analysis of four studies showed no relation between abnormal thyroid function and ADHD. Thus, the evidence does not support the use of tests of thyroid function to screen for ADHD.
- Analysis of seven imaging studies of the brain (computed tomography [CT], computerized axial tomography [CAT], and magnetic resonance imaging [MRI]) that were performed to detect morphologic differences in brain structures of children with ADHD yielded sparse and diverse evidence. Thus, none of the imaging procedures analyzed are considered useful as a screening or diagnostic tool for ADHD.
- Eight studies of electroencephalogram (EEG) patterns and ADHD found no serious EEG abnormalities in ADHD children, although many studies found significant differences in brain wave activity between ADHD children and normal controls. The heterogeneity of results across studies indicates that the EEG should not be routinely used as a screening tool for ADHD.
- Evidence from studies of neurological screening tests did not yield any clues to the etiology of ADHD. Thus, these tests are not deemed effective for screening ADHD.
- Continuous performance tests measure impulsivity, inattention, and vigilance. Statistical analysis of studies using these tests indicated that CPTs would not serve as useful screening tools for ADHD.

Future Research

- There is a need for continued work to gather data on prevalence of ADHD using the following factors, which are lacking in much of the work already done: DSM-IV, use of both genders as subjects, rates of ADHD—Primarily Inattentive Type, and wider-scale studies across regions of the country or across countries using the same criteria.
- Comparison studies are needed to assess the ability of broad-band behavior checklists to discriminate between clinical and nonclinical samples (the studies available at this time have only presented results of the ability of these tests to discriminate between referred and nonreferred samples). Clinically severe problems are present in both of these groups, as are subclinical problems.
- Continued work is needed in the area of magnetic resonance imaging and PET, when possible, to continue to explore structural and functional differences in the brains of children diagnosed with ADHD and each of the types of ADHD.

Availability of the Full Report

The full technical review from which this summary was taken was prepared by Technical Resources International, Inc., located in Rockville, Maryland. It was developed for AHCPR under contract No. 290-94-2024, and is expected to be available in late 1999.

When the technical review is available, printed copies may be obtained free of charge from the AHCPR Publications Clearinghouse by calling 1-800-358-9295. Requestors should ask for Technical Review No. 3, *Diagnosis of Attention-Deficit/Hyperactivity Disorder* (AHCPR Publication No. 99-0050). Internet users will be able to access the review online at: http://www.ahrq.gov/clinic/epcix.htm.

For more information on AHCPR's Evidence-Based Practice Initiative or the development of this report, contact the Center for Practice and Technology Assessment, Agency for Health Care Policy and Research, 6000 Executive Boulevard, Suite 310, Rockville, MD 20852; phone (301) 594-4015; fax (301) 594-4027.

AHCPR Publication No. 99-0049
Current as of October 1999

Early Detection of Developmental Dysplasia of the Hip

- *Clinical Practice Guideline*
- *Technical Report Summary*

Readers of this clinical practice guideline are urged to review the technical report to enhance the evidence-based decision-making process. The report is available on the Pediatrics electronic pages Web site at the following URL: http://www.pediatrics.org/cgi/content/full/105/4/e57.

Clinical Practice Guideline:
Early Detection of Developmental Dysplasia of the Hip

Author:

American Academy of Pediatrics
Subcommittee on Developmental
Dysplasia of the Hip
Committee on Quality Improvement

American Academy of Pediatrics
PO Box 927, 141 Northwest Point Blvd
Elk Grove Village, IL 60009-0927

Subcommittee on Developmental Dysplasia of the Hip
1999–2000

Michael J. Goldberg, MD, Chairperson

Theodore H. Harcke, MD
Section on Radiology
Anthony Hirsch, MD
Practitioner
Harold Lehmann, MD, PhD
Section on Epidemiology

Dennis R. Roy, MD
Section on Orthopaedics
Philip Sunshine, MD
Section on Perinatology

Consultant

Carol Dezateux, MB, MPH

Committee on Quality Improvement
1999–2000

Charles J. Homer, MD, MPH, Chairperson

Richard D. Baltz, MD
Gerald B. Hickson, MD
Paul V. Miles, MD

Thomas B. Newman, MD, MPH
Joan E. Shook, MD
William M. Zurhellen, MD

Betty A. Lowe, MD,
Liaison, National
Association of Children's
Hospitals and Related
Institutions (NACHRI)
Ellen Schwalenstocker,
MBA, Liaison, NACHRI
Michael J. Goldberg, MD,
Liaison, Council on Sections

Richard Shiffman, MD,
Liaison, Section on
Computers and Other
Technology
Jan Ellen Berger, MD,
Liaison, Committee on
Medical Liability
F. Lane France, MD,
Committee on Practice
and Ambulatory Medicine

Abstract

Developmental dysplasia of the hip is the preferred term to describe the condition in which the femoral head has an abnormal relationship to the acetabulum. Developmental dysplasia of the hip includes frank dislocation (luxation), partial dislocation (subluxation), instability wherein the femoral head comes in and out of the socket, and an array of radiographic abnormalities that reflect inadequate formation of the acetabulum. Because many of these findings may not be present at birth, the term *developmental* more accurately reflects the biologic features than does the term *congenital*. The disorder is uncommon. The earlier a dislocated hip is detected, the simpler and more effective is the treatment. Despite newborn screening programs, dislocated hips continue to be diagnosed later in infancy and childhood,[1-11] in some instances delaying appropriate therapy and leading to a substantial number of malpractice claims. The objective of this guideline is to reduce the number of dislocated hips detected later in infancy and childhood. The target audience is the primary care provider. The target patient is the healthy newborn up to 18 months of age, excluding those with neuromuscular disorders, myelodysplasia, or arthrogryposis.

Biologic Features and Natural History

Understanding the developmental nature of developmental dysplasia of the hip (DDH) and the subsequent spectrum of hip abnormalities requires a knowledge of the growth and development of the hip joint.[12] Embryologically, the femoral head and acetabulum develop from the same block of primitive mesenchymal cells. A cleft develops to separate them at 7 to 8 weeks' gestation. By 11 weeks' gestation, development of the hip joint is complete. At birth, the femoral head and the acetabulum are primarily cartilaginous. The acetabulum continues to develop postnatally. The growth of the fibrocartilaginous rim (the labrum) that surrounds the bony acetabulum deepens the socket. Development of the femoral head and acetabulum are intimately related, and normal adult hip joints depend on further growth of these structures. Hip dysplasia may occur in utero, perinatally, or during infancy and childhood.

The acronym DDH includes hips that are unstable. subluxated, dislocated (luxated), and/or have malformed acetabula. A hip is *unstable* when the tight fit between the femoral head and the acetabulum is lost and the femoral head is able to move within (subluxated) or outside (dislocated) the confines of the acetabulum. A *dislocation* is a complete loss of contact of the femoral head with the acetabulum. Dislocations are divided into 2 types: teratologic and typical.[12] *Teratologic dislocations* occur early in utero and often are associated with neuromuscular disorders, such as arthrogryposis and myelodysplasia, or with various dysmorphic syndromes. The *typical dislocation* occurs in an otherwise healthy infant and may occur prenatally or postnatally.

During the immediate newborn period, laxity of the hip capsule predominates, and, if clinically significant enough, the femoral head may spontaneously dislocate and relocate. If the hip spontaneously relocates and stabilizes within a few days, subsequent hip development usually is normal. If subluxation or dislocation persists, then structural anatomic changes may develop. A deep concentric position of the femoral head in the acetabulum is necessary for normal development of the hip. When not deeply reduced (subluxated), the labrum may become everted and flattened. Because the femoral head is not reduced into the depth of the socket, the acetabulum does not grow and remodel and, therefore, becomes shallow. If the femoral head moves further out of the socket (dislocation), typically superiorly and laterally, the inferior capsule is pulled upward over the now empty socket. Muscles surrounding the hip, especially the adductors, become contracted, limiting abduction of the hip. The hip capsule constricts; once this capsular constriction narrows to less than the diameter of the femoral head, the hip can no longer be reduced by manual manipulative maneuvers, and operative reduction usually is necessary.

The hip is at risk for dislocation during 4 periods: 1) the 12th gestational week, 2) the 18th gestational week, 3) the final 4 weeks of gestation, and 4) the postnatal period. During the 12th gestational week, the hip is at risk as the fetal lower limb rotates medially. A dislocation at this time is termed teratologic. All elements of the hip joint develop abnormally. The hip muscles develop around the 18th gestational week. Neuromuscular problems at this time, such as myelodysplasia and arthrogryposis, also lead to teratologic dislocations. During the final 4 weeks of pregnancy, mechanical forces have a role. Conditions such as oligohydramnios or breech position predispose to DDH.[13] Breech position occurs in ~3% of births, and DDH occurs more frequently in breech presentations, reportedly in as many as 23%. The frank breech position of hip flexion and knee extension places a newborn or infant at the highest risk. Postnatally, infant positioning such as swaddling, combined with ligamentous laxity, also has a role.

The true incidence of dislocation of the hip can only be presumed. There is no "gold standard" for diagnosis during the newborn period. Physical examination, plane radiography, and ultrasonography all are fraught with false-positive and false-negative results. Arthrography (insertion of contrast medium into the hip joint) and magnetic resonance imaging, although accurate for determining the precise hip anatomy, are inappropriate methods for screening the newborn and infant.

The reported incidence of DDH is influenced by genetic and racial factors, diagnostic criteria, the experience and training of the examiner, and the age of the child at the time of the examination. Wynne-Davies[14] reported an increased risk to subsequent children in the presence of a diagnosed dislocation (6% risk with healthy parents and an affected child, 12% risk with an affected parent, and 36% risk with an affected parent and 1 affected child). DDH is not always detectable at birth, but some newborn screening surveys suggest an incidence as high as 1 in 100 newborns with evidence of instability, and 1 to 1.5 cases of dislocation per 1000 newborns. The incidence of DDH is higher in girls. Girls are especially susceptible to the maternal hormone relaxin, which may contribute to ligamentous laxity with the resultant instability of the hip. The left hip is involved 3 times as commonly as the right hip, perhaps related to the left occiput anterior positioning of most non-breech newborns. In this position, the left hip resides posteriorly against the mother's spine, potentially limiting abduction.

Physical Examination

DDH is an evolving process, and its physical findings on clinical examination change.[12,15,16] The newborn must be relaxed and preferably examined on a firm surface. Considerable patience and skill are required. The physical examination changes as the child grows older. No signs are pathognomonic for a dislocated hip. The examiner must look for asymmetry. Indeed, bilateral dislocations are more difficult to diagnose than unilateral dislocations because symmetry is retained. Asymmetrical thigh or gluteal folds, better observed when the child is prone, apparent limb length discrepancy, and restricted motion, especially abduction, are significant, albeit not pathognomonic signs. With the infant supine and the pelvis stabilized, abduction to 75° and adduction to 30° should occur readily under normal circumstances.

The 2 maneuvers for assessing hip stability in the newborn are the Ortolani and Barlow tests. The Ortolani elicits the sensation of the dislocated hip reducing, and the Barlow detects the unstable hip dislocating from the acetabulum. The Ortolani is performed with the newborn supine and the examiner's index and middle fingers placed along the greater trochanter with the thumb placed along the inner thigh. The hip is flexed to 90° but not more, and the leg is held in neutral rotation. The hip is gently abducted while lifting the leg anteriorly. With this maneuver, a "clunk" is felt as the dislocated femoral head reduces into the acetabulum. This is a positive Ortolani sign. The Barlow provocative test is performed with the newborn positioned supine and the hips flexed to 90°. The leg is then gently adducted while posteriorly directed pressure is placed on the knee. A palpable clunk or sensation of movement is felt as the femoral head exits the acetabulum posteriorly. This is a positive Barlow sign. The Ortolani and Barlow maneuvers are performed 1 hip at a time. Little force is required for the performance of either of these tests. The goal is not to prove that the hip can be dislocated. Forceful and repeated examinations can break the seal between the labrum and the femoral head. These strongly positive signs of Ortolani and Barlow are distinguished from a large array of soft or equivocal physical findings present during the newborn period. High-pitched clicks are commonly elicited with flexion and extension and are inconsequential. A dislocatable hip has a rather distinctive clunk, whereas a subluxable hip is characterized by a feeling of looseness, a sliding movement, but without the true Ortolani and Barlow clunks. Separating true dislocations (clunks) from a feeling of instability and from benign adventitial sounds (clicks) takes practice and expertise. This guideline recognizes the broad range of physical findings present in newborns and infants and the confusion of terminology generated in the literature. By 8 to 12 weeks of age, the capsule laxity decreases, muscle tightness increases, and the Barlow and Ortolani maneuvers are no longer positive regardless of the status of the femoral head. In the 3-month-old infant, limitation of abduction is the most reliable sign associated with DDH. Other features that arouse suspicion include asymmetry of thigh folds, a positive Allis or Galeazzi sign (relative shortness of the femur with the hips and knees flexed), and discrepancy of leg lengths. These physical findings alert the examiner that abnormal relationships of the femoral head to the acetabulum (dislocation and subluxation) *may* be present.

Maldevelopments of the acetabulum alone (acetabular dysplasia) can be determined only by imaging techniques. Abnormal physical findings may be absent in an infant with acetabular dysplasia but no subluxation or dislocation. Indeed, because of the confusion, inconsistencies, and misuse of language in the literature (eg, an Ortolani sign called a click by some and a clunk by others), this guideline uses the following definitions.

- A *positive examination* result for DDH is the Barlow or Ortolani sign. This is the clunk of dislocation or reduction.
- An *equivocal examination* or *warning signs* include an array of physical findings that may be found in children with DDH, in children with another orthopaedic disorder, or in children who are completely healthy. These physical findings include asymmetric thigh or buttock creases, an apparent or true short leg, and limited abduction. These signs, used singly or in combination, serve to raise the pediatrician's index of suspicion and act as a threshold for referral. Newborn soft tissue hip clicks are not predictive of DDH[17] but may be confused with the Ortolani and Barlow clunks by some screening physicians and thereby be a reason for referral.

Imaging

Radiographs of the pelvis and hips have historically been used to assess an infant with suspected DDH. During the first few months of life when the femoral heads are composed entirely of cartilage, radiographs have limited value. Displacement and instability may be undetectable, and evaluation of acetabular development is influenced by the infant's position at the time the radiograph is performed. By 4 to 6 months of age, radiographs become more reliable, particularly when the ossification center develops in the femoral head. Radiographs are readily available and relatively low in cost.

Real-time ultrasonography has been established as an accurate method for imaging the hip during the first few months of life.[15,18–25] With ultrasonography, the cartilage can be visualized and the hip can be viewed while assessing the stability of the hip and the morphologic features of the acetabulum. In some clinical settings, ultrasonography can provide information comparable to arthrography (direct injection of contrast into the hip joint), without the need for sedation, invasion, contrast medium, or ionizing radiation. Although the availability of equipment for ultrasonography is widespread, accurate results in hip sonography require training and experience. Although expertise in pediatric hip ultrasonography is increasing, this examination may not always be available or obtained conveniently. Ultrasonographic techniques include *static evaluation* of the morphologic features of the hip, as popularized in Europe by Graf,[26] and a *dynamic evaluation,* as developed by Harcke[20] that assesses the hip for stability of the femoral head in the socket, as well as static anatomy. Dynamic ultrasonography yields more useful information. With both techniques, there is considerable interobserver variability, especially during the first 3 weeks of life.[7,27]

Experience with ultrasonography has documented its ability to detect abnormal position, instability, and dysplasia not evident on clinical examination. Ultrasonography during the first 4 weeks of life often reveals the presence of minor degrees of instability and acetabular immaturity. Studies[7,28,29] indicate that nearly all these mild early findings, which will not be apparent on physical examination, resolve spontaneously without treatment. Newborn screening with ultrasonography has required a high frequency of reexamination and results in a large number of hips being unnecessarily treated. One study[23] demonstrates that a screening process with higher false-positive results also yields increased prevention of late cases. Ultrasonographic screening of all infants at 4 to 6 weeks of age would be expensive, requiring considerable resources. This practice is yet to be validated by clinical trial. *Consequently, the use of ultrasonography is recommended as an adjunct to the clinical evaluation.* It is the technique of choice for clarifying a physical finding, assessing a high-risk infant, and monitoring DDH as it is observed or treated. Used in this selective capacity, it can guide treatment and may prevent overtreatment.

Preterm Infants

DDH may be unrecognized in prematurely born infants. When the infant has cardiorespiratory problems, the diagnosis and management are focused on providing appropriate ventilatory and cardiovascular support, and careful examination of the hips may be deferred until a later date. The most complete examination the infant receives may occur at the time of discharge from the hospital, and this single examination may not detect subluxation or dislocation. Despite the medical urgencies surrounding the preterm infant, it is critical to examine the entire child.

Methods for Guideline Development

Our goal was to develop a practice parameter by using a process that would be based whenever possible on available evidence. The methods used a combination of expert panel, decision modeling, and evidence synthesis[30] (see the Technical Report available on *Pediatrics electronic pages* at www. pediatrics.org). The predominant methods recommended for such evidence synthesis are generally of 2 types: a *data-driven* method and a *model-driven*[31,32] method. In data-driven methods, the analyst finds the best data available and induces a conclusion from these data. A model-driven method, in contrast, begins with an effort to define the context for evidence and then searches for the data as defined by that context. Data-driven methods are useful when the quality of evidence is high. A careful review of the medical literature revealed that the published evidence about DDH did not meet the criteria for high quality. There was a paucity of randomized clinical trials.[8] We decided, therefore, to use the model-driven method.

A decision model was constructed based on the perspective of practicing clinicians and determining the best strategy for screening and diagnosis. The target child was a full-term newborn with no obvious orthopaedic abnormalities. We focused on the various options available to the pediatrician* for the detection of DDH, including screening by physical examination, screening by ultrasonography, and episodic screening during health supervision. Because the

---

* In this guideline, the term *pediatrician* includes the range of pediatric primary care providers, eg, family practitioners and pediatric nurse practitioners.

detection of a dislocated hip usually results in referral by the pediatrician, and because management of DDH is not in the purview of the pediatrician's care, treatment options are not included. We also included in our model a wide range of options for detecting DDH during the first year of life if the results of the newborn screen are negative.

The outcomes on which we focused were a dislocated hip at 1 year of age as the major morbidity of the disease and avascular necrosis of the hip (AVN) as the primary complication of DDH treatment. AVN is a loss of blood supply to the femoral head resulting in abnormal hip development, distortion of shape, and, in some instances, substantial morbidity. Ideally, a gold standard would be available to define DDH at any point in time. However, as noted, no gold standard exists except, perhaps, arthrography of the hip, which is an inappropriate standard for use in a detection model. Therefore, we defined outcomes in terms of the *process of care*. We reviewed the literature extensively. The purpose of the literature review was to provide the probabilities required by the decision model since there were no randomized clinical trials. The article or chapter title and the abstracts were reviewed by 2 members of the methodology team and members of the subcommittee. Articles not rejected were reviewed, and data were abstracted that would provide evidence for the probabilities required by the decision model. As part of the literature abstraction process, the evidence quality in each article was assessed. A computer-based literature search, hand review of recent publications, or examination of the reference section for other articles ("ancestor articles") identified 623 articles; 241 underwent detailed review, 118 of which provided some data. Of the 100 ancestor articles, only 17 yielded useful articles, suggesting that our accession process was complete. By traditional epidemiologic standards,[33] the quality of the evidence in this set of articles was uniformly low. There were few controlled trials and few studies of the follow-up of infants for whom the results of newborn examinations were negative. When the evidence was poor or lacking entirely, extensive discussions among members of the committee and the expert opinion of outside consultants were used to arrive at a consensus. No votes were taken. Disagreements were discussed, and consensus was achieved.

The available evidence was distilled in 3 ways. First, estimates were made of DDH at birth in infants without risk factors. These estimates constituted the baseline risk. Second, estimates were made of the rates of DDH in the children with risk factors. These numbers guide clinical actions: rates that are too high might indicate referral or different follow-up despite negative physical findings. Third, each screening strategy (pediatrician-based, orthopaedist-based, and ultrasonography-based) was scored for the estimated number of children given a diagnosis of DDH at birth, at mid-term (4–12 months of age), and at late-term (12 months of age and older) and for the estimated number of cases of AVN incurred, assuming that all children given a diagnosis of DDH would be treated. These numbers suggest the best strategy, balancing DDH detection with incurring adverse effects.

The baseline estimate of DDH based on orthopaedic screening was 11.5/1000 infants. Estimates from pediatric screening were 8.6/1000 and from ultrasonography were 25/1000. The 11.5/1000 rate translates into a rate for not-at-risk boys of 4.1/1000 boys and a rate for not-at-risk girls of 19/1000 girls. These numbers derive from the facts that the relative risk—the rate in girls divided by the rate in boys across several studies—is 4.6 and because infants are split evenly between boys and girls, so .5 × 4.1/1000 + .5 × 19/1000 = 11.5/1000.[34,35] We used these baseline rates for calculating the rates in other risk groups. Because the relative risk of DDH for children with a positive family history (first-degree relatives) is 1.7, the rate for boys with a positive family history is 1.7 × 4.1 = 6.4/1000 boys, and for girls with a positive family history, 1.7 × 19 = 32/1000 girls. Finally, the relative risk of DDH for breech presentation (of all kinds) is 6.3, so the risk for breech boys is 7.0 × 4.1 = 29/1000 boys and for breech girls, 7.0 × 19 = 133/1000 girls. These numbers are summarized in Table 1.

These numbers suggest that boys without risk or those with a family history have the lowest risk; girls without risk and boys born in a breech presentation have an intermediate risk; and girls with a positive family history, and especially girls born in a breech presentation, have the highest risks. Guidelines, considering the risk factors, should follow these risk profiles. Reports of newborn screening for DDH have included various screening techniques. In some, the screening clinician was an orthopaedist, in others, a pediatrician, and in still others, a physiotherapist. In addition, screening has been performed by ultrasonography. In assessing the expected effect of each strategy, we estimated the newborn DDH rates, the mid-term DDH rates, and the late-term DDH rates for each of the 3 strategies, as shown in Table 2. We also estimated the rate of AVN for DDH treated before 2 months of age (2.5/1000 treated) and after 2 months of age (109/1000 treated). We could not distinguish the AVN rates for children treated between 2 and 12 months of age from those treated

TABLE 1. Relative and Absolute Risks for Finding a Positive Examination Result at Newborn Screening by Using the Ortolani and Barlow Signs

Newborn Characteristics	Relative Risk of a Positive Examination Result	Absolute Risk of a Positive Examination Result per 1000 Newborns With Risk Factors
All newborns	...	11.5
Boys	1.0	4.1
Girls	4.6	19
Positive family history	1.7	
Boys	...	6.4
Girls	...	32
Breech presentation	7.0	
Boys	...	29
Girls	...	133

TABLE 2. Newborn Strategy*

Outcome	Orthopaedist PE	Pediatrician PE	Ultrasonography
DDH in newborn	12	8.6	25
DDH at ~6 mo of age	.1	.45	.28
DDH at 12 mo of age or more	.16	.33	.1
AVN at 12 mo of age	.06	.1	.1

* PE indicates physical examination. Outcome per 1000 infants initially screened.

later. Table 2 gives these data. The total cases of AVN per strategy are calculated, assuming that all infants with positive examination results are treated.

Table 2 shows that a strategy using pediatricians to screen newborns would give the lowest newborn rate but the highest mid- and late-term DDH rates. To assess how much better an ultrasonography-only screening strategy would be, we could calculate a cost-effectiveness ratio. In this case, the "cost" of ultrasonographic screening is the number of "extra" newborn cases that probably include children who do not need to be treated. (The cost from AVN is the same in the 2 strategies.) By using these cases as the cost and the number of later cases averted as the effect, a ratio is obtained of 71 children treated neonatally because of a positive ultrasonographic screen for each later case averted. Because this number is high, and because the presumption of better late-term efficacy is based on a single study, we do not recommend ultrasonographic screening at this time.

Recommendations and Notes to Algorithm (Fig 1)

1. **All newborns are to be screened by physical examination.** The evidence[†] for this recommendation is good. The expert consensus[‡] is strong. Although initial screening by orthopaedists[§] would be optimal (Table 2), it is doubtful that if widely practiced, such a strategy would give the same good results as those published from pediatric orthopaedic research centers. **It is recommended that screening be done by a properly trained health care provider** (eg, physician, pediatric nurse practitioner, physician assistant, or physical therapist). (Evidence for this recommendation is strong.) A number of studies performed by properly trained nonphysicians report results indistinguishable from those performed by physicians.[36] The examination after discharge from the neonatal intensive care unit should be performed as a newborn examination with appropriate screening. **Ultrasonography of all newborns is not recommended.** (Evidence is fair; consensus is strong.) Although there is indirect evidence to support the use of ultrasonographic screening of all newborns, it is not advocated because it is operator-dependent, availability is questionable, it increases the rate of

---

† In this guideline, evidence is listed as good, fair, or poor based on the methodologist's evaluation of the literature quality. (See the Technical Report.)

‡ Opinion or consensus is listed as *strong* if opinion of the expert panel was unanimous or *mixed* if there were dissenting points of view.

§ In this guideline, the term *orthopaedist* refers to an orthopaedic surgeon with expertise in pediatric orthopaedic conditions.

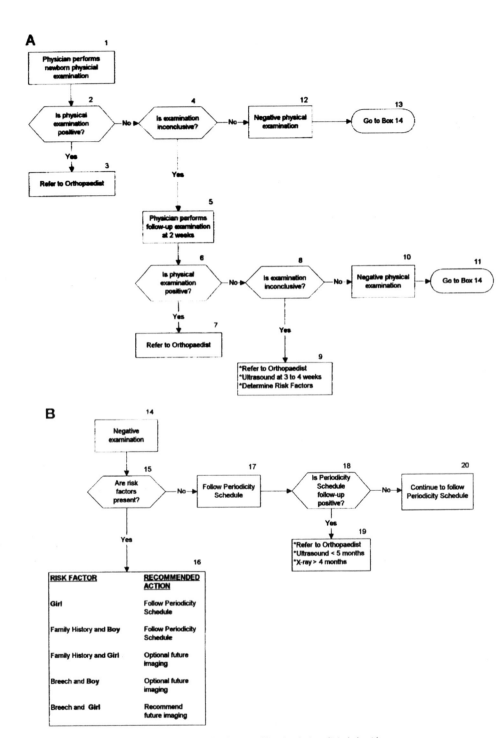

Fig 1. Screening for developmental hip dysplasia—clinical algorithm.

treatment, and interobserver variability is high. There are probably some increased costs. We considered a strategy of "no newborn screening." This arm is politically indefensible because screening newborns is inherent in pediatrician's care. The technical report details this limb through decision analysis. Regardless of the screening method used for the newborn, DDH is detected in 1 in 5000 infants at 18 months of age.[3] The evidence and consensus for newborn screening remain strong.

Newborn Physical Examination and Treatment

2. If a positive Ortolani or Barlow sign is found in the newborn examination, the infant should be referred to an orthopaedist. Orthopaedic referral is recommended when the Ortolani sign is unequivocally positive (a clunk). Orthopaedic referral is not recommended for any softly positive finding in the examination (eg, hip click without dislocation). The precise time frame for the newborn to be evaluated by the orthopaedist cannot be determined from the literature. However, the literature suggests that the majority of "abnormal" physical findings of hip examinations at birth (clicks and clunks) will resolve by 2 weeks; therefore, consultation and possible initiation of treatment are recommended by that time. The data recommending that all those with a positive Ortolani sign be referred to an orthopaedist are limited, but expert panel consensus, nevertheless, was strong, because pediatricians do not have the training to take full responsibility and because true Ortolani clunks are rare and their management is more appropriately performed by the orthopaedist.

If the results of the physical examination at birth are "equivocally" positive (ie, soft click, mild asymmetry, but neither an Ortolani nor a Barlow sign is present), then a follow-up hip examination by the pediatrician in 2 weeks is recommended. (Evidence is good; consensus is strong.) The available data suggest that most clicks resolve by 2 weeks and that these "benign hip clicks" in the newborn period do not lead to later hip dysplasia.[9,17,28,37] Thus, for an infant with softly positive signs, the pediatrician should reexamine the hips at 2 weeks before making referrals for orthopaedic care or ultrasonography. We recognize the concern of pediatricians about adherence to follow-up care regimens, but this concern regards all aspects of health maintenance and is not a reason to request ultrasonography or other diagnostic study of the newborn hips.

3. If the results of the newborn physical examination are positive (ie, presence of an Ortolani or a Barlow sign), ordering an ultrasonographic examination of the newborn is not recommended. (Evidence is poor; opinion is strong.) Treatment decisions are not influenced by the results of ultrasonography but are based on the results of the physical examination. The treating physician may use a variety of imaging studies during clinical management. **If the results of the newborn physical examination are positive, obtaining a radiograph of the newborn's pelvis**

and hips is not recommended (evidence is poor; opinion is strong), because they are of limited value and do not influence treatment decisions.

The use of triple diapers when abnormal physical signs are detected during the newborn period is not recommended. (Evidence is poor; opinion is strong.) Triple diaper use is common practice despite the lack of data on the effectiveness of triple diaper use; and, in instances of frank dislocation, the use of triple diapers may delay the initiation of more appropriate treatment (such as with the Pavlik harness). Often, the primary care pediatrician may not have performed the newborn examination in the hospital. The importance of communication cannot be overemphasized, and triple diapers may aid in follow-up as a reminder that a possible abnormal physical examination finding was present in the newborn.

2-Week Examination

4. **If the results of the physical examination are positive (eg, positive Ortolani or Barlow sign) at 2 weeks, refer to an orthopaedist.** (Evidence is strong; consensus is strong.) Referral is urgent but is not an emergency. Consensus is strong that, as in the newborn, the presence of an Ortolani or Barlow sign at 2 weeks warrants referral to an orthopaedist. An Ortolani sign at 2 weeks may be a new finding or a finding that was not apparent at the time of the newborn examination.

5. **If at the 2-week examination the Ortolani and Barlow signs are absent but physical findings raise suspicions, consider referral to an orthopaedist or request ultrasonography at age 3 to 4 weeks.** Consensus is mixed about the follow-up for softly positive or equivocal findings at 2 weeks of age (eg, adventitial click, thigh asymmetry, and apparent leg length difference). Because it is necessary to confirm the status of the hip joint, the pediatrician can consider referral to an orthopaedist or for ultrasonography if the constellation of physical findings raises a high level of suspicion. However, if the physical findings are minimal, continuing follow-up by the periodicity schedule with focused hip examinations is also an option, provided risk factors are considered. (See "Recommendations" 7 and 8.)

6. **If the results of the physical examination are negative at 2 weeks, follow-up is recommended at the scheduled well-baby periodic examinations.** (Evidence is good; consensus is strong.)

7. **Risk factors. If the results of the newborn examination are negative (or equivocally positive), risk factors may be considered.**[13,21,38–41] Risk factors are a study of thresholds to act.[42] Table 1 gives the risk of finding a positive Ortolani or Barlow sign at the time of the initial newborn screening. If this examination is negative, the absolute risk of there being a true dislocated hip is greatly reduced. Nevertheless, the data in Table 1 may influence the pediatrician to perform confirmatory evaluations. Action will

vary based on the individual clinician. The following recommendations are made (evidence is strong; opinion is strong):

- **Girl** (newborn risk of 19/1000). When the results of the newborn examination are negative or equivocally positive, hips should be reevaluated at 2 weeks of age. If negative, continue according to the periodicity schedule; if positive, refer to an orthopaedist or for ultrasonography at 3 weeks of age.
- **Infants with a positive family history of DDH** (newborn risk for boys of 9.4/1000 and for girls, 44/1000). When the results of the newborn examination in boys are negative or equivocally positive, hips should be reevaluated at 2 weeks of age. If negative, continue according to the periodicity schedule; if positive, refer to an orthopaedist or for ultrasonography at 3 weeks of age. In girls, the absolute risk of 44/1000 may exceed the pediatrician's threshold to act, and imaging with an ultrasonographic examination at 6 weeks of age or a radiograph of the pelvis at 4 months of age is recommended.
- **Breech presentation** (newborn risk for boys of 26/1000 and for girls, 120/1000). **For negative or equivocally positive newborn examinations, the infant should be reevaluated at regular intervals (according to the periodicity schedule) if the examination results remain negative.** Because an absolute risk of 120/1000 (12%) probably exceeds most pediatricians' threshold to act, imaging with an ultrasonographic examination at 6 weeks of age or with a radiograph of the pelvis and hips at 4 months of age is recommended. In addition, because some reports show a high incidence of hip abnormalities detected at an older age in children born breech, this imaging strategy remains an option for all children born breech, not just girls. These hip abnormalities are, for the most part, inadequate development of the acetabulum. Acetabular dysplasia is best found by a radiographic examination at 6 months of age or older. A suggestion of poorly formed acetabula may be observed at 6 weeks of age by ultrasonography, but the best study remains a radiograph performed closer to 6 months of age. Ultrasonographic newborn screening of all breech infants will not eliminate the possibility of later acetabular dysplasia.

8. Periodicity. **The hips must be examined at every well-baby visit according to the recommended periodicity schedule for well-baby examinations (2–4 days for newborns discharged in less than 48 hours after delivery, by 1 month, 2 months, 4 months, 6 months, 9 months, and 12 months of age).** If at any time during the follow-up period DDH is suspected because of an abnormal physical examination or by a parental complaint of difficulty diapering or abnormal appearing legs, the pediatrician must confirm that the hips are stable, in the sockets, and developing normally. Confirmation can be made by a focused physical examination when the infant is calm and relaxed, by consultation with another primary care pediatrician, by consultation with an orthopaedist, by ultrasonography if

the infant is younger than 5 months of age, or by radiography if the infant is older than 4 months of age. (Between 4 and 6 months of age, ultrasonography and radiography seem to be equally effective diagnostic imaging studies.)

Discussion

DDH is an important term because it accurately reflects the biologic features of the disorder and the susceptibility of the hip to become dislocated at various times. Dislocated hips always will be diagnosed later in infancy and childhood because not every dislocated hip is detectable at birth, and hips continue to dislocate throughout the first year of life. Thus, this guideline requires that the pediatrician follow *a process of care for the detection of DDH*. The process recommended for early detection of DDH includes the following:

- Screen all newborns' hips by physical examination.
- Examine all infants' hips according to a periodicity schedule and follow-up until the child is an established walker.
- Record and document physical findings.
- Be aware of the changing physical examination for DDH.
- If physical findings raise suspicion of DDH, or if parental concerns suggest hip disease, confirmation is required by expert physical examination, referral to an orthopaedist, or by an age-appropriate imaging study.

When this process of care is followed, the number of dislocated hips diagnosed at 1 year of age should be minimized. However, the problem of late detection of dislocated hips will not be eliminated. The results of screening programs have indicated that 1 in 5000 children have a dislocated hip detected at 18 months of age or older.[3]

Technical Report

The Technical Report is available from the American Academy of Pediatrics from several sources. The Technical Report is published in full-text on *Pediatrics electronic pages*. The objective was to create a recommendation to pediatricians and other primary care providers about their role as screeners for detecting DDH. The patients are a theoretical cohort of newborns. A model-based method using decision analysis was the foundation. Components of the approach include:

- Perspective: primary care provider
- Outcomes: DDH and AVN
- Preferences: expected rates of outcomes
- Model: influence diagram assessed from the subcommittee and from the methodology team with critical feedback from the subcommittee
- Evidence sources: Medline and EMBase (detailed in "Methods" section)
- Evidence quality: assessed on a custom, subjective scale, based primarily on the fit of the evidence in the decision model

The results are detailed in the "Methods" section. Based on the raw evidence and Bayesian hierarchical meta-analysis,[34,35] estimates for the incidence of DDH based on the type of screener (orthopaedist vs pediatrician); the odds ratio for DDH given risk factors of sex, family history, and breech presentation; and estimates for late detection and AVN were determined and are detailed in the "Methods" section and in Tables 1 and 2.

The decision model (reduced based on available evidence) suggests that orthopaedic screening is optimal, but because orthopaedists in the published studies and in practice would differ in pediatric expertise, the supply of pediatric orthopaedists is relatively limited, and the difference between orthopaedists and pediatricians is statistically insignificant, we conclude that pediatric screening is to be recommended. The place for ultrasonography in the screening process remains to be defined because of the limited data available regarding late diagnosis in ultrasonography screening to permit definitive recommendations.

These data could be used by others to refine the conclusion based on costs, parental preferences, or physician style. Areas for research are well defined by our model-based method. All references are in the Technical Report.

Research Questions

The quality of the literature suggests many areas for research, because there is a paucity of randomized clinical trials and case-controlled studies. The following is a list of possibilities:

1. Minimum diagnostic abilities of a screener. Although there are data for pediatricians in general, few, if any, studies evaluated the abilities of an individual examiner. What should the minimum sensitivity and specificity be, and how should they be assessed?
2. Intercurrent screening. There were few studies on systemic processes for screening after the newborn period.[2,43,44] Although several studies assessed postneonatal DDH, the data did not specify how many examinations were performed on each child before the abnormal result was found.
3. Trade-offs. Screening always results in false-positive results, and these patients suffer the adverse effects of therapy. How many unnecessary AVNs are we—families, physicians, and society—willing to tolerate from a screening program for every appropriately treated infant in whom late DDH was averted? This assessment depends on people's values and preferences and is not strictly an epidemiologic issue.
4. Postneonatal DDH after ultrasonographic screening. Although we concluded that ultrasonographic screening did not result in fewer diagnoses of postneonatal DDH, that conclusion was based on only 1 study.[36] Further study is needed.
5. Cost-effectiveness. If ultrasonographic screening reduces the number of postneonatal DDH diagnoses, then there will be a cost trade-off between

the resources spent up front to screen everyone with an expensive technology, as in the case of ultrasonography, and the resources spent later to treat an expensive adverse event, as in the case of physical examination-based screening. The level at which the cost per case of postneonatal DDH averted is no longer acceptable is a matter of social preference, not of epidemiology.

Acknowledgments

We acknowledge and appreciate the help of our methodology team, Richard Hinton, MD, Paola Morello, MD, and Jeanne Santoli, MD, who diligently participated in the literature review and abstracting the articles into evidence tables, and the subcommittee on evidence analysis.

We would also like to thank Robert Sebring, PhD, for assisting in the management of this process; Bonnie Cosner for managing the workflow; and Chris Kwiat, MLS, from the American Academy of Pediatrics Bakwin Library, who performed the literature searches.

References

1. Bjerkreim I, Hagen O, Ikonomou N, Kase T, Kristiansen T, Arseth P. Late diagnosis of developmental dislocation of the hip in Norway during the years 1980–1989. *J Pediatr Orthop B.* 1993;2:112–114

2. Clarke N, Clegg J, Al-Chalabi A. Ultrasound screening of hips at risk for CDH: failure to reduce the incidence of late cases. *J Bone Joint Surg Br.* 1989;71:9–12

3. Dezateux C, Godward C. Evaluating the national screening programme for congenital dislocation of the hip. *J Med Screen.* 1995;2:200–206

4. Hadlow V. Neonatal screening for congenital dislocation of the hip: a prospective 21-year survey. *J Bone Joint Surg Br.* 1988;70:740–743

5. Krikler S, Dwyer N. Comparison of results of two approaches to hip screening in infants. *J Bone Joint Surg Br.* 1992;74:701–703

6. Macnicol M. Results of a 25-year screening programme for neonatal hip instability. *J Bone Joint Surg Br.* 1990;72:1057–1060

7. Marks DS, Clegg J, Al-Chalabi AN. Routine ultrasound screening for neonatal hip instability: can it abolish late-presenting congenital dislocation of the hip? *J Bone Joint Surg Br.* 1994;76:534–538

8. Rosendahl K, Markestad T, Lie R. Congenital dislocation of the hip: a prospective study comparing ultrasound and clinical examination. *Acta Paediatr.* 1992;81:177–181

9. Sanfridson J, Redlund-Johnell I, Uden A. Why is congenital dislocation of the hip still missed? Analysis of 96,891 infants screened in Malmo 1956–1987. *Acta Orthop Scand.* 1991;62:87–91

10. Tredwell S, Bell H. Efficacy of neonatal hip examination. *J Pediatr Orthop.* 1981;1: 61–65

11. Yngve D, Gross R. Late diagnosis of hip dislocation in infants. *J Pediatr Orthop.* 1990;10:777–779

12. Aronsson DD, Goldberg MJ, Kling TF, Roy DR. Developmental dysplasia of the hip. *Pediatrics.* 1994;94:201–212

13. Hinderaker T, Daltveit AK, Irgens LM, Uden A, Reikeras O. The impact of intra-uterine factors on neonatal hip instability: an analysis of 1,059,479 children in Norway. *Acta Orthop Scand.* 1994;65:239–242

14. Wynne-Davies R. Acetabular dysplasia and familial joint laxity: two etiological factors in congenital dislocation of the hip: a review of 589 patients and their families. *J Bone Joint Surg Br.* 1970;52:704–716

15. De Pellegrin M. Ultrasound screening for congenital dislocation of the hip: results and correlations between clinical and ultrasound findings. *Ital J Orthop Traumatol.* 1991;17:547–553

16. Stoffelen D, Urlus M, Molenaers G, Fabry G. Ultrasound, radiographs, and clinical symptoms in developmental dislocation of the hip: a study of 170 patients. *J Pediatr Orthop B.* 1995;4:194–199

17. Bond CD, Hennrikus WL, Della Maggiore E. Prospective evaluation of newborn soft tissue hip clicks with ultrasound. *J Pediatr Orthop.* 1997;17:199–201

18. Bialik V, Wiener F, Benderly A. Ultrasonography and screening in developmental displacement of the hip. *J Pediatr Orthop B.* 1992;1:51–54

19. Castelein R, Sauter A. Ultrasound screening for congenital dysplasia of the hip in newborns: its value. *J Pediatr Orthop.* 1988;8:666–670

20. Clarke NMP, Harcke HT, McHugh P, Lee MS, Borns PF, MacEwen GP. Real-time ultrasound in the diagnosis of congenital dislocation and dysplasia of the hip. *J Bone Joint Surg Br.* 1985;67:406–412

21. Garvey M, Donoghue V, Gorman W, O'Brien N, Murphy J. Radiographic screening at four months of infants at risk for congenital hip dislocation. *J Bone Joint Surg Br.* 1992;74:704–707

22. Langer R. Ultrasonic investigation of the hip in newborns in the diagnosis of congenital hip dislocation: classification and results of a screening program. *Skeletal Radiol.* 1987;16:275–279

23. Rosendahl K, Markestad T, Lie RT. Ultrasound screening for developmental dysplasia of the hip in the neonate: the effect on treatment rate and prevalence of late cases. *Pediatrics.* 1994;94:47–52

24. Terjesen T. Ultrasound as the primary imaging method in the diagnosis of hip dysplasia in children aged <2 years. *J Pediatr Orthop B.* 1996;5:123–128

25. Vedantam R, Bell M. Dynamic ultrasound assessment for monitoring of treatment of congenital dislocation of the hip. *J Pediatr Orthop.* 1995;15:725–728

26. Graf R. Classification of hip joint dysplasia by means of sonography. *Arch Orthop Trauma Surg.* 1984;102:248–255

27. Berman L, Klenerman L. Ultrasound screening for hip abnormalities: preliminary findings in 1001 neonates. *Br Med J (Clin Res Ed).* 1986;293:719–722

28. Castelein R, Sauter A, de Vlieger M, van Linge B. Natural history of ultrasound hip abnormalities in clinically normal newborns. *J Pediatr Orthop.* 1992;12:423–427

29. Clarke N. Sonographic clarification of the problems of neonatal hip stability. *J Pediatr Orthop.* 1986;6:527–532

30. Eddy DM. The confidence profile method: a Bayesian method for assessing health technologies. *Operations Res.* 1989;37:210–228

31. Howard RA, Matheson JE. Influence diagrams. In: Matheson JE, ed. *Readings on the Principles and Applications of Decision Analysis.* Menlo Park, CA: Strategic Decisions Group; 1981:720–762

32. Nease RF, Owen DK. Use of influence diagrams to structure medical decisions. *Med Decis Making.* 1997;17:265–275

33. Guyatt GH, Sackett DL, Sinclair JC, Hayward R, Cook DJ, Cook RJ. Users' guide to the medical literature, IX: a method for grading health care recommendations. *JAMA.* 1995;274:1800–1804

34. Gelman A, Carlin JB, Stern HS, Rubin DB. *Bayesian Data Analysis.* London, UK: Chapman and Hall; 1997

35. Spiegelhalter D, Thomas A, Best N, Gilks W. *BUGS 0.5: Bayesian Inference Using Gibbs Sampling Manual, II.* Cambridge, MA: MRC Biostatistics Unit, Institute of Public Health; 1996. Available at: http://www.mrc-bsu.cam.ac.uk/bugs/software/software.html

36. Fiddian NJ, Gardiner JC. Screening for congenital dislocation of the hip by physiotherapists: results of a ten-year study. *J Bone Joint Surg Br.* 1994;76:458–459

37. Dunn P, Evans R, Thearle M, Griffiths H. Witherow P. Congenital dislocation of the hip: early and late diagnosis and management compared. *Arch Dis Child.* 1992;60:407–414

38. Holen KJ, Tegnander A, Terjesen T, Johansen OJ, Eik-Nes SH. Ultrasonographic evaluation of breech presentation as a risk factor for hip dysplasia. *Acta Paediatr.* 1996;85:225–229

39. Jones D, Powell N. Ultrasound and neonatal hip screening: a prospective study of "high risk" babies. *J Bone Joint Surg Br.* 1990;72:457–459

40. Teanby DN, Paton RW. Ultrasound screening for congenital dislocation of the hip: a limited targeted programme. *J Pediatr Orthop.* 1997;17:202–204

41. Tonnis D, Storch K, Ulbrich H. Results of newborn screening for CDH with and without sonography and correlation of risk factors. *J Pediatr Orthop.* 1990;10:145–152

42. Pauker SG, Kassirer JP. The threshold approach to clinical decision making. *N Engl J Med.* 1980;302:1109–1117

43. Bower C, Stanley F, Morgan B, Slattery H, Stanton C. Screening for congenital dislocation of the hip by child-health nurses in western Australia. *Med J Aust.* 1989;150:61–65

44. Franchin F, Lacalendola G, Molfetta L, Mascolo V, Quagliarella L. Ultrasound for early diagnosis of hip dysplasia. *Ital J Orthop Traumatol.* 1992;18:261–269

Addendum to References for the DDH Guideline

New information is generated constantly. Specific details of this report must be changed over time.

New articles (additional articles 1–7) have been published since the completion of our literature search and construction of this Guideline. These articles taken alone might seem to contradict some of the Guideline's estimates as detailed in the article and in the Technical Report. However, taken in context with the literature synthesis carried out for the construction of this Guideline, our estimates remain intact and no conclusions are obviated.

Additional Articles

1. Bialik V, Bialik GM, Blazer S, Sujov P, Wiener F, Berant M. Developmental dysplasia of the hip: a new approach to incidence. *Pediatrics.* 1999;103:93–99

2. Clegg J, Bache CE, Raut VV. Financial justification for routine ultrasound screening of the neonatal hip. *J Bone Joint Surg.* 1999;81-B:852–857

3. Holen KJ, Tegnander A, Eik-Nes SH, Terjesen T. The use of ultrasound in determining the initiation in treatment in instability of the hips in neonates. *J Bone Joint Surg.* 1999;81-B:846-851

4. Lewis K, Jones DA, Powell N. Ultrasound and neonatal hip screening: the five-year results of a prospective study in high risk babies. *J Pediatr Orthop.* 1999;19:760–762

5. Paton RW, Srinivasan MS, Shah B, Hollis S. Ultrasound screening for hips at risk in developmental dysplasia: is it worth it? *J Bone Joint Surg.* 1999;81-B:255–258

6. Sucato DJ, Johnston CE, Birch JG, Herring JA, Mack P. Outcomes of ultrasonographic hip abnormalities in clinically stable hips. *J Pediatr Orthop.* 1999;19:754–759

7. Williams PR, Jones DA, Bishay M. Avascular necrosis and the aberdeen splint in developmental dysplasia of the hip. *J Bone Joint Surg.* 1999;81-B:1023–1028

Technical Report Summary:
Developmental Dysplasia of the Hip

Authors:

Harold P. Lehmann, MD, Phd; Richard Hinton, MD, MPH;
Paola Morello, MD; and Jeanne Santoli, MD
in conjunction with the
American Academy of Pediatrics
Subcommittee on Developmental
Dysplasia of the Hip

American Academy of Pediatrics
PO Box 927, 141 Northwest Point Blvd
Elk Grove Village, IL 60009-0927

Abstract

Objective. To create a recommendation for pediatricians and other primary care providers about their role as screeners for detecting developmental dysplasia of the hip (DDH) in children.

Patients. Theoretical cohorts of newborns.

Method. Model-based approach using decision analysis as the foundation. Components of the approach include the following:

Perspective: Primary care provider.

Outcomes: DDH, avascular necrosis of the hip (AVN).

Options: Newborn screening by pediatric examination; orthopaedic examination; ultrasonographic examination; orthopaedic or ultrasonographic examination by risk factors. Intercurrent health supervision-based screening.

Preferences: 0 for bad outcomes, 1 for best outcomes.

Model: Influence diagram assessed by the Subcommittee and by the methodology team, with critical feedback from the Subcommittee.

Evidence Sources: Medline and EMBASE search of the research literature through June 1996. Hand search of sentinel journals from June 1996 through March 1997. Ancestor search of accepted articles.

Evidence Quality: Assessed on a custom subjective scale, based primarily on the fit of the evidence to the decision model.

Results. After discussion, explicit modeling, and critique, an influence diagram of 31 nodes was created. The computer-based and the hand literature searches found 534 articles, 101 of which were reviewed by 2 or more readers. Ancestor searches of these yielded a further 17 articles for evidence abstraction. Articles came from around the globe, although primarily Europe, British Isles, Scandinavia, and their descendants. There were 5 controlled trials, each with a sample size less than 40. The remainder were case series. Evidence was available for 17 of the desired 30 probabilities. Evidence quality ranged primarily between one third and two thirds of the maximum attainable score (median: 10–21; interquartile range: 8–14).

Based on the raw evidence and Bayesian hierarchical meta-analyses, our estimate for the incidence of DDH revealed by physical examination performed by pediatricians is 8.6 per 1000; for orthopaedic screening, 11.5; for ultrasonography, 25. The odds ratio for DDH, given breech delivery, is 5.5; for female sex, 4.1; for positive family history, 1.7, although this last factor is not statistically significant. Postneonatal cases of DDH were divided into mid-term (younger than 6 months of age) and late-term (older than 6 months of age). Our estimates for the mid-term rate for screening by pediatricians is 0.34/1000 children screened; for orthopaedists, 0.1; and for ultrasonography, 0.28. Our estimates for late-term DDH rates are 0.21/1000 newborns screened by pediatricians; 0.08, by orthopaedists; and 0.2 for ultrasonography. The rates of AVN for children referred before 6 months of age is estimated at 2.5/1000 infants referred. For those referred after 6 months of age, our estimate is 109/1000 referred infants.

The decision model (reduced, based on available evidence) suggests that orthopaedic screening is optimal, but because orthopaedists in the published studies and in practice would differ, the supply of orthopaedists is relatively limited, and the difference between orthopaedists and pediatricians is statistically insignificant, we conclude that pediatric screening is to be recommended. The place of ultrasonography in the screening process remains to be defined because there are too few data about post-neonatal diagnosis by ultrasonographic screening to permit definitive recommendations. These data could be used by others to refine the conclusions based on costs, parental preferences, or physician style. Areas for research are well defined by our model-based approach. *Pediatrics* 2000;105(4). URL: http://www. pediatrics.org/cgi/content/full/105/4/e57; keywords: *developmental dysplasia of the hip, avascular necrosis of the hip, newborn.*

I. Guideline Methods

A. Decision Model

The steps required to build the model were taken with the Subcommittee as a whole, with individuals in the group, and with members of the methodology team. Agreement on the model was sought from the Subcommittee as a whole during face-to-face meetings.

1. Perspective

Although there are a number of perspectives to take in this problem (parental, child's, societal, and payer's), we opted for the view of the practicing clinician: What are the clinician's obligations, and what is the best strategy for the clinician? This choice of perspective meant that the focus would be on screening for developmental dysplasia of the hip (DDH) and obviated the need to review the evidence for efficacy or effectiveness of specific strategies.

2. Context

The target child is a full-term newborn with no obvious orthopaedic abnormalities. Children with such findings would be referred to an orthopaedist, obviating the need for a practice parameter.

3. Options

We focused on the following options: screening by physical examination (PE) at birth by a pediatrician, orthopaedist, or other care provider; ultrasonographic screening at birth; and episodic screening during health supervision. Treatment options are not included.

We also included in our model a wide range of options for managing the screening process during the first year of life when the newborn screening was negative.

4. Outcomes

Our focus is on dislocated hips at 1 year of age as the major morbidity of the disease and on avascular necrosis of the hip (AVN), as the primary sentinel complication of DDH therapy.

Ideally, we would have a "gold standard" that would define DDH at any point in time, much as cardiac output can be obtained from a pulmonary-artery catheter. However, no gold standard exists. Therefore, we defined our outcomes in terms of the process of care: a pediatrician and an ultrasonographer perform initial or confirmatory examinations and refer the patient, whereas the orthopaedist treats the patient. It is the treatment that has the greatest effect on postneonatal DDH or on complications, so we focus on that intermediate outcome, rather than the orthopaedist's stated diagnosis. We operationalized the definitions of these outcomes for use in abstracting the data from articles. A statement that a "click" was found on PE was considered to refer to an intermediate result, unless the authors defined their "click" in terms of our definition of a positive examination. Dynamic ultrasonographic examinations include those of Harcke et al, and static refers primarily to that of Graf. The radiologic focus switches from ultrasonography to plain radiographs after 4 months of age, in keeping with the development of the femoral head.

5. Decision Structure

We used an influence diagram to represent the decision model. In this representation, nodes refer to actions to be taken or to states of the world (the patient) about which we are uncertain. We devoted substantial effort to the construction of a model that balanced the need to represent the rich array of possible screening pathways with the need to be parsimonious. We constructed the master influence diagram and determined its construct validity through consensus by the Subcommittee before data abstraction. However, the available evidence could specify only a portion of the diagram. The missing components suggest research questions that need to be posed.

6. Probabilities

The purpose of the literature review was to provide the probabilities required by the decision model. The initial number of individual probabilities was 55. (Sensitivity and specificity for a single truth-indicator pair are counted as a single probability because they are garnered from the same table.) Although this is a large number of parameters, the structure of the model helped the team of readers. As 1 reader said, referring to the influence diagram, "Because we did the picture together, it was easy to find the parameters." What follows are some operational rules for matching the data to our parameters. The list is not complete. If an orthopaedic clinic worked at case finding, we used our judgment to determine whether to accept such reports as representing a population incidence.

Risk factors were included generally only if a true control group was used for comparison. For postneonatal diagnoses, no study we reviewed included the examination of all children without DDH, say, 1 year of age, so there is always the possibility of missed cases (false-negative diagnoses) in the screen, which leads to a falsely elevated estimate of the denominator. For studies originating in referral clinics, the data on the reasons for referrals were not usable for our purposes.

7. Preferences

Ideally, we would have cost data for the options, as well as patient data on the human burden of therapy and of DDH itself. We have deferred these assessments to later research. Therefore, we assigned a preference score of

0 to DDH at 1 year of age and 1 to its absence; for AVN, we assigned 0 for presence at 1 year of age and 1 for absence at 1 year of age.

B. Literature Review

For the literature through May 1995, the following sources were searched: Books in Print, CAT-LINE, Current Contents, EMBASE, Federal Research in Progress, Health Care Standards, Health Devices Alerts, Health Planning and Administration, Health Services/Technology Assessment, International Health Technology Assessment, and Medline. Medline and EMBASE were searched through June 1996. The search terms used in all databases included the following: hip dislocation, congenital; hip dysplasia; congenital hip dislocation; developmental dysplasia; ultrasonography/ adverse effects; and osteonecrosis. Hand searches of leading orthopaedic journals were performed for the issues from June 1996 to March 1997. The bibliographies of journals accepted for use in formulating the practice parameter also were perused.

The titles and the abstracts were then reviewed by 2 members of the methodology team to determine whether to accept or reject the articles for use. Decisions were reviewed by the Subcommittee, and conflicts were adjudicated. Similarly, articles were read by pairs of reviewers; conflicts were resolved in discussion.

The focus of the data abstraction process was on data that would provide evidence for the probabilities required by the decision model.

As part of the literature abstraction process, the evidence quality in each article was assessed. The scoring process was based on our decision model and involved traditional epidemiologic concerns, like outcome definition and bias of ascertainment, as well as influence–diagram-based concerns, such as how well the data fit into the model.

Cohort definition: Does the cohort represented by the denominator in the study match a node in our influence diagram? Does the cohort represented by the numerator match a node in our influence diagram? The closer the match, the more confident we are that the reported data provide good evidence of the conditional probability implied by the arrow between the corresponding nodes in the influence diagram.

Path: Does the implied path from denominator to numerator lead through 1 or more nodes of the influence diagram? The longer the path, the more likely that uncontrolled biases entered into the study, making us less confident about accepting the raw data as a conditional probability in our model. Assignment and comparison: Was there a control group? How was assignment made to experimental or control arms? A randomized, controlled study provides the best quality evidence.

Follow-up: Were patients with positive and negative initial findings followed up? The best studies should have data on both.

Outcome definition: Did the language of the out-come definitions (PE, orthopaedic examination, ultrasonography, and radiography) match ours, and, in particular, were PE findings divided into 3 categories or 2? The closer the definition to ours, the more we could pool the data. Studies with only 2 categories do not help to distinguish clicks from "clunks."

Ascertainment: When the denominator represented more than 1 node, to what degree was the denominator a mix of nodes? The smaller the contamination, the more confident we were that the raw data represented a desired conditional probability.

Results: Did the results fill an entire table or were data missing? This is related to the follow-up category but is more general.

C. Synthesis of Evidence

There are 3 levels of evidence synthesis.

1. Listing evidence for individual probabilities
2. Summarizing evidence across probabilities
3. Integrating the pooled evidence for individual probabilities into the decision model

A list of evidence for an individual probability (or arc) is called an *evidence table* and provides the reader a look at the individual pieces of data. The probabilities are summarized in 3 ways: by averaging, by averaging weighted by sample size (pooled), and by meta-analysis. We chose Bayesian meta-analytic techniques, which allow the representation of *prior belief* in the evidence and provide an explicit portrayal of the uncertainty of our conclusions. The framework we used was that of a hierarchical Bayesian model, similar to the random effects model in traditional meta-analysis. In this hierarchical model, each study has its own parameter, which, in turn, is sampled from a wider population parameter. Because there are 2 stages (ie, population to sample and sample to observation), and, therefore, the population parameter of interest is more distant from the data, the computed estimates in the population parameters are, in general, less certain (wider confidence interval) than simply pooling the data across studies. This lower certainty is appropriate in the DDH content area because the studies vary so widely in their raw estimates because of the range in time and geography over which they were performed. In the Bayesian model, the observations were assumed to be Poisson distributed, given the study DDH rates. Those rates, in turn, were assumed to be Gamma distributed, given the population rate. The prior belief on that rate was set as Gamma ($\propto$, ß), with mean $\propto$/ß, and variance $\propto$/ß^2 (as defined in the BUGS software). In this parameterization, $\propto$ has the semantics closest to that of location, and ß has the semantics of certainty: the higher its value, the narrower the distribution and the more certain we are of the estimate. The parameter, $\propto$, was modeled as Exponential (1), and ß, as Gamma (0.01, 1), with a mean of 0.01. Together, these correspond to a prior belief in the rate of a mean of 100 per 1000, and a standard deviation (SD) of 100, representing ignorance of the true rate.

As an example of interpretation, for pediatric newborn screening, the posterior $\propto$ was 1.46, and the posterior ß was 0.17, to give a posterior rate of 8.6/1000, with a variance of 50, or an SD of 7.1. The value of ß rose from 0.01 to 0.17, indicating a higher level of certainty.

The Bayesian confidence interval is the narrowest interval that contains 95% of the area under the posterior-belief curve. The confidence interval for the prior curve is 2.53 to 370. The confidence interval for the posterior curve is 0.25 to 27.5, a significant shrinking and increase in certainty but still broad.

The model for the odds ratios is more complicated and is based on the Oxford data set and analysis in the BUGS manual.

D. Thresholds

In the course of discussions about results, the Subcommittee was surveyed about the acceptable risks of DDH for different levels of interventions.

E. Recommendations

Once the evidence and thresholds were obtained, a decision tree was created from the evidence available and was reviewed by the Subcommittee. In parallel, a consensus guideline (flowchart) was created. The Subcommittee evaluated whether evidence was available for links within the guidelines, as well as their strength of consensus. The decision tree was evaluated to check consistency of the evidence with the conclusions.

F. "Cost"-Effectiveness Ratios

To integrate the results, we defined cost-effectiveness ratios, in which cost was excess neonatal referrals or excess cases of AVNs, and *effectiveness* was a decrease in the number of later cases. The decision tree from section E ("Recommendations") was used to calculate the expected outcomes for each of pediatric, orthopaedic, and ultrasonographic strategies. Pediatric strategy was used as the baseline, because its neonatal screening rate was the lowest. The cost-effectiveness ratios then were calculated as the quotient of the difference in cost and the difference in effect.

Results

A. Articles

The peak number of articles is for 1992, with 10 articles. The articles are from sites all over the world, although the Nordic, Anglo-Saxon, and European communities and their descendants are the most represented.

B. Evidence

By traditional epidemiologic standards, the quality of evidence in this set of articles is uniformly low. There are few controlled trials and few studies in which infants with negative results on their newborn examinations are followed up. (A number of studies attempted to cover all possible places where an affected child might have been ascertained.)

We found data on all chance nodes, for a total of 298 distinct tables. *Decision* nodes were poorly represented: beyond the neonatal strategy, there were almost no data clarifying the paths for the diagnosis children after the newborn period. Thus, although communities like those in southeast Norway have a postnewborn screening program, it is unclear what the program was, and it was unclear how many examination results were normal before a child was referred to an orthopaedist.

The mode is a score of 10, achieved in 16 give a sense of the "weight" of the data. articles. The median is 9.9, with an interquartile range of 8 to 14, suggesting that articles with scores below 8 are poor sources of evidence. Note that the maximum achievable quality score is 21, so half the articles do not achieve half the maximum quality score.

Graphing evidence quality against publication year suggests an improvement in quality over time, as shown in Fig 9, but the linear fit through the data is statistically indistinguishable from a flat line. (A nonparametric procedure yields the same conclusion).

The studies include 5 in which a comparative arm was designed into the study. The remainder are divided between prospective and retrospective studies. Surprisingly, the evidence quality is not higher in the former than in the latter (data not shown).

Of the 298 data tables, half the data tables relate to the following:

• probabilities of DDH in different screening strategies
• relative risk of DDH, given risk factors
• the incidence of postneonatal DDH, and
• the incidence of AVN.

The remainder of our discussion will focus on these probabilities.

C. Evidence Tables

The evidence table details are found in the appendix of the full technical report.

1. Newborn Screening

a. Pediatric Screening

There were 51 studies, providing 57 arms, for pediatric screening. However, of these, 17 were unclear on how the intermediate examinations were handled, and, unsurprisingly, their observed rates of positivity (clicks) were much higher than the studies that distinguished 3 categories, as we had specified. Therefore, we included only the 34 studies that used 3 categories.

For pediatric screening, the rate is about 8 positive cases per 1000 examinations. The rates are distributed almost uniformly between 0 and 20 per 1000. All studies represent a large experience: a total of 2 149 972 subjects. Although their methods may not have been the best, the studies demand attention simply because of their size.

In looking for covariates or confounding variables, we studied the relationship between positivity rate and the independent variables, year of publication, evidence quality, and sample size. Year and evidence quality show a positive effect: the higher the year (slope: 0.2; $P \leq .018$) or evidence quality (slope: 0.6; $P \leq .046$), the higher the observed rate. A model with both factors has evidence that suggests that most of the effect is in the factor, year (slope for year: 0.08; $P \leq .038$; slope for quality of evidence: 0.49; $P \leq .09$). Note that a regression using evidence quality is improper, because our evidence scale is not properly ratio (eg, the distance between 6 and 7 is not necessarily equivalent to the distance between 14 and 15), but the regression is a useful exploratory device.

b. Orthopaedic Screening

Evidence was found in 25 studies. Three studies provided 2 arms each.

The positivity rate for orthopaedic screening is between 7 and 11/1000. One outlier study, with an observed rate of more than 300/1000, skews the unweighted and meta-analytic averages. The estimate (between 7.1 and 11) is just below that of pediatric screening and is statistically indistinguishable. Note, however, that a fair number of studies have rates near 22/1000 or higher.

Unlike with pediatric screening, there are no correlations with other factors.

c. Ultrasonographic Screening

Evidence was found in 17 studies, each providing a single arm.

The rate for ultrasonographic screening is 20/1000 or more. Although the estimates are sensitive to pooling and to the outlier, the positivity rate is clearly higher than in either PE strategy. There are no correlating factors. In particular, studies that use the Graf method 2 or those that use the method of Harcke et al show comparable rates.

2. Postneonatal Cases

We initially were interested in all postneonatal diagnoses of DDH. However, the literature did not provide data within the narrow time frames initially specified for our model. Based on the data that were available, we considered 3 classes of postneonatal DDH: DDH diagnosed after 12 months of age ("late-term"), DDH diagnosed between 6 and 12 months of age ("mid-term"), and DDH diagnosed before 6 months of age. There were few data for the latter group, which often was combined with the newborn screening programs. Therefore, we collected data on only the first 2 groups.

a. After Pediatric Screening

Evidence was found in 24 studies. The study by Dunn and O'Riordan provided 2 arms. It is difficult to discern an estimate rate for mid-term DDH, because the study by Czeizel et al is such an outlier, with a rate of 3.73/1000, and because the weighted and unweighted averages also differ greatly. The meta-analytic estimate of 0.55/1000 seems to be an upper limit.

The late-term rate is easier to estimate at ~0.3/1000. Although it is intuitive that the late-term rate should be lower than the mid-term rate, our data do not allow us to draw that conclusion.

b. After Orthopaedic Screening

There were only 4 studies. The rates were comparable for mid- and late-term: 0.1/1000 newborns. A meta-analytic estimate was not calculated.

c. After Ultrasonographic Screening

Only 1 study, by Rosendahl et al is available; it reported rates for infants with and without initial risk factors (eg, family history and breech presentation). The mid-term rate was 0.28/1000 newborns in the non-risk group, and the late-term rate was 0/1000 in the same group.

3. AVN After Treatment

For these estimates, we grouped together all treatments, because from the viewpoint of the referring primary care provider, orthopaedic treatment is a "black box:" A literature synthesis that teased apart the success and complications of particular *therapeutic* strategies is beyond the scope of the present study.

The complication rate should depend only on the age of the patient at time of orthopaedic referral and on the type of treatment received. We report on the complication rates for children treated before and after 12 months of age.

a. After Early Referral

There were 17 studies providing evidence. Infants were referred to orthopaedists during the newborn period in each study except 2. In the study by Pool et al, infants were referred during the newborn period and before 2 months of age; in the study by Sochart and Paton, infants were referred between 2 weeks and 2 months of age.

The range of AVN rates per 1000 infants referred was huge, from 0 to 123. The largest rate occurred in the study by Pool et al, a sample-based study that included later referrals. Its evidence quality was 8, within the 7 to 13 interquartile range of the other studies in this group. As in earlier tables, the meta-analytic estimate lies between the average and weighted (pooled) average of the studies.

b. After Later Referral

Evidence was obtained from 6 studies. Some of the studies included children referred during the newborn period or during the 2-week to 2-month period, but even in these, the majority of infants were referred later during the first year of life.

There were no outlier rates, although the highest rate (216/1000 referred children) occurred in the study with the oldest referred children in the sample with children referred who were older than 12 months of age). One study contributed 5700 patients to the analysis, more than half of the 9270 total, so its AVN rate of 27/1000 brought the unweighted rate of 116/1000 to 54. A meta-analytic estimate was not computed.

4. Risk Factors

A number of factors are known to predispose infants to DDH. We sought evidence for 3 of these: sex, obstetrical position at birth, and family history. Studies were included in these analyses only if a control group could be ascertained from the available study data.

The key measure is the odds ratio, an estimate of the relative risk. The meaning of the odds ratio is that if the DDH rate for the control group is known, then the DDH rate for the at-risk group is the product of the control-group DDH rate and the odds ratio for the risk factor. An odds ratio statistically significantly greater than 1 indicates that the factor is a risk factor.

The Bayesian meta-analysis produces estimates between the average of the odds ratios and the pooled odds ratio and is, therefore, the estimate we used in our later analyses.

a. Female

The studies were uniform in discerning a risk to girls ~4 times that of boys for being diagnosed with DDH. This risk was seen in all 3 screening environments.

b. Breech

The studies for breech also were confident in finding a risk for breech presentation, on the order of fivefold. One study found breech presentation to be protective, but the study was relatively small and used ultrasonography rather than PE as its outcome measure.

c. Family History

Although some studies found family history to be a risk factor, the range was wide. The confidence intervals for the pooled odds ratio and for the Bayesian analysis contained 1.0, suggesting that family history is *not* an independent risk factor for DDH. However, because of traditional concern with this risk factor, we kept it in our further considerations.

D. Evidence Summary and Risk Implications

To bring all evidence tables together, we constructed a summary table, which contains the estimates we chose for our recommendations. The intervals are asymmetric, in keeping with the intuition that rates near zero cannot be negative, but certainly can be very positive.

Risk factors are based on the pediatrician population rate of 8.6 labeled cases of DDH per 1000 infants screened. In the Subcommittee's discussion, 50/1000 was a cutoff for automatic referral during the newborn period. Hence, girls born in the breech position are classified in a separate category for newborn strategies than infants with other risk factors.

If we use the orthopaedists' rate as our baseline, numbers suggest that boys without risks or those with a family history have the lowest risk; girls without risks and boys born in the breech presentation have an intermediate risk; and girls with a positive family history, and especially girls born in the breech presentation, have the highest risks. Guidelines that consider risk factors should follow these risk profiles.

E. Decision Recommendations

With the evidence synthesized, we can estimate the expected results of the target newborn strategies for postneonatal DDH and AVN.

If a case of DDH is observed in an infant with an initially negative result of screening by an orthopaedist in a newborn screening program, that case is "counted" against the orthopaedist strategy.

The numbers are combined using a simple decision tree, which is not the final tree represented by our influence diagram but is a tree that is supported by our evidence. The results show that pediatricians diagnose fewer newborns with DDH and perhaps have a higher postneonatal DDH rate than orthopaedists but one that is comparable to ultrasonography (acknowledging that our knowledge of postneonatal DDH revealed by ultrasonographic screening is limited). The AVN rates are comparable with pediatrician and ultrasonographic screening and less than with orthopaedist screening.

F. Cost-Effectiveness Ratios

In terms of excess neonatal referrals, the ratios suggest that there is a trade-off: for every case that these strategies detect beyond the pediatric strategy, they require more than 7000 or 16 000 extra referrals, respectively.

Discussion

A. Summary

We derived 298 evidence tables from 118 studies culled from a larger set of 624 articles. Our literature review captured most in our model-based approach, if not all, of the past literature on DDH that was usable. The decision model (reduced based on available evidence) suggests that orthopaedic screening is optimal, but because orthopaedists in the published studies and in practice would differ, the supply of orthopaedists is relatively limited, and the difference between orthopaedists and pediatricians is relatively small, we conclude that pediatric screening is to be recommended. The place of ultrasonography in the screening process remains to be defined because there are too few data about postneonatal diagnosis by ultrasonographic screening to permit definitive recommendations.

Our conclusions are tempered by the uncertainties resulting from the wide range of the evidence. The confidence intervals are wide for the primary parameters. The uncertainties mean that, even with all the evidence collected from the literature, we are left with large doubts about the values of the different parameters.

Our data do not bear directly on the issue about the earliest point that any patient destined to have DDH will show signs of the disease. Our use of the terms *mid-term* and *late-term* DDH addresses that ignorance.

Our conclusions about other areas of the full decision model are more tentative because of the paucity of data about the effectiveness of periodicity examinations. Even the studies that gave data on mid-term and late-term case findings by pediatricians were sparse in their details about how the screening was instituted, maintained, or followed up.

Our literature search was weakest in addressing the European literature, where results about ultrasonography are more prevalent. We found, however, that many of the seminal articles were republished in English or in a form that we could assess.

B. Specific Issues

1. Evidence Quality

Our measure of evidence quality is unique, although it is based on solid principles of study design and decision modeling. In particular, our measure was based on the notion that if the data conform poorly to how we need to use it, we downgrade its value.

However, throughout the analyses, there was never a correlation with the results of a study (in terms of the values of outcomes) and with evidence quality, so we never needed to use the measure for weighting the values of the outcome or for culling articles from our review. Had this been so, the measures would have needed further scrutiny and validation.

2. Outliers

Perhaps the true surrogates for study quality were the outlying values of outcomes. In general, however, there were few cases in which the outliers were clearly the result of poor-quality studies. One example is that of the outcomes of pediatric screening ($1\rightarrow3$), in which the DDH rates in studies using only 2 categories were generally higher than those that explicitly specified 3 levels of outcomes.

Our general justification for using estimates that excluded outliers is that the outliers so much drove the results that they dominated the conclusion out of proportion to their sample sizes. As it is, our estimates have wide ranges.

3. Newborn Screening

The set of studies labeled "pediatrician screening" includes studies with a variety of examiners. We could not estimate the sensitivity and specificity of pediatricians' examinations versus those of other primary care providers versus orthopaedists. There are techniques for extracting these measures from agreement studies, but they are beyond the scope of the present study. It is intuitive that the more cases that one examines, the better an examiner one will be, regardless of professional title.

We were surprised that the results did not show a clear difference in results between the Graf and Harcke et al ultrasonographic examinations. Our data make no statement about the relative advantages of these methods for following up children or in addressing treatment.

4. Postneonatal Cases

As mentioned, our data cannot say when a postneonatal case is established or, therefore, the best time to screen children. We established our initial age categories for postneonatal cases based on biology, treatment changes, and optimal imaging and examination strategies. It is frustrating that the data in the literature are not organized to match this pathophysiological way of thinking about DDH. Similarly, as mentioned, the lack of details by authors on the methods of intercurrent screening means that we cannot recommend a preferred method for mid-term or late-term screening.

5. AVN

We used AVN as our primary marker for treatment morbidity. We acknowledge that the studies we grouped together may reflect different philosophies and results of orthopaedic practice. The hierarchical meta-analysis treats every study as an individual case, and the wide range in our confidence intervals reflects the uncertainty that results in grouping disparate studies together.

C. Comments on Methods

This study is unique in its strong use of decision modeling at each step in the process. In the end, our results are couched in traditional terms (estimated rates of disease or morbidity outcomes), although the context is relatively non-traditional: attaching the estimates to strategies rather than to treatments. In this, our study is typical of an *effectiveness* study, which studied results in the real world, rather than of an *efficacy* study, which examines the biological effects of a treatment.

We made strong and recurrent use of the Bayesian hierarchical meta-analysis. A review of the tables will confirm that the Bayesian results were in the same "ballpark" as the average and pooled average estimates and had a more solid grounding.

The usual criticism of using Bayesian methods is that they depend on prior belief. The usual response is to show that the final estimates are relatively insensitive to the prior belief. In fact, for the screening strategies, a wide range of prior beliefs had no effect on the estimate. However, the prior belief used for the screening strategies—with a mean of 100 cases/1000 with a variance of 100— was too broad for the postneonatal case and AVN analyses; when data were sparse, the prior belief overwhelmed the data. For instance, in late-term DDH revealed by orthopaedic screening (53 30), in an analysis not shown, the posterior estimate from the 4 studies was a rate of 0.345 cases per 1000, despite an average and a pooled average on the order of 0.08. Four studies were insufficient to overpower a prior belief of 100.

D. Research Issues

The place of ultrasonography in DDH screening needs more attention, as does the issue of intercurrent pediatrician screening. In the latter case, society and health care systems must assess the effectiveness of education and the "return on investment" for educational programs. The place of preferences— of the parents, of the clinician—must be established.

We hope that the framework we have delineated— of a decision model and of data—can be useful in these future research endeavors.

The Neurodiagnostic Evaluation of the Child With a First Simple Febrile Seizure

- *Clinical Practice Guideline*
- *Technical Report Summary*

Readers of this clinical practice guideline are urged to review the technical report to enhance the evidence-based decision-making process. For a copy of the technical report, call Carla Herrerias, MPH, at the Academy, at 800/433-9016, ext 4317.

Clinical Practice Guideline:
The Neurodiagnostic Evaluation of the Child
With a First Simple Febrile Seizure

Author:

Subcommittee on Febrile Seizures
Provisional Committee on Quality Improvement

American Academy of Pediatrics
PO Box 927, 141 Northwest Point Blvd
Elk Grove Village, IL 60009-0927

Subcommittee on Diagnosis and Treatment of Febrile Seizures 1992–1995

Thomas A. Riemenschneider, MD, Chairman

Robert J. Baumann, MD
Patricia K. Duffner, MD

John L. Green, MD
Sanford Schneider, MD

Consultants:

James R. Cooley, MD,
  Clinical Algorithm
David L. Coulter, MD
Patricia K. Crumrine, MD
Sandra D'Angelo, PhD,
  Methodology Consultant
W. Edwin Dodson, MD

John M. Freeman, MD
Michael Kohrman, MD
James O. McNamara, MD
Karin B. Nelson, MD
N. Paul Rosman, MD
Shlomo Shinnar, MD

Provisional Committee on Quality Improvement 1993–1996

David A. Bergman, MD, Chairman

Richard D. Baltz, MD
James R. Cooley, MD
John B. Coombs, MD
Lawrence F. Nazarian, MD

Thomas A. Riemenschneider, MD
Kenneth B. Roberts, MD
Daniel W. Shea, MD

Liaison Representatives:

Michael J. Goldberg, MD
  Sections Liaison
Charles J. Homer, MD, MPH
  Section on Epidemiology

Thomas F. Tonniges, MD
  AAP Board of Directors

Abstract

The American Academy of Pediatrics and its Provisional Committee on Quality Improvement, in collaboration with experts from the Section on Neurology, general pediatricians, consultants in the fields of neurology and epilepsy, and research methodologists, developed this practice parameter.

This parameter provides recommendations for the neurodiagnostic evaluation of a child with a first simple febrile seizure. These recommendations derive from both a thorough review of the literature and expert consensus. Interventions of direct interest include lumbar puncture, electroencephalography, blood studies, and neuroimaging. The methods and results of the literature review and data analyses can be found in the technical report that is available from the American Academy of Pediatrics. This parameter is designed to assist pediatricians by providing an analytic framework for the evaluation and treatment of this condition. It is not intended to replace clinical judgment or establish a protocol for all patients with this condition. It rarely will be the only appropriate approach to the problem.

Definition of the Problem

This practice parameter provides recommendations for the neurodiagnostic evaluation of neurologically healthy infants and children between 6 months and 5 years of age who have had their first simple febrile seizures and present within 12 hours of the event. This practice parameter is not intended for patients who have had complex febrile seizures (prolonged, focal, and/or recurrent), nor does it pertain to those children with previous neurologic insults, known central nervous system abnormalities, or histories of afebrile seizures.

Target Audience and Practice Setting

This practice parameter is intended for use by pediatricians, family physicians, child neurologists, neurologists, emergency physicians, and other providers who treat children for febrile seizures.

Interventions of Direct Interest

1. Lumbar puncture;

2. Electroencephalography (EEG);

3. Blood studies—serum electrolytes, calcium, phosphorus, magnesium, and blood glucose, and a complete blood count (CBC); and

4. Neuroimaging—skull radiographs, computed tomography (CT), and magnetic resonance imaging.

Background

A febrile seizure is broadly defined as a seizure accompanied by fever without central nervous system infection, occurring in infants and children between 6 months and 5 years of age. Febrile seizures occur in 2% to 5% of all children and, as such, make up the most common convulsive event in children younger than 5 years of age. In 1976, Nelson and Ellenberg,[1] using data from the National Collaborative Perinatal Project, further defined febrile seizures as being either simple or complex. Simple febrile seizures were defined as primary generalized seizures lasting less than 15 minutes and not recurring within 24 hours. Complex febrile seizures were defined as focal, prolonged (>15 minutes), and/or occurring in a flurry. Those children who had simple febrile seizures had no evidence of increased mortality, hemiplegia, or mental retardation. During follow-up evaluation, the risk of epilepsy after a simple febrile seizure was shown to be only slightly higher than that of the general population, whereas the chief risk associated with simple febrile seizures was recurrence in one third of the children. The report concluded that simple febrile seizures are benign events with excellent prognoses, a conclusion reaffirmed in the 1980 National Institutes of Health Consensus Statement.[2]

Despite progress in understanding febrile seizures and the development of consensus statements about their diagnostic evaluation and management, a review of practice patterns of pediatricians indicates that a wide variation persists in physician interpretation, evaluation, and treatment of children with febrile seizures.[3]

This parameter is not intended for the evaluation of patients who have had complex febrile seizures, previous neurologic insults, or known brain abnormalities. The parameter also does not address treatment.

The expected outcomes of this practice parameter include the following.

1. Optimizing practitioner understanding of the scientific basis for the neurodiagnostic evaluation of children with simple febrile seizures;

2. Using a structured framework to aid the practitioner in decision making;

3. Optimizing evaluation of the child who has had a simple febrile seizure by ensuring that underlying diseases such as meningitis are detected, minimizing morbidity, and enabling the practitioner to reassure the anxious parents and child; and

4. Reducing costs of physician and emergency department visits, hospitalizations, and unnecessary testing.

Methodology

Two hundred three medical journal articles addressing the diagnosis and evaluation of febrile seizures were identified. Each article was subjected to formal, semistructured review by committee members. These completed reviews, as well as the original articles, were then reexamined by epidemiologic consultants to identify those population-based studies limited to children with simple febrile seizures that examined the usefulness of specific diagnostic studies. Given the scarcity of such studies, data from hospital-based studies and comparable groups were also reviewed. Tables were constructed using data from 28 articles. A second literature search failed to disclose pertinent articles containing data on brain imaging in children with febrile seizures.

A summary of the technical report describing the analyses used to prepare this parameter begins on page 167.

Recommendations

Lumbar Puncture

Recommendation. **The American Academy of Pediatrics (AAP) recommends, on the basis of the published evidence and consensus, that after the first seizures with fever in infants younger than 12 months, performance of a lumbar puncture be strongly considered, because the clinical signs and symptoms associated with meningitis may be minimal or absent in this age** group. **In a child between 12 and 18 months of age, a lumbar puncture should be considered, because clinical signs and symptoms of meningitis may be subtle. In a child older than 18 months, although a lumbar puncture is not routinely warranted, it is recommended in the presence of meningeal signs and symptoms (ie, neck stiffness and Kernig and Brudzinski signs), which are usually present with meningitis, or for any child whose history or examination result suggests the presence of intracranial infection. In infants and children who have had febrile seizures and have received prior antibiotic treatment, clinicians should be aware that treatment can mask the signs and symptoms of meningitis. As such, a lumbar puncture should be strongly considered.**

The clinical evaluation of young febrile children requires skills that vary among examiners. Moreover, published data do not address the quantification of such skills adequately. Because this practice parameter is for practitioners with a wide range of training and experience, the committee chose a conservative approach with an emphasis on the value of lumbar puncture in diagnosing meningitis.

The committee recognizes the diversity of opinion regarding the need for routine lumbar puncture in children younger than 18 to 24 months with first febrile seizures. In approximately 13% to 16% of children with meningitis, seizures are the presenting sign of disease, and in approximately 30% to 35% of these children (primarily children younger than 18 months), meningeal signs and symptoms may be lacking.[4,5] On the basis of published evidence, cerebrospinal fluid is more likely to be abnormal in children initially seen with fevers and seizures who have had: (1) suspicious findings on physical and/or neurologic examinations (particularly meningeal signs); (2) complex febrile seizures; (3) physician visits within 48 hours before the seizures; (4) seizures on arrival to emergency departments; (5) prolonged postictal states (typically most children with simple febrile seizures recover quickly); and (6) initial seizures after 3 years of age.[6,7] An increased risk of failure to diagnose meningitis occurs in children: (1) younger than 18 months who may show no signs and symptoms of meningitis; (2) who are evaluated by a less-experienced health care provider; or (3) who may be unavailable for follow-up.[5-8] A recognized source of fever, eg, otitis media, does not exclude the presence of meningitis. All recommendations, including those for lumbar puncture, are also given in the Algorithm.

EEG

Recommendation. **The AAP recommends, based on the published evidence and consensus, that EEG not be performed in the evaluation of a neurologically healthy child with a first simple febrile seizure.**

No published study demonstrates that EEG performed either at the time of presentation after a simple febrile seizure or within the following month will predict the occurrence of future afebrile seizures. Although the incidence of abnormal EEGs increases over time after a simple febrile seizure, no evidence exists that abnormal EEGs after the first febrile seizure are predictive for either the risk of recurrence of febrile seizures or the development of epilepsy. Even studies that have included children with complex febrile seizures and/or those with preexisting neurologic disease (a group at higher risk of having epilepsy develop) have not shown EEG to be predictive of the development of epilepsy.[9–10]

Blood Studies

Recommendation. **On the basis of published evidence,[7,8,11] the AAP recommends that the following determinations not be performed routinely in the evaluation of a child with a first simple febrile seizure: serum electrolytes, calcium, phosphorus, magnesium, CBC, or blood glucose.**

There is no evidence to suggest that routine blood studies are of benefit in the evaluation of the child with a first febrile seizure. Although some children initially seen with febrile seizures are dehydrated and have abnormal serum electrolyte values, their conditions should be identifiable by obtaining appropriate histories and performing careful physical examinations. A blood glucose determination, although not routinely needed, should be obtained if the child has a prolonged period of postictal obtundation. CBCs may be useful in the evaluation of fever, particularly in young children, because the incidence of bacteremia in children younger than 2 years of age with or without febrile seizures is the same.[12]

When fever is present, the decision regarding the need for laboratory testing should be directed toward identifying the source of the fever rather than as part of the routine evaluation of the seizure itself.

Neuroimaging

Recommendation. **On the basis of the available evidence and consensus, the AAP recommends that neuroimaging not be performed in the routine evaluation of the child with a first simple febrile seizure.**

The literature does not support the use of skull films in the evaluation of the child with a first febrile seizure.[7,13] Although no data have been published that either support or negate the need for CT or magnetic resonance imaging in the evaluation of children with simple febrile seizures, extrapolation of data from the literature on the use of CT in children who have generalized epilepsy has shown that clinically important intracranial structural abnormalities in this patient population are uncommon.[14,15]

Conclusion

Physicians evaluating infants or young children after first simple febrile seizures should direct their evaluations toward the diagnosis of the causes of the children's fevers. A lumbar puncture should be strongly considered in a child younger than 12 months and should be considered in children between 12 and 18 months of age. In children older than 18 months, the decision to do a lumbar puncture rests on the clinical suspicion of meningitis. The seizure usually does not require further evaluation — specifically EEG, blood studies, or neuroimaging.

The practice parameter, "The Neurodiagnostic Evaluation of the Child With a First Simple Febrile Seizure," was reviewed by the appropriate committees and sections of the AAP, including the Chapter Review Group, a focus group of office-based pediatricians representing each AAP district: Gene R. Adams, MD; Robert M. Corwin, MD; Lawrence C. Pakula, MD; Barbara M. Harley, MD; Howard B. Weinblatt, MD; Thomas J. Herr, MD; Kenneth E. Mathews, MD; Diane Fuquay, MD; Robert D. Mines, MD; and Delosa A Young, MD. Comments were also solicited from relevant outside organizations. The clinical algorithm was developed by Michael Kohrman, MD, Buffalo Children's Hospital, and James R. Cooley, MD, Harvard Community Health Plan.

The supporting data analyses are contained in the summary of the technical report, which begins on page 167.

References

1. Nelson KB, Ellenberg JH. Predictors of epilepsy in children who have experienced febrile seizures. *N Engl J Med.* 1976;295:1029–1033

2. Consensus statement. Febrile seizures: long-term management of children with fever-associated seizures. *Pediatrics.* 1980;66:1009–1012

3. Hirtz DG, Lee YJ, Ellenberg JH, Nelson KB. Survey on the management of febrile seizures. *Am J Dis Child.* 1986;140:909–914

4. Ratcliffe JC, Wolf SM. Febrile convulsions caused by meningitis in young children. *Ann Neurol.* 1977;1:285–286

5. Rutter N, Smales OR. Role of routine investigations in children presenting with their first febrile convulsion. *Arch Dis Child.* 1977;52:188–191

6. Joffe A, McCormick M, DeAngelis C. Which children with febrile seizures need lumbar puncture? A decision analysis approach. *Am J Dis Child.* 1983;137:1153–1156

7. Jaffe M, Bar-Joseph G, Tirosh E. Fever and convulsions—indications for laboratory investigations. *Pediatrics.* 1981;57:729–731

8. Gerber MA, Berliner BC. The child with a "simple" febrile seizure: appropriate diagnostic evaluation. *Am J Dis Child.* 1981;135:431–433

9. Frantzen E, Lennox-Butchthal M, Nygaard A. Longitudinal EEG and clinical study of children with febrile convulsions. *Electroencephalogr Clin Neurophysiol.* 1968;24:197–212

10. Thorn I. The significance of electroencephalography in febrile convulsions. In: Akimoto H, Kazamatsuri H, Seino M, Ward A, eds. *Advances in Epileptology: XIIIth Epilepsy International Symposium.* New York, NY: Raven Press; 1982:93–95

11. Heijbel J, Blom S, Bergfors PG. Simple febrile convulsions: a prospective incidence study and an evaluation of investigations initially needed. *Neuropaediatrie.* 1980;11:45–56

12. Chamberlain JM, Gorman RL. Occult bacteremia in children with simple febrile seizures. *Am J Dis Child.* 1988;142:1073–1076

13. Nealis GT, McFadden SW, Asnes RA, Ouellette EM. Routine skull roentgenograms in the management of simple febrile seizures. *J Pediatr.* 1977;90:595–596

14. Yang PJ, Berger PE, Cohen ME, Duffner PK. Computed tomography and childhood seizure disorders. *Neurology.* 1979;29:1084–1088

15. Bachman DS, Hodges FJ, Freeman JM. Computerized axial tomography in chronic seizure disorders of childhood. *Pediatrics.* 1976;58:828–832

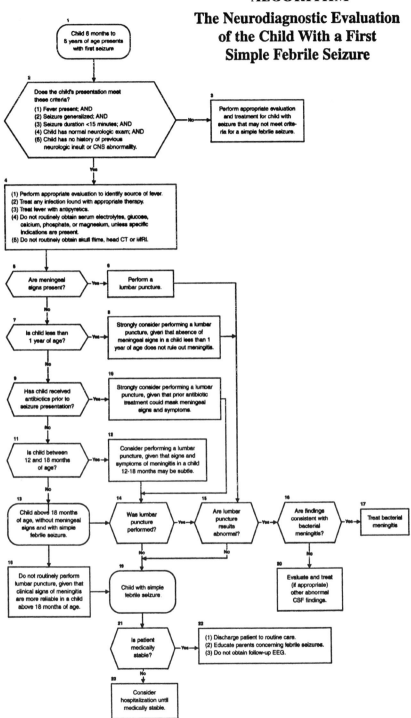

ALGORITHM

The Neurodiagnostic Evaluation of the Child With a First Simple Febrile Seizure

1 Child 6 months to 5 years of age presents with first seizure

2 Does the child's presentation meet these criteria?
(1) Fever present; AND
(2) Seizure generalized; AND
(3) Seizure duration <15 minutes; AND
(4) Child has normal neurologic exam; AND
(5) Child has no history of previous neurologic insult or CNS abnormality.

3 Perform appropriate evaluation and treatment for child with seizure that may not meet criteria for a simple febrile seizure. — No

4
(1) Perform appropriate evaluation to identify source of fever.
(2) Treat any infection found with appropriate therapy.
(3) Treat fever with antipyretics.
(4) Do not routinely obtain serum electrolytes, glucose, calcium, phosphate, or magnesium, unless specific indications are present.
(5) Do not routinely obtain skull films, head CT or MRI.

5 Are meningeal signs present? — Yes → **6** Perform a lumbar puncture.

7 Is child less than 1 year of age? — Yes → **8** Strongly consider performing a lumbar puncture, given that absence of meningeal signs in a child less than 1 year of age does not rule out meningitis.

9 Has child received antibiotics prior to seizure presentation? — Yes → **10** Strongly consider performing a lumbar puncture, given that prior antibiotic treatment could mask meningeal signs and symptoms.

11 Is child between 12 and 18 months of age? — Yes → **12** Consider performing a lumbar puncture, given that signs and symptoms of meningitis in a child 12-18 months may be subtle.

13 Child above 18 months of age, without meningeal signs and with simple febrile seizure.

14 Was lumbar puncture performed? — Yes → **15** Are lumbar puncture results abnormal? — Yes → **16** Are findings consistent with bacterial meningitis? — Yes → **17** Treat bacterial meningitis

18 Do not routinely perform lumbar puncture, given that clinical signs of meningitis are more reliable in a child above 18 months of age.

19 Child with simple febrile seizure.

20 Evaluate and treat (if appropriate) other abnormal CSF findings.

21 Is patient medically stable? — Yes → **22**
(1) Discharge patient to routine care.
(2) Educate parents concerning febrile seizures.
(3) Do not obtain follow-up EEG.

23 Consider hospitalization until medically stable.

Technical Report Summary:
The Neurodiagnostic Evaluation of the Child
With a First Simple Febrile Seizure

Authors:

Robert J. Baumann, MD
Sandra L. D'Angelo, PhD

University of Kentucky
Lexington, Kentucky

consultants to the Subcommittee on Simple Febrile Seizures

American Academy of Pediatrics
PO Box 927, 141 Northwest Point Blvd
Elk Grove Village, IL 60009-0927

Subcommittee on Diagnosis and Treatment of Febrile Seizures 1992 – 1995

Thomas A. Riemenschneider, MD, Chairman

Robert J. Baumann, MD   John L. Green, MD
Patricia K. Duffner, MD   Sanford Schneider, MD

In Consultation With:

David L. Coulter, MD
Patricia K. Crumrine, MD
Sandra D'Angelo, PhD (methodology consultant)
W. Edwin Dodson, MD
John M. Freeman, MD
Michael Kohrman, MD
James O. McNamara, MD
Karin B. Nelson, MD
N. Paul Rosman, MD
Shlomo Shinnar, MD

Provisional Committee on Quality Improvement 1993 – 1995

David A. Bergman, MD, Chairman

Richard D. Baltz, MD   Lawrence F. Nazarian, MD
James R. Cooley, MD   Thomas A. Riemenschneider, MD
John B. Coombs, MD   Kenneth B. Roberts, MD
Michael J. Goldberg, MD   Daniel W. Shea, MD
  Sections Liaison   Thomas F. Tonniges, MD
Charles J. Homer, MD, MPH   AAP Board of Directors Liaison
  Section on Epidemiology Liaison

Introduction

The scope of the practice parameter that is supported by this technical report was limited to the initial neurodiagnostic evaluation (within 12 hours of the event) of neurologically normal children with simple febrile seizures. Febrile seizures are a common problem in clinical practice, occurring in 2.7% of children in the British Birth Cohort study. Febrile seizures are also the most common epileptic events in children younger than 5 years. The subcommittee's efforts were focused on the large subgroup of children (88%)[1] who have simple febrile seizures because in the view of most clinicians and on the basis of the epidemiologic evidence, this is a relatively homogeneous clinical grouping in terms of age, clinical presentation, course, and outcome. It is appropriate, therefore, to help clinicians develop a common neurodiagnostic approach for their evaluation.

Definition of the Problem

Children younger than 5 years who experience their first seizure in association with a fever are commonly divided into three groups. Children with simple febrile seizures make up the largest group. The second group includes children whose seizures are secondary to a central nervous system (CNS) infection (symptomatic febrile seizures). In the third group, children whose seizures are neither simple nor secondary to CNS infection are classified as having complex febrile seizures.

The practice parameter supported by this technical report contains recommendations for the initial neurodiagnostic evaluation of a child who has experienced a simple febrile seizure. The parameter requires all of the following factors for inclusion: Children who were between 6 months and 5 years at the time of the seizure. Seizures were single, isolated, and generalized; associated with a fever in the absence of a CNS infection; and lasted less than 15 minutes. The study excluded any children experiencing focal or complex seizures or flurries of seizures, or children who had experienced a previous neurologic insult or who were not neurologically normal on examination.

This definition of a simple febrile seizure corresponds to that in usual clinical practice and is also supported by the analysis of data from the Collaborative Perinatal Project of the National Institute of Neurological and Communicative Disorders and Stroke. In that project, Nelson and Ellenberg analyzed the data of 1706 children aged 7 years who had had one or more febrile seizures. The risk of epilepsy (afebrile seizures) was significantly higher for children whose neurological development was not normal before the seizure, whose seizure occurred before 6 months of age, whose seizure lasted longer than 15 minutes, or who had more than one febrile seizure per day. Most recently Verity and Golding examined the records for 398 children who had had at least one febrile seizure. Follow-up continued until age 10 years. They found a higher rate of epilepsy after a complex febrile convulsion (lasting longer than 15 minutes, focal or multiple seizures) than after a simple febrile convulsion. The available data indicated that these children experienced adverse neurologic outcomes (such as early mortality or mental retardation) at rates similar to those of their peers. Nevertheless, their rate for single or repeated afebrile seizures (epilepsy is defined as having two or more afebrile seizures) exceeded that of the general age-matched population. The study concluded that children with simple febrile seizures demonstrated a higher rate for afebrile seizures than that seen in the base population but had a lower rate than subjects who experienced complex febrile seizures.

The Commission on Epidemiology and Prognosis of the International League Against Epilepsy, which published a "Guidelines for Epidemiologic Studies on Epilepsy," suggested that the definition of febrile seizure include "childhood after age 1 month." No maximum age or definition of the duration of childhood was given. This Panel agreed that epidemiologic studies should examine the outcomes of febrile seizures among infants younger than 6 months as well as children older than 5 years. Nevertheless, existing studies as well as common clinical practice suggest that the practice parameter be limited to patients older than 6 months and younger than 5 years of age.

Selection of Interventions

The subcommittee further limited the parameter to the study of commonly used neurodiagnostic tests. These tests were evaluated on their potential to help the clinician decide whether children: had experienced a simple febrile seizure (as opposed to a complex or symptomatic febrile seizure) or were likely to have subsequent afebrile seizures or other adverse outcomes.

The following tests were included:
1. Lumbar puncture (to diagnose CNS infection).
2. Electroencephalography (EEG [to predict the likelihood of future afebrile seizures]).
3. Blood chemistries (to discover potential metabolic etiologies for the seizure).
4. Imaging studies of the head and brain, including skull x-ray films, computed tomography (CT), and magnetic resonance imaging (MRI) (to identify brain lesions).

Methods

In an attempt to discover all pertinent articles, a Medline search was performed by staff of the American Academy of Pediatrics. An additional search from the Epilepsy Foundation of America using their database was also performed. Other articles that were obtained from bibliographies were suggested by subcommittee members; 203 articles were identified. Each article was reviewed by a subcommittee member using a semistructured review form. The completed forms and the articles were reviewed again by the epidemiologic consultants with the assistance of a graduate student.

The goal of this search was to identify population-based studies limited to patients with well-defined simple febrile seizures and in which neurodiagnostic tests were employed. The subcommittee attempted to use the method of Eddy and Woolf to develop these guidelines. Such a rigorous analysis requires well-designed population-based or case-comparison studies. The studies must adhere to a consistent definition of the study group, in this instance children with simple febrile seizures (as previously defined). The diagnostic test of interest must be applied in a standard way to all eligible subjects. The subjects must then be followed up for a sufficient period of time to discover important outcomes.

None of the previously cited population-based studies were designed to investigate the utility of neurodiagnostic testing. In all three studies, tests were selectively requested based on the physician's clinical judgment. Further retrospective analysis is unlikely to be fruitful.

Given the scarcity of population-based studies, data from hospital and clinic series were also analyzed. These studies had the following methodological problems.

Subject Selection. Most studies recruited subjects from clinics, emergency departments, or hospital admissions. The selection factors that influenced the constitution of these patient groups were difficult, if not impossible, to characterize. Moreover children from these patient groups usually have substantially higher rates of adverse outcomes than do children in population-based studies.

Disease Definition. Many studies either failed to define their criteria for febrile seizures, used a definition different from that used in the practice parameter, or did not rigorously follow any specific definition. Often there was no attempt to exclude (or at least identify) children with preexisting neurological disease.

Uniformity of Neurodiagnostic Testing. Many studies failed to apply the test(s) to all eligible subjects, raising serious questions about subject selection. An excess of positive tests and adverse outcomes could be expected based on physicians who exempt "healthier" children from testing.

Duration of Follow-up. Few studies had an extended follow-up period. The number of subjects experiencing afebrile seizures increases with age. Although the optimal duration of follow-up is uncertain, in the Rochester, Minnesota study most subjects were found to have experienced a seizure by age 9 years.

The consultants presented the abstracted data from 28 articles in tabular form, subsequently eliminating nine of them. These do not contain studies suitable for meta-analysis.

The subcommittee was concerned with the use of MRI and CT in evaluating children with febrile seizures. Because the initial literature search did not discover any suitable articles using these technologies, another literature search was conducted using MRI and CT MeSH terms, but again no pertinent articles were located.

Many articles not included in the study were reviews, commentaries, or editorials that lacked original data. Some of these articles reported disorders other than simple febrile seizures or intermingled children with simple seizures with children who were not neurologically normal or who had had complex febrile seizures. An additional 13 studies were eliminated because they did not define "febrile seizure" or used a definition different from that of the subcommittee.

Subcommittee Recommendations and Levels of Evidence

Recommendations were made based on the quality of scientific evidence. In the absence of high-quality scientific evidence, subcommittee consensus or a combination of evidence and consensus was used as the basis for recommendations.

Clinical options are actions for which the Panel failed to find compelling evidence for or against. A health care provider may or may not wish to implement clinical options, depending on the child.

No recommendation was made when scientific evidence was lacking and there was no compelling reason to make an expert judgment.

Panel Recommendations

Lumbar Puncture

The goal of lumbar puncture is to identify children with CNS infection. A positive spinal fluid examination can have obvious treatment implications. In addition if the seizure is associated with an intracranial infection, the child is considered to have a symptomatic febrile seizure. Lumbar puncture with spinal fluid examination is not an effective neurodiagnostic technique for evaluating the febrile seizure per se.

An important concern is the number of children presenting with fever and seizures who have meningitis (for example, 4/119, or 3.4% [Heijbel et al], 28/562, or 5% [Jaffe et al], 13/241, or 5.4% [Joffe et al], 21/878, or 2.4% [Rossi et al], 6/328, or 1.8% [Rutter and Smales]). In the study by Jaffe et al, children with simple febrile seizures were less likely (2/323) to have meningitis than those with complex febrile seizures (26/239). None of the subjects with simple febrile seizures and 6 subjects with complex febrile seizures had bacterial meningitis. The previously described rates of meningitis (except those for the study by Heijbel et al) include children admitted to emergency departments or the hospital and thus are unlikely to typify the populations from which they come and are likely to vary with the factors that influence emergency department and hospital utilization.

Reviewing the emergency room records for 241 children who had a first seizure with fever and underwent lumbar puncture, Joffe et al found that the following five items were important in determining those with and without meningitis:

1) visiting a physician within 48 hours of the seizure, 2) seizure activity at the time of arrival in the emergency room, 3) a focal seizure, 4) suspicious findings on physical examination (rash or petechiae, cyanosis, hypotension, or grunting respirations), and 5) abnormal neurological examination results (stiff neck, increased tone, deviated eyes, ataxia, no response to voice, inability to fix and follow, no response to painful stimuli, positive doll's eye sign, floppy muscle tone, nystagmus, or bulging or tense fontanel).

Clearly the clinical evaluation of young febrile children requires skills that vary between examiners. Moreover, published data do not adequately address the quantification of such skills. Therefore the subcommittee relied on expert opinion and Panel consensus. Since this practice parameter is for practitioners with a wide range of training and experience, the committee chose a conservative approach with an emphasis on the value of lumbar puncture in diagnosing meningitis. This was not intended to ignore the occurrence of false-negative results (for example, Rutter and Smales found 2/310 false-negative spinal fluid examinations).

In the absence of other data, the Panel reviewed studies in which children with fever and seizures presented to medical institutions. The study of Heijbel et al was population-based, but lumbar puncture was performed selectively in 47 of 107 subjects.

EEG

The primary purpose of EEG in the evaluation of the children with simple febrile seizures is to predict the risk of future afebrile seizures. The subcommittee searched for but could not find a definitive study. In such a population-based study, EEGs would be obtained on children shortly after they experience their first simple seizure, with the EEG pattern being correlated with subsequent seizure occurrence. The study from Macedonia by Sofijanov et al seems to approximate this pattern. Initial EEG data were published; follow-up data, however, are not yet available. In this study 18% of 376 subjects with first febrile seizures had paroxysmal abnormalities on EEG, which were more likely when the seizure was either focal or lasted longer than 15 minutes (not a simple febrile seizure).

Given the high rate of simple febrile seizures and the low rate of subsequent afebrile seizures, obtaining routine EEGs would require a large number of tests to identify a small number of children destined to have these seizures. For example, in the British Birth Cohort study, only 2.6% of children who had experienced their first simple febrile seizure subsequently had a single afebrile seizure before their 10th birthday. Only 1.6% of the children had two or more afebrile seizures (ie, epilepsy). A number of well-known studies included patients with both simple and focal febrile seizures and did not exclude subjects with preexisting neurological disability. The results for subjects with simple febrile seizures from the published data could not be isolated. Heijbel et al limited their study to simple febrile seizures. Their two subjects who subsequently developed epilepsy had normal initial EEGs. Interpretation of their data is complicated by the small number of subjects (n=107) and the elimination of 5 potential subjects because they had epileptiform EEG activity interictally. These 5 subjects were not characterized further so it is unknown whether they fit the clinical criteria for having experienced simple febrile seizures. No follow-up data were given for these 5 children and follow-up was limited to 3 years for the other subjects. Koyama et al evaluated 133 subjects from a population of 490 children with a history of febrile seizures. It is unclear if the 133 subjects are typical of the 490. Moreover, the EEGs were obtained months after the initial seizure; 32% of the subjects had abnormal EEGs—in 9% of the subjects the abnormalities were paroxysmal compared with 7% of the control group (who had had EEGs for "other medical reasons"). Follow-up data were not available.

The study of Heijbel is population-based. Some of its limitations are discussed above. Without other population-based data, the Panel reviewed studies in which relatively large numbers of children with fever and seizures presented to medical institutions. In some studies only a subset of subjects had EEGs, introducing the additional issue of selection bias.

Blood Chemistries

In a population-based study that included 107 children with simple febrile seizures, Heijbel et al retrospectively reviewed the routine blood chemistries requested by the treating physicians. They found no clinically important abnormalities in serum calcium (n=92), phosphorus (n=85), or glucose (n=56) levels. One child with a low glucose level was reportedly asymptomatic on follow-up.

Other studies were hospital-based. For 100 consecutive admissions Gerber and Berliner reported normal values of serum glucose (n=82), calcium (n=58), electrolytes, and urea nitrogen.[7] The five children with elevated glucose levels were asymptomatic. Thirteen children had minimally reduced calcium levels (8.3 to 8.9 mg/dL) and were asymptomatic. Jaffe et al reviewed 323 records of children with simple febrile seizures. Three children had abnormalities (one each hyponatremia, hypocalcemia, and hypokalemia) and the authors thought that the abnormalities could have been anticipated on clinical grounds independent of the occurrence of the simple febrile seizure. One child was a compulsive water drinker, one had "florid" rickets, and one had dehydration due to gastroenteritis. Rutter and Smales[9] reviewed 328 children admitted to the hospital after their first febrile convulsion and found that determinations for serum sugar, calcium, urea, electrolytes, and blood counts were "commonly performed but were unhelpful." Among 269 subjects who had blood glucose measurements they found hyperglycemia to be common (14%) but clinically unimportant. The child who was hypoglycemic on admission (glucose level, 30 mg/dL) subsequently had a normal fasting blood glucose level; of the 232 children who had serum calcium determinations, three of the four children with levels below 8.0 mg/dL were normal on further evaluation and the fourth child was lost to follow-up.

Four authors determined that in their subjects with simple febrile seizures, the routine blood chemistries performed did not alter patient management in an important way. The child's clinical condition and underlying illness determined the need for routine blood chemistries. Otherwise, the management of a child after a simple febrile seizure was not improved.

Neuroimaging

To our knowledge, no study has been done in which children with simple febrile seizures have undergone imaging. We also searched (without success) for a related imaging study involving otherwise normal children after a first seizure. Three studies reviewing skull x-ray films in children with febrile seizures concluded that skull x-ray films were not of value.

Long-term Treatment of the Child With Simple Febrile Seizures

- *Clinical Practice Guideline*
- *Technical Report Summary*

Readers of this clinical practice guideline are urged to review the technical report to enhance the evidence-based decision-making process. The report is available on the *Pediatrics electronic pages* Web site at the following URL: http://www.pediatrics.org/cgi/content/full/103/6/e86.

Clinical Practice Guideline:
Long-term Treatment of the Child With
Simple Febrile Seizures

Author:

Subcommittee on Febrile Seizures
Committee on Quality Improvement

American Academy of Pediatrics
PO Box 927, 141 Northwest Point Blvd
Elk Grove Village, IL 60009-0927

Subcommittee on Febrile Seizures
1998–1999

Patricia K. Duffner, MD, Chairperson

Robert J. Baumann, MD,
  Methodologist
Peter Berman, MD

John L. Green, MD
Sanford Schneider, MD

Consultants:

Carole S. Camfield, MD,
  FRCP(C)
Peter R. Camfield, MD,
  FRCP(C)
David L. Coulter, MD
Patricia K. Crumrine, MD
W. Edwin Dodson, MD

John M. Freeman, MD
Arnold P. Gold, MD
Gregory L. Holmes, MD
Michael Kohrman, MD
Karin B. Nelson, MD
N. Paul Rosman, MD
Shlomo Shinnar, MD

Committee on Quality Improvement
1998–1999

David A. Bergman, MD, Chairperson

Richard D. Baltz, MD
James R. Cooley, MD
Gerald B. Hickson, MD

Paul V. Miles, MD
Joan E. Shook, MD
William M. Zurhellen, MD

Liaisons:

Betty A. Lowe, MD
  National Association for
  Children's Hospitals and
  Related Institutions
Shirley Girouard, PhD, RN
  National Association for
  Children's Hospitals and
  Related Institutions
Michael J. Goldberg, MD
  AAP Sections

Charles J. Homer, MD
  AAP Section on
  Epidemiology
Jan E. Berger, MD
  AAP Committee on
  Medical Liability
Jack T. Swanson, MD
  AAP Committee on Practice
  and Ambulatory Medicine

Acknowledgments

The Committee on Quality Improvement and Subcommittee on Febrile Seizures appreciate the expertise of Richard N. Shiffman, MD, Center for Medical Informatics, Yale School of Medicine, for his input and analysis in development of this practice guideline. Comments were also solicited and received from organizations such as the American Academy of Family Physicians, the American Academy of Neurology, the Child Neurology Society, and the American College of Emergency Physicians.

Abstract

The Committee on Quality Improvement, Subcommittee on Febrile Seizures, of the American Academy of Pediatrics, in collaboration with experts from the Section on Neurology, general pediatricians, consultants in the fields of child neurology and epilepsy, and research methodologists, developed this practice parameter. This guideline provides recommendations for the treatment of a child with simple febrile seizures. These recommendations are derived from a thorough search and analysis of the literature. The methods and results of the literature review can be found in the accompanying technical report. This guideline is designed to assist pediatricians by providing an analytic framework for the treatment of children with simple febrile seizures. It is not intended to replace clinical judgment or establish a protocol for all patients with this condition. It rarely will be the only appropriate approach to the problem.

The technical report entitled "Treatment of the Child With Simple Febrile Seizures" provides in-depth information on the studies used to form guideline recommendations. A complete bibliography is included as well as evidence tables that summarize data extracted from scientific studies. This report also provides pertinent evidence on the individual therapeutic agents studied including study results and dosing information. Readers of this clinical practice guideline are urged to review the technical report to enhance the evidence-based decision-making process. The report is available on the *Pediatrics electronic pages* website at the following URL: http://www.pediatrics.org/cgi/content/full/103/6/e86.

Definition of the Problem

This practice parameter provides recommendations for therapeutic intervention in neurologically healthy infants and children between 6 months and 5 years of age who have had one or more simple febrile seizures. A simple febrile seizure is defined as a brief (<15 minutes) generalized seizure that occurs only once during a 24-hour period in a febrile child who does not have an intracranial infection or severe metabolic disturbance. This practice parameter is not intended for patients who have had complex febrile seizures (prolonged, ie, >15 minutes, focal, or recurrent in 24 hours), nor does it pertain to children with previous neurologic insults, known central nervous system abnormalities, or a history of afebrile seizures.

Target Audience and Practice Setting

This practice parameter is intended for use by pediatricians, family physicians, child neurologists, neurologists, emergency physicians, and other health care professionals who treat children with febrile seizures.

Possible Therapeutic Interventions

Possible therapeutic approaches to a child with simple febrile seizures include continuous anticonvulsant therapy with agents such as phenobarbital, valproic acid, carbamazepine, or phenytoin; intermittent therapy with antipyretic agents or diazepam; or no anticonvulsant therapy.

Background

For a child who has experienced a simple febrile seizure, there are potentially 2 major adverse outcomes that may theoretically be altered by an effective therapeutic agent. These are the occurrence of subsequent febrile seizures or afebrile seizures, including epilepsy. The risk of having recurrent simple febrile seizures varies, depending on age. Children younger than 12 months at the time of their first simple febrile seizure have approximately a 50% probability of having recurrent febrile seizures. Children older than 12 months at the time of their first event have approximately a 30% probability of a second febrile seizure; of those that do have a second febrile seizure, 50% have a chance of having at least 1 additional recurrence.[1]

Children with simple febrile seizures have only a slightly greater risk for developing epilepsy by the age of 7 years than the 1% risk of the general population.[2,3] Children who have had multiple simple febrile seizures and are younger than 12 months at the time of the first febrile seizure are at the highest risk, but, even in this group, generalized afebrile seizures develop by age 25 in only 2.4%.[4] No study has demonstrated that treatment for simple febrile seizures can prevent the later development of epilepsy. Furthermore, there is no evidence that simple febrile seizures cause structural damage and no evidence that children with simple febrile seizures are at risk for cognitive decline.[5]

Despite the frequency of febrile seizures (approximately 3%), there is no unanimity of opinion about therapeutic interventions.[3] The following recommendations are based on an analysis of the risks and benefits of continuous or intermittent therapy in children with simple febrile seizures. The recommendations reflect an awareness of the very low risk that a simple febrile seizure poses to the individual child and the large number of children who have this type of seizure at some time in early life.[1,3-5] To be commensurate, a proposed therapy would need to be exceedingly low in risks and adverse effects, inexpensive, and highly effective.

The expected outcomes of this practice parameter include the following:

1. Optimize practitioner understanding of the scientific basis for using or avoiding various proposed treatments for children with simple febrile seizures.

2. Improve the health of children with simple febrile seizures by avoiding therapies with high potential for side effects and no demonstrated ability to improve children's eventual outcomes.

3. Reduce costs by avoiding therapies that will not demonstrably improve children's long-term outcomes.

4. Help the practitioner educate caregivers about the low risks associated with simple febrile seizures.

Methodology

More than 300 medical journal articles reporting studies of the natural history of simple febrile seizures or the therapy of these seizures were reviewed and abstracted. Emphasis was placed on articles that differentiated simple febrile seizures from other types of febrile seizures, articles that carefully matched treatment and control groups, and articles that described adherence to the drug regimen. Tables were constructed from 62 articles that best fit these criteria. **A more comprehensive review of the literature on which this report is based can be found in the technical report. The technical report also contains dosing information.**

Benefits and Risks of Continuous Anticonvulsant Therapy

Phenobarbital

Phenobarbital is effective in preventing the recurrence of simple febrile seizures.[6-8] In a controlled, double-blind study, daily therapy with phenobarbital reduced the rate of subsequent febrile seizures from 25 per 100 subjects per year to 5 per 100 subjects per year.[6]

The adverse effects of phenobarbital include behavioral problems such as hyperactivity and hypersensitivity reactions.[6,9-11]

Valproic Acid

In randomized, controlled studies, only 4% of children taking valproate as opposed to 35% of control subjects had a subsequent febrile seizure. Therefore, valproic acid seems to be at least as effective in preventing recurrent, simple febrile seizures as phenobarbital and significantly more effective than placebo. [7,12,13] Drawbacks to therapy with valproic acid include its rare association with fatal hepatotoxicity (especially in children younger than 3 years who also are at greatest risk for febrile seizures), thrombocytopenia, weight loss and gain, gastrointestinal disturbances, and pancreatitis.[14]

Carbamazepine

Carbamazepine has not been shown to be effective in preventing the recurrence of simple febrile seizures.[9]

Phenytoin

Phenytoin has not been shown to be effective in preventing the recurrence of simple febrile seizures.[15]

Benefits and Risks of Intermittent Oral Therapy

Antipyretic Agents

Antipyretic agents, in the absence of anticonvulsants, are not effective in preventing recurrent febrile seizures.[6,16]

Diazepam

A double-blind, controlled study in patients with a history of febrile seizures demonstrated that administration of oral diazepam (given at the time of a fever) could reduce the recurrence of febrile seizures. Children with a history of febrile seizures were given oral diazepam or a placebo at the time of fever. There was a 44% reduction in the risk of febrile seizures per person-year with diazepam.[17] A potential drawback to intermittent medication is that a seizure could occur before a fever is noticed. Adverse effects of oral diazepam include lethargy, drowsiness, and ataxia.[17] The sedation associated with this therapy could mask evolving signs of a central nervous system infection.

Summary

The Subcommittee has determined that a simple febrile seizure is a benign and common event in children between the ages of 6 months and 5 years. Most children have an excellent prognosis. Although there are effective therapies that could prevent the occurrence of additional simple febrile seizures, the potential adverse effects of such therapy are not commensurate with the benefit. In situations in which parental anxiety associated with febrile seizures is severe, intermittent oral diazepam at the onset of febrile illness may be effective in preventing recurrence. There is no convincing evidence, however, that any therapy will alleviate the possibility of future epilepsy (a relatively unlikely event). Antipyretics, although they may improve the comfort of the child, will not prevent febrile seizures.

Recommendation

Based on the risks and benefits of the effective therapies, neither continuous nor intermittent anticonvulsant therapy is recommended for children with 1 or more simple febrile seizures. The American Academy of Pediatrics recognizes that recurrent episodes of febrile seizures can create anxiety in some parents and their children, and, as such, appropriate education and emotional support should be provided.

References

1. Nelson KB, Ellenberg JH. Prognosis in children with febrile seizures. *Pediatrics.* 1978; 61:720–727
2. Nelson KB, Ellenberg JH. Predictors of epilepsy in children who have experienced febrile seizures. *N Engl J Med.* 1976;295:1029–1033
3. Verity CM, Golding J. Risk of epilepsy after febrile convulsions: a national cohort study. *Br Med J.* 1991;303:1373–1376
4. Annegers JF, Hauser WA, Shirts SB, Kurland LT. Factors prognostic of unprovoked seizures after febrile convulsions. *N Engl J Med.* 1987;316:493–498
5. Ellenberg JH, Nelson KB. Febrile seizures and later intellectual performance. *Arch Neurol.* 1978;35:17–21
6. Camfield PR, Camfield CS, Shapiro SH, Cummings C. The first febrile seizure: antipyretic instruction plus either phenobarbital or placebo to prevent recurrence. *J Pediatr.* 1980; 97:16–21
7. Wallace SJ, Smith JA. Successful prophylaxis against febrile convulsions with valproic acid or phenobarbitone. *Br Med J.* 1980;280:353–380

8. Wolf SM. The effectiveness of phenobarbital in the prevention of recurrent febrile convulsions in children with and without a history of pre-, peri-, and postnatal abnormalities. *Acta Paediatr Scand.* 1977;66:585–587

9. Antony JH, Hawke S. Phenobarbital compared with carbamazepine in prevention of recurrent febrile convulsions. *Am J Dis Child.* 1983;137:892–895

10. Knudsen FU, Vestermark S. Prophylactic diazepam or phenobarbitone in febrile convulsions: a prospective, controlled study. *Arch Dis Child.* 1978;53:660–663

11. Vining EPG, Mellits ED, Dorsen MM, et al. Psychologic and behavioral effects of antiepileptic drugs in children: a double-blind comparison between phenobarbital and valproic acid. *Pediatrics.* 1987;80:165–174

12. Marmelle NM, Plasse JC, Revol M, Gilly R. Prevention of recurrent febrile convulsions: a randomized therapeutic assay: sodium valproate, phenobarbital and placebo. *Neuropediatrics.* 1984;15:37–42

13. Ngwane E, Bower B. Continuous sodium valproate or phenobarbitone in the prevention of "simple" febrile convulsions. *Arch Dis Child.* 1980;55:171–174

14. Dreifuss FE. Valproic acid toxicity. In: Levy RH, Mattson RH, Meldrum BS, eds. *Antiepileptic Drugs.* New York, NY: Raven Press; 1995:641–648

15. Bacon CJ, Hierons AM, Mucklow JC, Webb J, Rawlins MD, Weightman D. Placebo-controlled study of phenobarbitone and phenytoin in the prophylaxis in febrile convulsions. *Lancet.* 1981;2:600–604

16. Uhari M, Rantala H, Vainionpaa L, Kurttila R. Effect of acetaminophen and of low intermittent doses of diazepam on prevention of recurrence of febrile seizures. *J Pediatr.* 1995;126:991–995

17. Rosman NP, Colton T, Labazzo J, et al. A controlled trial of diazepam administered during febrile illnesses to prevent recurrence of febrile seizures. *N Engl J Med.* 1993;329:79–84

Technical Report Summary: Treatment of the Child With Simple Febrile Seizures

Author:

Robert J. Baumann, MD

American Academy of Pediatrics
PO Box 927, 141 Northwest Point Blvd
Elk Grove Village, IL 60009-0927

Abstract

Overview

Simple febrile seizures that occur in children ages 6 months to 5 years are common events with few adverse outcomes. Those who advocate therapy for this disorder have been concerned that such seizures lead to additional febrile seizures, to epilepsy, and perhaps even to brain injury. Moreover, they note the potential for such seizures to cause parental anxiety. We examined the literature to determine whether there was demonstrable benefit to the treatment of simple febrile seizures and whether such benefits exceeded the potential side effects and risks of therapy. The therapeutic approaches considered included continuous anticonvulsant therapies, intermittent therapy, or no anticonvulsant therapy.

Methods

This analysis focused on the neurologically healthy child between 6 months and 5 years of age whose seizure is brief (<15 minutes), generalized, and occurs only once during a 24-hour period during a fever. Children whose seizures are attributable to a central nervous system infection and those who have had a previous afebrile seizure or central nervous system abnormality were excluded. A review of the current literature was conducted using articles obtained through searches in MEDLINE and additional databases. Articles were obtained following defined criteria and data abstracted using a standardized literature review form. Abstracted data were summarized into evidence tables.

Results

Epidemiologic studies demonstrate a high risk of recurrent febrile seizures but a low, though increased, risk of epilepsy. Other adverse outcomes either don't occur or occur so infrequently that their presence is not convincingly demonstrated by the available studies. Although daily anticonvulsant therapy with phenobarbital or valproic acid is effective in decreasing recurrent febrile seizures, the risks and potential side effects of these medications outweigh this benefit. No medication has been shown to prevent the future onset of recurrent afebrile seizures (epilepsy). The use of intermittent diazepam with fever after an initial febrile seizure is likely to decrease the risk of another febrile seizure, but the rate of side effects is high although most families find the perceived benefits to be low. Although antipyretic therapy has other benefits, it does not prevent additional simple febrile seizures.

Conclusions

The Febrile Seizures Subcommittee of the American Academy of Pediatrics' Committee on Quality Improvement used the results of this analysis to derive evidence-based recommendations for the treatment of simple febrile seizures. The outcomes anticipated as a result of the analysis and development of the practice guideline include: 1) to optimize practitioner understanding of the scientific basis for using or avoiding various proposed treatments for children with simple febrile seizures; 2) to improve the health of children with simple febrile seizures by avoiding therapies with high potential for side effects and no demonstrated ability to improve children's eventual outcomes; 3) to reduce costs by avoiding therapies that will not demonstrably improve children's long-term outcomes; and 4) to help the practitioner educate caregivers about the low risks associated with simple febrile seizures. *Key words: febrile seizures, epilepsy, valproic acid, carbamazepine, phenytoin, diazepam, phenobarbital, sodium valproate, pyridoxine.*

The debate over whether children with recurrent febrile seizures benefit from anticonvulsant therapy began early in this century. An important advance was the identification of the subgroup of children with simple febrile seizures; a subgroup that is large, remarkably homogeneous, and healthy at 7- and 10-year follow-ups. Furthermore, the recognition of such favorable outcomes has accentuated the need to balance the risk of any treatment with an expected benefit. Epidemiologic studies helped to identify this subgroup, demonstrated their predominantly favorable outcomes, and confirmed what has long been known: febrile seizures are common events. Of youngsters in a British birth cohort, 2.7% had febrile seizures, 88% of whom had simple febrile seizures.

Definition of the Problem

This parameter is limited to children with simple febrile seizures defined as neurologically healthy infants and children between 6 months and 5 years of age whose seizure is brief (<15 minutes), generalized, and occurs only once during a 24-hour period in a febrile child. This definition is easily applied in the usual clinical circumstances and has the additional advantages of encompassing most children with febrile seizures and defining a relatively homogeneous group of patients. This practice parameter excludes children whose seizures are attributable to a central nervous system infection (symptomatic febrile seizures) and those who have had a previous afebrile seizure or central nervous system abnormality (secondary febrile seizures).

Background

Proponents of therapy for simple febrile seizures have worried that repeated simple febrile seizures will lead to more febrile seizures and possibly to afebrile seizures (epilepsy). They also have been apprehensive that these seizures will cause brain injury and thus diminish intelligence or impair motor coordination.

A child who has experienced a single simple febrile seizure is likely to experience another. As epidemiologic data indicate, this recurrence rate is strongly age-related. The younger the child at the time of the first event, the more likely there will be subsequent events. In the National Collaborative Perinatal Project (NCPP), half the subjects with onset of febrile seizures during the first year versus approximately 30% with onset after the first year had one or more additional febrile seizures. This project included 1706 prospectively studied children with febrile seizures from approximately 54 000 pregnancies.

The risk of experiencing a single afebrile seizure or two or more afebrile seizures (defined as epilepsy) is elevated when comparing children with simple febrile seizures with the general age-matched population. In the NCPP, the risk factors for epilepsy after a febrile seizure were a positive family history of afebrile seizures, preexisting neurologic abnormality, and a complicated initial febrile seizure. Interestingly, the age at first febrile seizure and the number of febrile seizures did not alter this risk. At age 7 years, only 1.9% of children with simple febrile seizures and negative family histories of epilepsy had experienced a single afebrile seizure, and epilepsy had developed in 0.9%. The comparable figures for study children who never experienced a febrile seizure were 0.9% for a single afebrile seizure and 0.5% for epilepsy. Similar rates were seen in the large British cohort study that included all surviving neonates born in the United Kingdom during 1 week in April 1970. These children were followed until age 10 years, and 305 had an initial simple febrile seizure. Of the 305 children, 8 (2.6%) subsequently had an afebrile seizure and epilepsy eventually developed in 5 (1.6%). The comparable number with epilepsy among the 14 278 children who never had febrile seizures was 53 (0.4%).

Although the risk of epilepsy among children with simple febrile seizures is elevated, the rate is still low, and the number of children in any given study is small. These numbers provide some understanding of the difficulty of designing a population-based study to determine if any treatment for the prevention of simple febrile seizures would subsequently prevent the development of epilepsy.

Investigators have attempted to look at this issue. The Kaiser Foundation Hospitals in Southern California studied 400 children who had febrile seizures (identified from lumbar puncture reports). They divided the children into three study groups: those who received phenobarbital daily, those who received phenobarbital only with fever, and those who received no therapy. Follow-up lasted a mean of 6.3 years. No difference was found in the rate of afebrile seizures. This study included children with complex as well as simple febrile seizures, many children did not receive the prescribed medication (approximately one third), and the study was small and could have missed a statistically valid effect.

In another study, 289 children with febrile seizures were randomized to rectal diazepam prophylaxis at the onset of any fever or rectal diazepam therapy during any febrile seizure. At age 14 years, there was no difference in intelligence, coordination, or occurrence of epilepsy between the two groups. The number of study patients was small, there are questions regarding compliance, and patients with complex and simple febrile seizures were included.

Evidence for adverse outcomes other than epilepsy has been sought. The NCPP had the benefit of longitudinal examination of a predefined group of children. No evidence of death in relation to asymptomatic febrile seizures was found, and examination of the children revealed no evidence for the development of motor deficits. There also has been concern about cognitive deficits in relation to febrile seizures. The NCPP found no effect on intelligence among 431 children with febrile seizures who were compared with their siblings. Comparisons of children with simple febrile seizures with the general population also have found no adverse effect. Smith and Wallace believed that they found an adverse effect of repeated febrile seizures on intelligence as measured by the Griffith Mental Development Scale. Because they studied children with simple and complex febrile seizures, it is possible that underlying neurologic disease predisposed to further seizures and to lower scores on retesting.

Methods

Pertinent articles previously obtained by a medline search and a search of the Epilepsy Foundation of America database 4 were reviewed and supplemented by references suggested by members of the Committee and the Committee's consultants. More than 300 articles were reviewed.

The goal of the review was to identify articles that met the following criteria:

- The study children had simple febrile seizures that were convincingly differentiated from afebrile seizures and other types of febrile seizures.
- The subjects with simple febrile seizures were reasonably representative of children with simple febrile seizures.
- A suitable control group was included in the study. Preference was given to blinded protocols.

Continuous Anticonvulsant Therapy

Phenobarbital

There are several studies in which phenobarbital administered daily successfully prevented recurrent febrile seizures. Camfield and associates randomized 79 children who had had a first simple febrile seizure to receive phenobarbital at 5 mg/kg per day in a single dose or a placebo. Compliance was monitored by use of the urine fluorescence of a riboflavin additive and by measurements of serum phenobarbital levels. There was a significant difference in the incidence of recurrent febrile seizures between the phenobarbital recipients (2/39 [5%]) and the placebo group (10/40 [25%]). Neither parents nor investigators knew which subjects received the active drug. Investigators found no significant difference in IQ (using Stanford-Binet or Bayley Scales) between the placebo and phenobarbital groups after 8 to 12 months of therapy. Nevertheless, phenobarbital was demonstrated to decrease memory and concentration in proportion to higher serum phenobarbital levels. Transient sleep disturbances and daytime fussiness were more common among phenobarbital recipients, but by 1 year, the two groups were indistinguishable. This was partially accounted for by

4 children receiving phenobarbital whose side effects resolved after the dosage was reduced.

In a controlled trial comparing phenobarbital (5 mg/kg per day) with phenytoin (8 mg/kg per day) and placebo, Bacon and associates also found phenobarbital to be effective. In younger children, the febrile seizure recurrence rate was 9% (2/22) for phenobarbital recipients versus 44% (12/27) placebo recipients. This trial included subjects with complicated febrile seizures who were stratified proportionally into the three groups. The study had major problems with compliance. All phenobarbital-treated children with a recurrence for whom drug levels were obtained at the time of recurrence had a plasma level <15 mg/L. Interestingly the reported behavioral changes were similar in the subjects treated with phenobarbital and a placebo.

Mamelle et al compared phenobarbital (3 to 4 mg/kg per day), valproate (30 to 40 mg/kg per day in 2 doses), and placebo in a randomized single-blind study of infants with a first simple febrile seizure. They found significantly fewer recurrences in the valproate (1/22 [4.5%]) and phenobarbital (4/21 [19%]) groups compared with the placebo group (9/26 [35%]). Compliance was measured by serum drug levels. Only 5 subjects were removed from therapy because of side effects; all were described as having agitation and all were receiving phenobarbital. Other studies, some with designs that were less rigorous, also found phenobarbital to be effective, including the previously mentioned Kaiser Foundation study.

Not all studies have found phenobarbital to be effective. Heckmatt et al found recurrent febrile seizures in 14 (19%) of 73 control subjects, 10 (11%) of 88 children for whom phenobarbital was prescribed, and 4 (8%) of 49 who actually took the prescribed phenobarbital (4 to 5 mg/kg per day in divided doses). These last 4 subjects had plasma phenobarbital levels >16 mg/L at the time of recurrence. Although the differences between the treatment groups are not statistically important, they seem to suggest that an effect favoring phenobarbital might have been evident had the numbers been larger or the duration of the study longer.

Children who had complicated febrile seizures analyzed by intention to treat experienced no difference in recurrence rate between phenobarbital-treated subjects and controls. The study described a poor rate of compliance and seemed to show that a medication is not effective if parents are unable to administer it. Early in the study when compliance was high, 56% of phenobarbital recipients (4 to 5 mg/kg once per day) and 35% of placebo recipients were reported to have side effects. The study found that the mean IQ was 8.4 points lower in the phenobarbital group than in the placebo group (95% CI: $-3.3 - -3.5$, $P = .0057$) at the end of the 2-year study, with an IQ differential that persisted 6 months after the taper of medication had begun. The analysis of these data was complicated by the low compliance rates, the fact that 24 (26%) of 94 placebo recipients and 53 (64%) of 83 phenobarbital recipients were prescribed phenobarbital after the study ended, and the inclusion of subjects with complicated febrile seizures.

Phenobarbital is associated with impairment of short-term memory and concentration and worsening of behavior. Most data on the effects of phenobarbital have been obtained from adults or from children with epilepsy. The drug's effect seems most prominent at the onset of therapy. The reported effect in children with simple febrile seizures varies among studies. In the study by Camfield et al, parents were only aware of side effects early in the study, but higher serum levels were associated with decreased memory concentration. Smith and Wallace found no effect of therapy but believed that repeated seizures in children with complicated febrile seizures were associated with lower mental development scores. Wolf and Forsythe reported hyperactivity in 46 (42%) of 109 children treated with phenobarbital (initial dose, 3 to 4 mg/kg per day, adjusted to give a serum level of 10 to 15 $\mu g/mL$) for febrile seizures compared with 21 (17.5%) of 120 not receiving phenobarbital. As in other studies, a substantial rate of improvement was noted in both groups with time. When 25 children from each group were extensively tested, no cognitive differences could be detected.

Valproic Acid

A number of studies have demonstrated the effectiveness of this agent in preventing recurrent febrile seizures. The study by Mamelle et al typifies the studies that found valproic acid to be more effective than phenobarbital. Although no severe adverse effects are described among the children participating in the febrile seizure trials, the numbers in these trials are small. Valproic acid therapy is associated with fatal hepatotoxicity, pancreatitis, renal toxicity, hematopoietic disturbances, and other problems.

Carbamazepine

Carbamazepine was not effective for febrile seizures in preliminary trials and, thus, has not been studied widely. In a double-blind trial of carbamazepine (20 mg/kg per day in twice daily doses) vs phenobarbital (4 to 5 mg/kg per day) involving children with complicated febrile seizures, Antony and Hawke reported recurrent febrile seizures in 9 (47%) of 19 carbamazepine recipients and 2 (10%) of 21 phenobarbital recipients.

Phenytoin

As with carbamazepine, preliminary studies showed no evidence that phenytoin was effective for febrile seizures, so it has not been studied extensively. In a randomized, controlled study of children with simple and complex febrile seizures, the recurrence rate in the phenytoin group (8 mg/kg per day) of younger children was 33% (9/27) compared with 9% (2/22) for the phenobarbital group (5 mg/kg per day) and 44% (12/27) for the equivalent placebo group.

Intermittent Therapy

Antipyretic Agents

Because simple febrile seizures occur only in conjunction with a fever, it has seemed logical to try to prevent these seizures by using aggressive antipyretic therapy. In the randomized, double-blind study by Camfield and associates, all subjects received detailed instruction about temperature control, including antipyretic use with any rectal temperature higher than 37.2°C (99°F). Ten (25%) of 40 subjects using only temperature control had recurrences compared with 2 (5%) of 39 receiving continuous phenobarbital. A randomized, controlled trial using a complicated study design with placebo, low-dose diazepam, and acetaminophen also found no evidence that acetaminophen prevented recurrent febrile seizures. In this protocol, the diazepam-treated children who had previously experienced a febrile seizure received a rectal diazepam solution (if they weighed <7 kg, they received 2.5 mg; if 7 to 15 kg, 5 mg; and if >15 kg, 10 mg) followed in 6 hours by 0.2 mg/kg three times a day whenever they were febrile. The antipyretic treatment group received 10 mg/kg of acetaminophen four times per day.

In children hospitalized after a simple febrile seizure, Schnaiderman et al found that acetaminophen (15 to 20 mg/kg per dose) given every 4 hours did not prevent a second febrile seizure during that admission any better than giving acetaminophen sporadically. The two groups also had the same frequency, duration, and height of temperature elevations. There is no evidence that aggressive antipyretic therapy prevents recurrent febrile seizures.

Diazepam

The use of intermittent diazepam prophylaxis for febrile seizures is well-reported in the literature. Autret and colleagues, in a randomized, controlled multicenter study, found that oral diazepam (0.5 mg/kg initially, then 0.2 mg/kg every 12 hours) was no more effective than a placebo in preventing recurrent febrile seizures. Most of the children had simple febrile seizures, and the data were analyzed by intention to treat. Recurrence was experienced by 15 (16%) of 93 children in the diazepam group compared with 18 (20%) of 92 children in the placebo group. Although parents "were instructed verbally, in writing, and by demonstration," there were major problems with compliance. In children with recurrences, only 1 (7%) of/15 diazepam recipients and 7 (39%) of 18 placebo recipients received the medication or placebo as prescribed. The difference between these two groups is significant. The reasons that the subjects did not receive their assigned treatment included the following: 1) 7 in each group had a seizure as the first sign of illness, 2) 5 parents in the diazepam group and 4 in the placebo group did not give the medication, and 3) 2 children in the diazepam group would not take their medication. Because 14 (93%) of the 15 children for whom diazepam was prescribed who had a recurrence had not received their prescribed medication, these data demonstrate that a treatment is not effective if parents cannot or will not administer it before the febrile seizure occurs. The only noted side effect was hyperactivity, which was significantly more frequent in the diazepam group (138 vs 34 days).

By contrast, in a similarly well-designed, randomized, double-blind, placebo-controlled trial, Rosman et al found oral diazepam to be significantly more effective than placebo when analyzed by intention to treat. A 44% reduction in the risk of febrile seizures per person-year occurred with diazepam. Children in the diazepam group had 675 febrile episodes and 41 febrile seizures, of which 7 occurred while receiving the study medication. Comparable figures for the placebo group were 526 febrile episodes and 72 febrile seizures, of which 38 occurred while receiving the placebo. These investigators describe febrile seizures as "highly upsetting" to the parent population, which may have influenced adherence. Not surprisingly, they found that a higher rate of side effects accompanied their subjects' better compliance. Of the diazepam recipients, 59 (39%) had at least one "moderate" side effect and a similar number had a "mild" side effect.

The Management of Acute Gastroenteritis in Young Children

- *Clinical Practice Guideline*
- *Technical Report Summary*

Readers of this clinical practice guideline are urged to review the technical report to enhance the evidence-based decision-making process. For a copy of the technical report, call Carla Herrerias, MPH, at the Academy, at 800/433-9016, ext 4317.

Clinical Practice Guideline:
The Management of Acute
Gastroenteritis in Young Children

Author:

Subcommittee on Acute Gastroenteritis
Provisional Committee on Quality Improvement

American Academy of Pediatrics
PO Box 927, 141 Northwest Point Blvd
Elk Grove Village, IL 60009-0927

Subcommittee on Acute Gastroenteritis
1992–1995

Lawrence F. Nazarian, MD, Chairman

James H. Berman, MD

Gail Brown, MD, MPH

Peter A. Margolis, MD, PhD

David O. Matson, MD, PhD

Juhling McClung, MD

Larry K. Pickering, MD

John D. Snyder, MD

Provisional Committee on Quality Improvement
1993–1995

David A. Bergman, MD, Chairman

Richard D. Baltz, MD

James R. Cooley, MD

John B. Coombs, MD

Lawrence F. Nazarian, MD

Thomas A. Riemenschneider, MD

Kenneth B. Roberts, MD

Daniel W. Shea, MD

Liaison Representatives:

Michael J. Goldberg, MD
    Section Liaison
Charles J. Homer, MD, MPH
    Section on Epidemiology

Thomas F. Tonniges, MD
    AAP Board of Directors

Abstract

This practice parameter formulates recommendations for health care providers about the management of acute diarrhea in children ages 1 month to 5 years. It was developed through a comprehensive search and analysis of the medical literature. Expert consensus opinion was used to enhance or formulate recommendations where data were insufficient.

The Provisional Committee on Quality Improvement of the American Academy of Pediatrics (AAP) selected a subcommittee composed of pediatricians with expertise in the fields of gastroenterology, infectious diseases, pediatric practice, and epidemiology to develop the parameter. The subcommittee, the Provisional Committee on Quality Improvement, a review panel of practitioners, and other groups of experts within and outside the AAP reviewed and revised the parameter. Three specific management issues were considered: (1) methods of rehydration, (2) refeeding after rehydration, and (3) the use of antidiarrheal agents. Main outcomes considered were success or failure of rehydration, resolution of diarrhea, and adverse effects from various treatment options. A comprehensive bibliography of literature on gastroenteritis and diarrhea was compiled and reduced to articles amenable to analysis.

Oral rehydration therapy was studied in depth; inconsistency in the outcomes measured in the studies interfered with meta-analysis but allowed for formulation of strong conclusions. Oral rehydration was found to be as effective as intravenous therapy in rehydrating children with mild to moderate dehydration and is the therapy of first choice in these patients. Refeeding was supported by enough comparable studies to permit a valid meta-analysis. Early refeeding with milk or food after rehydration does not prolong diarrhea; there is evidence that it may reduce the duration of diarrhea by approximately half a day and is recommended to restore nutritional balance as soon as possible. Data on antidiarrheal agents were not sufficient to demonstrate efficacy; therefore, the routine use of antidiarrheal agents is not recommended, because many of these agents have potentially serious adverse effects in infants and young children.

This practice parameter is not intended as a sole source of guidance in the treatment of acute gastroenteritis in children. It is designed to assist pediatricians by providing an analytic framework for the evaluation and treatment of this condition. It is not intended to replace clinical judgment or to establish a protocol for all patients with this condition. It rarely will provide the only appropriate approach to the problem. A technical report describing the analyses used to prepare this guideline and a patient education brochure are available through the American Academy of Pediatrics.

Background

Although most children with gastroenteritis who live in developed countries have mild symptoms and little or no dehydration, a substantial number will have more severe disease. In the United States, an average of 220 000 children younger than 5 years are hospitalized each year with gastroenteritis, accounting for more than 900 000 hospital days. Approximately 9% of all hospitalizations of children younger than 5 years are because of diarrhea.[1] In addition, approximately 300 children younger than 5 years die each year of diarrhea and dehydration (R. I. Glass, written communication, February 1995). Clinicians should be aware that young infants who were premature and children of teenaged mothers who have not completed high school, had little or no prenatal care, and belong to minority groups are at higher risk of death caused by diarrhea (R. I. Glass, written communication, February 1995).

In the United States, the incidence of diarrhea in children younger than 3 years has been estimated to be 1.3 to 2.3 episodes per child per year; rates in children attending day care centers are higher.[2] Hospitalization and outpatient care for pediatric diarrhea result in direct costs of more than $2.0 billion per year.[3-5] There are also indirect costs to families. Surveys show that many health care providers do not follow recommended procedures for management of this disorder.[6] This practice parameter is intended to present current knowledge about the optimal treatment of children with diarrhea.

Children Covered by the Parameter

In this practice parameter, acute gastroenteritis is defined as diarrheal disease of rapid onset, with or without accompanying symptoms and signs, such as nausea, vomiting, fever, or abdominal pain. Although the emphasis of this parameter is on diarrhea, vomiting can be an important component of gastroenteritis and is addressed specifically below. These recommendations apply to children 1 month to 5 years of age who live in developed countries and who have no previously diagnosed disorders, including immunodeficiency, affecting major organ systems. Episodes of diarrhea lasting longer than 10 days, diarrhea accompanying failure to thrive, and vomiting with no accompanying diarrhea are not addressed. Although most patients meeting the criteria of this parameter will have viral or self-limited bacterial diarrhea, children with bacterial dysentery or protozoal disease can be treated according to the principles presented herein but may benefit from specific antimicrobial therapy.

Outcomes Studied

The major outcomes studied in this analysis of management options were success or failure of rehydration, resolution of diarrhea, and adverse effects of antidiarrheal agents.

Target Audience and Settings

This parameter was designed to aid physicians, nurse practitioners, physician assistants, nurses, and other health care providers who care for children with acute diarrheal disease in outpatient and inpatient settings. It is meant to guide treatment of such children; clinical judgment guided by the special circumstances of each situation will determine the ultimate care of any individual child and may vary from the management outlined herein.

Sources of Information

Ideally, medical information and recommendations are derived from well-designed, properly analyzed scientific studies. When such data are not available on a given subject, consensus may be obtained from experts in the field. In this parameter, three specific topics have received in-depth analysis: rehydration, reintroduction of feeding, and the use of medications designed to influence diarrhea and to provide symptomatic relief. These issues were chosen because of their importance in the management of diarrhea, because there is evidence that practitioners need more information in these areas, and because data are available for study.

In researching these key aspects of the management of acute gastroenteritis, references were identified through MEDLINE searches using the terms *gastroenteritis*, *diarrhea*, and *diarrhea, infantile* to provide an initial, broad database of articles. In addition, specific MEDLINE searches were conducted for various antidiarrheal agents. To supplement the MEDLINE results, articles also were obtained from a number of other sources, including personal files of subcommittee members, bibliographies of articles identified through the computer search, the Centers for Disease Control and Prevention report on management of acute diarrhea in children,[7] the *Federal Register* notice,[8] and a petition to the Food and Drug Administration from the consumer group Public Citizen (written communication, January 1993). More than 4000 articles were included on the original list; after evaluation for relevance and validity, 230 articles were selected for complete review.

Sufficient randomized trials with similar outcomes performed in developed countries were available on early refeeding to allow the combining of results for meta-analysis. Many controlled studies on oral rehydration therapy (ORT) in developed countries were available, but the outcomes of these studies varied;

it was not possible to combine their results quantitatively. Many trials on ORT performed in developing countries were available but were not included in this analysis. Few studies on specific antidiarrheal agents were available, although the committee examined reports on drug therapy from developing as well as developed countries. Recommendations have been drawn from analysis of available literature and have been augmented by expert consensus opinion. The sources and validity of data underlying the committee's conclusions are indicated. Further details on the literature review and analyses are available in the technical report. A summary of the technical report follows this practice parameter.

Other clinical decisions must be addressed when treating children with gastroenteritis, eg, when to obtain stool cultures, the appropriate use of antibiotics, and the prevention of diarrhea. Extensive evaluation of these issues has not been included as part of this parameter. For additional information, the reader is referred to the general review articles that address many of these issues in detail.

Rehydration and Refeeding:
Scientific Background

ORT

Recommendation. **ORT is the preferred treatment of fluid and electrolyte losses caused by diarrhea in children with mild to moderate dehydration** (based on evaluation of controlled clinical trials documenting the effectiveness of ORT; an explanation of what constitutes a recommendation can be found in the technical report).

Replacement of fluid and electrolyte losses is the critical central element of effective treatment of acute diarrhea. Beginning with initial studies conducted 150 years ago, investigators have demonstrated that stool losses of water, sodium, potassium, chloride, and base must be restored to ensure effective rehydration.[9-11] Approximately 60 years ago, intravenous (IV) therapy became the first successful routine method of administration of fluid and electrolytes and was widely accepted as the standard form of rehydration therapy.[12] The treatment of diarrhea was advanced further in the mid-1960s with the discovery of coupled transport of sodium and glucose (or other small, organic molecules), providing scientific justification for ORT as an alternative to IV therapy.[12]

ORT has obvious potential advantages over IV therapy; it is less expensive and can be administered in many settings, including at home by family members. The first studies comparing oral glucose-electrolyte solutions with standard IV therapy were conducted successfully in patients with cholera in Bangladesh and India in the late 1960s.[13,14] The solutions used were similar to the oral rehydration salt solution recommended by the World Health Organization and the United Nations Children's Fund that has been used successfully throughout the world for more than 20 years.

During the past decade, a series of studies from developed countries has proved the effectiveness of ORT compared with IV therapy in children with diarrhea from causes other than cholera.[15–19] These studies evaluated glucose-electrolyte ORT solutions with sodium concentrations ranging from 50 to 90 mmol/L compared with rapidly administered IV therapy. These ORT solutions successfully rehydrated more than 90% of dehydrated children and had lower complication rates than those for IV therapy.[15] The cost of ORT, when hospitalization can be spared, is substantially less than that of IV therapy,[17] but the frequency of stools, duration of diarrhea, and rate of weight gain are similar with both therapies.[15–19]

A variety of oral solutions are available in the United States (Table 1). Those most readily available commercially and used most commonly have sodium concentrations ranging from 45 to 50 mmol/L, which is at or just less than the lower concentration of the solutions studied. Although these products are best suited for use as maintenance solutions, they can rehydrate satisfactorily otherwise healthy children who are mildly or moderately dehydrated.[15,16,20] Glucose-electrolyte solutions such as these, which are formulated on physiologic principles, must be distinguished from other popular but nonphysiologic liquids that have been used inappropriately to treat children with diarrhea (Table 2). These beverages have inappropriately low electrolyte concentrations for ORT use and are hypertonic, owing to their high carbohydrate content.[6] Parents should be discouraged from using nonphysiologic solutions to treat children with diarrhea.

TABLE 1. Composition of Representative Glucose-Electrolyte Solutions*

Solution	CHO, mmol/L	Na, mmol/L	K, mmol/L	Base, mmol/L	Osmolality
Naturalyte (unlimited beverage)	140	45	20	48	265
Pediatric electrolyte (NutraMax)	140	45	20	30	250
Pedialyte (Ross)	140	45	20	30	250
Infalyte (formerly Ricelyte; Mead Johnson)	70	50	25	30	200
Rehydralyte (Ross)	140	75	20	30	310
WHO/UNICEF oral rehydration salts†	111	90	20	30	310

* Adapted from Snyder J. The continuing evolution of oral therapy for diarrhea. *Semin Pediatr Infect Dis.* 1994;5:231–235. CHO, carbohydrate; Na, sodium; K, potassium; WHO, World Health Organization; UNICEF, United Nations Children's Fund.
† Available from Jaianas Bros Packaging Co, 2533 SW Blvd, Kansas City, MO 64108.

TABLE 2. Composition of Representative Clear Liquids Not Appropriate for Oral Rehydration Therapy*

Liquid	CHO, mmol/L	Na, mmol/L	K, mmol/L	Base, mmol/L	Osmolality
Cola	700 (F,G)	2	0	13	750
Apple juice	690 (F,G,S)	3	32	0	730
Chicken broth	0	250	8	0	500
Sports beverage	255 (S,G)	20	3	3	330

* Adapted from Snyder J. The continuing evolution of oral therapy for diarrhea. *Semin Pediatr Infect Dis.* 1994;5:231–235. CHO, carbohydrate; F, fructose; G, glucose; K, potassium; Na, sodium; S, sucrose.

Although glucose-electrolyte ORT is extremely effective in replacing fluid and electrolyte losses, it has no effect on stool volume or the duration of diarrhea. To address this limitation, investigators have administered cereal-based solutions that include naturally occurring food polymers from starch, simple proteins, and a variety of other substrates. Starch and simple proteins provide more cotransport molecules with little osmotic penalty, thus increasing fluid and electrolyte uptake by enterocytes and reducing stool losses.[21,22] The best studied of these solutions contain rice, 50 g/L, instead of glucose. These solutions are not the same as rice water, which has a low concentration of glucose and glucose polymers and is used inappropriately in some parts of the United States, nor are they the same as a commercial product that derives its carbohydrates from glucose polymers purified from rice. Cereal-based ORT can reduce stool volume by more than 30% in children with toxicogenic diarrhea and by close to 20% in those with nontoxicogenic diarrhea.[22] Cereal- or rice powder–based solutions are not presently available commercially; early refeeding, however, can provide similar benefits (see below).

Hypo-osmolar solutions containing glucose polymers to supply transport molecules also have been developed (Table 1). These solutions have shown no appreciable additional benefit compared with the standard glucose-electrolyte oral solution.[23]

Early Feeding of Appropriate Foods

Recommendation. **Children who have diarrhea and are not dehydrated should continue to be fed age-appropriate diets. Children who require rehydration should be fed age-appropriate diets as soon as they have been rehydrated** (based on evaluation of controlled clinical studies documenting the benefits of early feeding of liquid and solid foods).

Optimal oral therapy regimens have incorporated early feeding of age-appropriate foods as an integral component. When used with glucose-electrolyte ORT, early feeding can reduce stool output as much as cereal-based ORT can.[24,25] A variety of early feeding regimens have been studied, including human milk,[26-29] diluted and full-strength animal milk and animal milk formulas,[26,27,29-31] diluted and full-strength lactose-free formulas,[26,32,33] and staple food diets with milk.[28,30,31,34-37] These studies have demonstrated that unrestricted diets do not worsen the course or symptoms of mild diarrhea[27,28] and can decrease stool output[32,36,37] compared with ORT or IV therapy alone. The literature from developed countries on early refeeding[27,32,34,35] allows for meta-analysis, which shows that the duration of diarrhea may be reduced by 0.43 days (95% confidence interval, -0.74 to -0.12). Although these beneficial effects are modest, of major importance is the added benefit of improved nutrition with early feeding.[32,33]

A meta-analysis was performed to evaluate the use of lactose-containing feedings in children with diarrhea and concluded that 80% or more of children with acute diarrhea can tolerate full-strength milk safely.[38] Although reduction in intestinal brush-border lactase levels is often associated with diarrhea,[39] most infants with decreased lactase levels will not have clinical signs or symptoms of malabsorption.[7,39] Infants fed human milk can be nursed safely during episodes of diarrhea.[26] Full-strength animal milk or animal milk formula usually is well tolerated by children who have mild, self-limited diarrhea.[27,38] The combination of milk with staple foods, such as cereal, is an appropriate and well-tolerated regimen for children who are weaned.[28,30,34-37] In the past, the American Academy of Pediatrics (AAP) recommended gradual reintroduction of milk-based formulas or cow's milk in the management of acute diarrhea, beginning with diluted mixtures.[40] This recommendation has been reevaluated in light of recent data. If children are monitored to identify the few in whom signs of malabsorption develop, a regular age-appropriate diet, including full-strength milk, can be used safely.

The question of which foods are best for refeeding has been an issue of continuing study. Although agreement is not universal, clinical experience based on controlled clinical trials suggests that certain foods, including complex carbohydrates (rice, wheat, potatoes, bread, and cereals), lean meats, yogurt, fruits, and vegetables, are better tolerated.[24,25,36,37] Fatty foods or foods high in simple sugars (including tea, juices, and soft drinks) should be avoided.[7] Note that this is not the classic BRAT diet, which consists of bananas, rice, applesauce, and toast. Although these foods can be tolerated, this limited diet is low in energy density, protein, and fat.

Rehydration and Refeeding:
Management Guidelines

The following therapeutic recommendations are based on the evaluation of available literature augmented by expert opinion, as described in previous sections. These recommendations are presented in schematic form in the algorithm.

General Considerations

Evaluation of Dehydration

Available published data have provided rigorous justification for the principles of ORT for diarrhea. Successful implementation of ORT starts with an evaluation of the child's degree of dehydration. Guidelines for assessment of dehydration and rehydration are listed in Table 3. If an accurate recent weight is available, determination of the percentage of weight lost is an objective measure of dehydration. Capillary refill time can be a helpful adjunctive measure to determine the degree of dehydration.[41] Although refill can be affected by fever, ambient temperature, and age,[42] the clinician should consider delayed capillary refill to be a sign of significant dehydration until proven otherwise. Urinary output and specific gravity are helpful measures to confirm the degree of dehydration and to determine that rehydration has been achieved. Parents should be taught the natural history of diarrhea and the signs of dehydration.

Electrolyte Measurement

Most episodes of dehydration caused by diarrhea are isonatremic, and serum electrolyte determinations are unnecessary. Electrolyte levels should be measured in moderately dehydrated children whose histories or physical findings are inconsistent with straightforward diarrheal episodes and in all severely dehydrated children. Clinicians should be aware of the features of hypernatremic dehydration, which can lead to neurologic damage and which requires special rehydration techniques. This condition can result from ingestion of hypertonic liquids (boiled milk and homemade solutions to which salt is added) or the loss of hypotonic fluids in the stool or urine. Irritability and fever may be present, and a doughy feel to the skin is a distinctive feature. The typical loose skin and tenting of the skin associated with the more common isotonic and hypotonic dehydration may not be present. In children receiving IV therapy, electrolyte levels should be measured initially and as therapy progresses. ORT can be used effectively in the treatment of both hypernatremic and hyponatremic dehydration, as well as isonatremic dehydration.

TABLE 3. Assessment of Dehydration*

Variable	Mild, 3%–5%	Moderate, 6%–9%	Severe, ≥10%
Blood pressure	Normal	Normal	Normal to reduced
Quality of pulses	Normal	Normal or slightly decreased	Moderately decreased
Heart rate	Normal	Increased	Increased†
Skin turgor	Normal	Decreased	Decreased
Fontanelle	Normal	Sunken	Sunken
Mucous membranes	Slightly dry	Dry	Dry
Eyes	Normal	Sunken orbits	Deeply sunken orbits
Extremities	Warm, normal capillary refill	Delayed capillary refill	Cool, mottled
Mental status	Normal	Normal to listless	Normal to lethargic or comatose
Urine output	Slightly decreased	<1 mL/kg/h	<<1 mL/kg/h
Thirst	Slightly increased	Moderately increased	Very thirsty or too lethargic to indicate

* Adapted from Duggan et al.[7] See text regarding hypernatremic dehydration. The percentages of body weight reduction that correspond to different degrees of dehydration will vary among authors. The critical factor in assessment is the determination of the patient's hemodynamic and perfusion status. If a clinician is unsure of the category into which a patient falls, it is recommended that therapy for the more severe category be used.

† Bradycardia may appear in severe cases

Vomiting

Vomiting occurs frequently in the course of acute gastroenteritis and sometimes may be the only manifestation. Almost all children who have vomiting and dehydration can be treated with ORT.[7] The key to therapy is to administer small volumes of a glucose-electrolyte solution frequently. Studies have indicated that therapy can be initiated with 5-mL (1-teaspoon) aliquots given every 1 to 2 minutes. Although this technique is labor intensive, it can be done by a parent and will deliver 150 to 300 mL/h.

As dehydration and electrolyte imbalance are corrected by the repeated administration of small amounts of the solution, vomiting often decreases in frequency. As the vomiting lessens, larger amounts of the solution can be given at longer intervals. When rehydration is achieved, other fluids, including milk, as well as food, may be introduced.

The use of a nasogastric tube is another option in a child with frequent vomiting; continuous rather than bolus infusion of ORT solution can result in improved absorption of fluid and electrolytes. Nasogastric infusion also can be used as a temporary expedient while IV access is being sought; however, nasogastric infusion should not be used in a comatose patient or in a child who may have ileus or an intestinal obstruction.

The committee did not evaluate the use of antiemetic drugs. Consensus opinion is that antiemetic drugs are not needed. Physicians who feel that antiemetic therapy is indicated in a given situation should be aware of potential adverse effects.

If vomiting continues despite efforts to administer an oral rehydrating solution, IV hydration is indicated, with return to the oral route when vomiting abates.

Refusal to Take an Oral Rehydrating Solution

Experience gained from more than 25 years of ORT use indicates that children who are dehydrated rarely refuse ORT; however, those who are not dehydrated may refuse the solution because of its salty taste. Children with mild diarrhea and no dehydration should be fed regular diets and do not require glucose-electrolyte solutions. As long as it is clear to the physician and parents that the child is not dehydrated and is in stable condition or showing improvement, special solutions need not be added to the regular feeding routine; however, young children should be given more fluids than usual during an episode of diarrhea.

Some practical techniques exist to induce reluctant children to drink glucose-electrolyte solutions. Administering the solution in small amounts at first may allow the child to get accustomed to the taste. Some commercial solutions have flavors added that do not alter their basic composition but may make them more palatable. Glucose-electrolyte solutions can be frozen into an ice-pop form, which may appeal to some children.

IV Therapy

Clinical studies strongly emphasize ORT; yet the clinician must know when and how to administer IV therapy, which maintains an important role in the treatment of children with diarrhea. All children who are severely dehydrated and in a state of shock or near shock require immediate and vigorous IV therapy. Children who are moderately dehydrated and who cannot retain oral liquids because of persistent vomiting also should receive fluids by the IV route, as should children who are unconscious or have ileus. Administration of ORT is labor intensive, requiring care givers who can administer small amounts of fluid at frequent intervals. If such personnel are not available, IV therapy is indicated.

Clinicians must evaluate a child's condition in light of the circumstances. If staff are skilled in IV administration and are unable to devote time to oral rehydration, and if reliable parents are not available, insertion of an IV line will be more expedient. Facility in IV therapy should not lead automatically to its use. Because children may show considerable improvement after periods of IV therapy, a child who is not severely dehydrated may be able to go home and complete rehydration orally, if proper follow-up is available, after receiving IV fluids for several hours in an emergency department or a similar facility.

The committee emphasizes the need for clinicians to recognize the advantages and disadvantages of both ORT and IV therapy in selecting the best treatment for an individual patient in a specific setting.

Costs

The major factor affecting the cost of rehydrating a child is the setting in which therapy occurs, with the expense increasing as one moves from home to office to emergency department or hospital ward. Oral rehydration is better suited to less-intensive levels of care, but clinicians must be certain that adequate assistance and supervision are available to provide effective therapy. If appropriate assistance is not available, a child may require hospital care for ORT. Clinicians should document the requirements of these patients to justify the need for such services to insurers.

Specific Therapy

The treatment of a child with diarrhea is directed primarily by the degree of dehydration present.

No Dehydration

ORT. Although ORT has been used to replace ongoing stool losses in children with mild diarrhea and no dehydration by giving 10 mL/kg for each stool,[7] these children are the least likely to take ORT, in part because of the salty taste of the solutions. If the stool output remains modest, a supplemental glucose-electrolyte solution may not be required if age-appropriate feeding is continued and fluid consumption is encouraged.

Feeding. Continued age-appropriate feeding, with the foods discussed above and increased fluid intake, may be the only therapy required if hydration is normal, which is the case in most US children with diarrhea. Infants should continue to drink human milk or regular strength formula. Older children may continue to drink milk.

Mild Dehydration (3% to 5%)

ORT. Dehydration should be corrected by giving 50 mL/kg ORT plus replacement of continuing losses during a 4-hour period.[7] Replacement of continuing losses from stool and emesis is accomplished by giving 10 mL/kg for each stool;[7]

also, emesis volume is estimated and replaced. Reevaluation of hydration and replacement of losses should occur at least every 2 hours.

Feeding. As soon as dehydration is corrected, feeding should begin and should follow the guidelines given above.

Moderate Dehydration (6% to 9%)

ORT. Dehydration is corrected by giving 100 mL/kg ORT plus replacement of continuing losses during a 4-hour period. Rapid restoration of the circulating volume helps correct acidosis and improves tissue perfusion, which aids the early refeeding process. At the end of each hour of rehydration, hydration should be assessed, and continuing stool and emesis losses should be calculated with the total added to the amount remaining to be given. This task may be accomplished best in a supervised setting, such as an emergency department, urgent-care facility, or physician's office.

Feeding. When rehydration is complete, feeding should be resumed and should follow the guidelines given above.

Severe Dehydration (≥10%)

Severe dehydration causes shock or a near-shock condition and is a medical emergency. The key to the treatment of the severely dehydrated child is bolus IV therapy with a solution such as normal saline or Ringer's lactate. A common recommendation is to give 20 mL/kg of body weight during a 1-hour period; however, larger quantities and much shorter periods of administration may be required.

Electrolyte levels must be determined in children with severe dehydration. Frequent clinical reevaluation is critical. If the patient does not respond to rapid bolus rehydration, the clinician should consider the possibility of an underlying disorder, including, but not limited to, septic shock, toxic shock syndrome, myocarditis, myocardiopathy, or pericarditis.

For appropriate guidance in treating these critically ill patients, the reader is referred to comprehensive reviews.[43-45]

ORT. When the patient's condition has stabilized and mental status is satisfactory, ORT may be instituted, with the IV line kept in place until it is certain that IV therapy is no longer needed.

Feeding. When rehydration is complete, feeding should be resumed and should follow the guidelines given above.

Therapy With Antidiarrheal Compounds

Drugs are used to alter the course of diarrhea by decreasing stool water and electrolyte losses, shortening the course of illness, or relieving discomfort. Passage of a formed stool is not in itself a measure of successful therapy, because water can remain high in formed stools. Such cosmetic changes may give patients or their families a false sense of security, causing a delay in seeking more effective therapy.

A variety of pharmacologic agents have been used to treat diarrhea. These compounds may be classified by their mechanisms of action, which include: (1) alteration of intestinal motility, (2) alteration of secretion, (3) adsorption of toxins or fluid, and (4) alteration of intestinal microflora. Some agents may have more than one mechanism of action. Many of the agents have systemic toxic effects that are augmented in infants and children or in the presence of diarrheal disease; most are not approved for children younger than 2 or 3 years. Few published data are available to support the use of most antidiarrheal agents to treat acute diarrhea, especially in children. For the purposes of this review, these drugs have been grouped for analysis by their proposed mechanisms of action. Agents for which there are sufficient available data are considered individually. Table 4 lists generic and brand names of the drugs commonly used to treat persons with diarrhea.

Recommendation. **As a general rule, pharmacologic agents should not be used to treat acute diarrhea** (based on limited studies and strong committee consensus).

TABLE 4. Medications Used to Relieve Symptoms in Patients With Acute Diarrhea*

Alteration of intestinal motility
    Opiates
        Loperamide (Imodium, Imodium-AD, Maalox Antidiarrhea, Pepto Diarrhea Control)
        Difenoxin and atropine (Motofen)†
        Diphenoxylate and atropine (Lomotil)†
        Tincture of opium (paregoric)†
Alteration of secretion
    Bismuth subsalicylate (Pepto-Bismol)
Adsorption of toxins and water
    Attapulgite (Diasorb, Donnagel, Kaopectate, Rheaban)
Alteration of intestinal microflora
    Lactobacillus (Pro-Bionate, Superdophilus)

* The actual formulations marketed under these trade names change frequently. More changes are anticipated in the near future based on Food and Drug Administration rulings. Other medications with similar mechanisms of action may be available.

† Requires prescription.

Drugs That Alter Intestinal Motility

Loperamide

Loperamide is a piperadine derivative, chemically related to meperidine, which decreases transit velocity and may increase the ability of the gut to retain fluid. Loperamide also may inhibit calmodulin, a protein involved in intestinal transport. Loperamide is more specific for the μ-opiate receptors of the gut and thus has fewer of the effects on the central nervous system associated with other opiates.[46] Under certain controlled conditions, it also has been shown to have antisecretory properties, but this effect was not seen in an adult volunteer model of acute gastroenteritis.[47] Well-designed clinical trials in both adults and children have demonstrated some beneficial effects of loperamide in the treatment of acute diarrhea.[47-49] Loperamide, when used in conjunction with oral rehydration, reduced the volume of stool losses and shortened the course of disease in children 3 months to 3 years of age. These effects, although statistically significant, were not clinically significant, and the small number of studies makes it difficult to combine them in a meaningful way. In addition, many of the studies and case reports involving children have shown unacceptably high rates of side effects, including lethargy, ileus, respiratory depression, and coma, especially in infants.[7,48,50-55] Death also has been associated with loperamide therapy.[51]

Recommendation. **Loperamide is not recommended to treat acute diarrhea in children** (based on limited scientific evidence that the risks of adverse effects of loperamide outweigh its limited benefits in reducing stool frequency, and on strong committee consensus).

Other Opiates

Few data support the use of other opiate analogues or opiate and atropine combinations (Table 4) to treat diarrhea in children. The potential for toxic side effects is a major concern.[49,56-59] Opiates can produce respiratory depression, altered mental status, and ileus. These drugs pose an additional danger to individuals with fever, toxemia, or bloody stools, because they have been shown to worsen the course of diarrhea in patients with shigellosis,[60] antimicrobial-associated colitis,[61] and diarrhea caused by *Escherichia coli* 0157:H7.[62]

Recommendation. **Opiates as well as opiate and atropine combination drugs are contraindicated in the treatment of acute diarrhea in children** (based on limited scientific evidence and strong committee consensus).

Anticholinergic Agents

Parasympatholytic agents have been used in the treatment of acute gastroenteritis to decrease the cramping associated with diarrhea. They exert their effect on gastrointestinal tract smooth muscle by decreasing motility and reducing tone. Few data are available to document the efficacy of these agents in children with diarrhea. A placebo-controlled trial of the drug mepenzolate bromide in adults failed to demonstrate a positive effect, and many anticholinergic side effects were reported.[63] A dry mouth, the most frequently observed side effect, may alter the clinical evaluation of dehydration. Infants and young children are especially susceptible to the toxic effects of anticholinergic drugs.[64] Coma, respiratory depression, and paradoxical hyperexcitability have been reported.[64]

Recommendation. **Anticholinergic agents are not recommended in the management of diarrhea in children** (based on limited scientific evidence and strong committee consensus).

Alteration of Secretion

Bismuth Subsalicylate

Bismuth subsalicylate, as well as bismuth subnitrate and bismuth subgallate, has been used as adjunctive therapy for acute diarrhea. The mechanism of action of these compounds is uncertain, although laboratory studies have shown that bismuth subsalicylate inhibits intestinal secretion caused by enterotoxicogenic *E coli* and cholera toxins.[65] Controlled trials have demonstrated that bismuth subsalicylate reduced the frequency of unformed stools and increased stool consistency in adults with traveler's diarrhea[66] and in volunteers receiving the Norwalk virus.[67] A controlled clinical trial in children with acute diarrhea demonstrated that the administration of bismuth subsalicylate was associated with a decreased duration of diarrhea and a decreased frequency of unformed stools.[68] A second controlled trial in children receiving only oral therapy for acute diarrhea found that bismuth subsalicylate administration was associated with a shorter duration of diarrhea, decreased total stool output, decreased need for intake of an oral rehydration solution, and reduced hospitalization,[69] although criteria for hospital discharge were not standardized in this study. Overall, the beneficial effects have been modest, and the treatment regimen involves a dose every 4 hours for 5 days. Salicylate absorption after ingestion of a bismuth subsalicylate compound has been reported in adults[70] and children.[71] Insufficient data exist as to the risk of Reye syndrome associated with this compound; such a risk is of at least theoretical concern. Bismuth-associated encephalopathy and other toxic effects have been reported after the long-term ingestion of high doses of bismuth-containing compounds.[72]

Recommendation. **The routine use of bismuth subsalicylate is not recommended in the treatment of children with acute diarrhea** (based on limited scientific evidence that the benefit of bismuth subsalicylate is modest in most children with diarrhea because of concerns about toxic effects, and on committee consensus; further studies may demonstrate a therapeutic role for this agent).

Adsorption of Fluid and Toxins

Adsorbents

Several antidiarrheal compounds are reported to work by adsorbing bacterial toxins and by binding water to reduce the number of bowel movements and to improve stool consistency. Kaolin-pectin, fiber, and activated charcoal are classified in this category, but the only such agent currently used widely is attapulgite. No conclusive evidence is available to show that these agents reduce the duration of diarrhea, stool frequency, or stool fluid losses.[50] Disadvantages include adsorption of nutrients, enzymes, and antibiotics in the intestine.[73]

Recommendation. **Adsorbents are not recommended for the treatment of diarrhea in children** (based on limited scientific evidence and committee consensus; efficacy has not been shown, although major toxic effects are not a concern).

Alteration of Intestinal Microflora

Lactobacillus

Lactobacillus is administered to patients with acute diarrhea to alter the composition of the intestinal flora.[74] Normally, saccharolytic bacteria in the intestine ferment dietary carbohydrates that have not been absorbed completely, causing a decrease in pH that produces short-chain fatty acids and deters intestinal pathogens. The short-chain fatty acids are absorbed through the colonic mucosa and facilitate absorption of water. When a patient has diarrhea, the fecal flora are diminished, production of short-chain fatty acids is reduced, and colonic absorption of water is impaired.[75] There is no consistent evidence that administration of *Lactobacillus*-containing compounds alters the course of diarrhea.[76,77] The supplementation of infant formula with *Bifidobacterium bifidum* and *Streptococcus thermophilus* has been shown to reduce the incidence of acute diarrhea and rotavirus shedding in hospitalized infants.[78] Two studies of young children demonstrated a reduction in the duration of diarrhea caused by rotavirus associated with the administration of *Lactobacillus GG*.[79,80] Additional research is needed in the area of bacterial interference using *Lactobacillus*-containing compounds.[77]

Recommendation. ***Lactobacillus*-containing compounds currently are not recommended in the treatment of acute diarrhea in children** (based on limited scientific evidence and committee consensus; efficacy has not been shown, although toxic effects are not a concern).

Newer Treatments for Diarrhea

Several medications have shown promise in the treatment of acute diarrhea on an experimental basis, mostly in studies involving adults. These include derivatives of berberine,[81] nicotinic acid, clonidine,[82] chloride channel blockers,[83] calmodulin inhibitors,[84] octreotide acetate,[85] and nonsteroidal antiinflammatory drugs. All of these agents must be considered experimental at this time.

Other Agents

A variety of drugs not discussed herein are used in clinical practice to treat diarrhea. Little evidence exists regarding their safety or efficacy; therefore, they cannot be recommended.

Research Issues

In developing this practice parameter, the committee reviewed a large body of literature, but only a fraction was amenable to rigorous scientific analysis. Only the issue of refeeding was supported by a sufficient number of comparable studies to allow meta-analysis. The systematic evaluation of the evidence for the remaining questions points to areas that need more research. In particular, the usefulness of drug therapy for acute gastroenteritis needs to be examined more closely. In developed countries, studies of ORT that focus on factors such as barriers to implementation, costs, and acceptability to parents and health care providers would help facilitate its use.

The practice parameter, "The Management of Acute Gastroenteritis in Young Children," was reviewed by the appropriate committees and sections of the AAP, including the Chapter Review Group, a focus group of office-based pediatricians representing each AAP district: Gene R. Adams, MD; Robert M. Corwin, MD; Lawrence C. Pakula, MD; Barbara M. Harley, MD; Howard B. Weinblatt, MD; Thomas J. Herr, MD; Kenneth E. Mathews, MD; Diane Fuquay, MD; Robert D. Mines, MD; and Delosa A. Young, MD. Comments also were solicited from relevant outside medical organizations. The clinical algorithm was developed by James R. Cooley, MD, Harvard Community Health Plan.

References

1. Cicirello HG, Glass RI. Current concepts of the epidemiology of diarrheal diseases. *Semin Pediatr Infect Dis.* 1994;5:163–167

2. Pickering LK, Hadler SC. Management and prevention of infectious diseases in day care. In: Feigin RD, Cherry JC, eds. *Textbook of Pediatric Infectious Diseases.* Philadelphia: WB Saunders; 1992:2308–2334

3. Glass RI, Ho MS, Lew J, Lebaron CW, Ing D. Cost-benefit studies of rotavirus vaccine in the United States. In: Sack DA, Freij L, eds. *Prospects for Public Health Benefits in Developing Countries From New Vaccines Against Enteric Infections.* Swedish Agency Research Cooperation With Developing Countries; 1990;2:102–107. Conference Report

4. Avendano P, Matson DO, Long J, Whitney S, Matson CC, Pickering LK. Costs associated with office visits for diarrhea in infants and toddlers. *Pediatr Infect Dis J.* 1993;12:897–902

5. Matson DO, Estes MK. Impact of rotavirus infection at a large pediatric hospital. *J Infect Dis.* 1990;162:598–604

6. Snyder JD. Use and misuse of oral therapy for diarrhea: comparison of US practices with American Academy of Pediatrics' recommendations. *Pediatrics.* 1991;87:28–33

7. Duggan C, Santosham M, Glass RI. The management of acute diarrhea in children: oral rehydration, maintenance, and nutritional therapy. *MMWR.* 1992;41(RR-16):1–20

8. 51.83 *Federal Register* 16138

9. Pratt EL. Development of parenteral fluid therapy. *J Pediatr.* 1984;104:581–584

10. Powers GF. A comprehensive plan of treatment for the so-called intestinal intoxication of children. *Am J Dis Child.* 1926;32:232–257

11. Darrow DC, Pratt EL, Flett J Jr, et al. Disturbances of water and electrolytes in infantile diarrhea. *Pediatrics.* 1949;3:129–156

12. Hirschhorn NJ. The treatment of acute diarrhea in children: an historical and physiological perspective. *Am J Clin Nutr.* 1980;33:637–663

13. Hirschhorn NJ, Kinzie JL, Sachar DB, et al. Decrease in net stool output in cholera during intestinal perfusion with glucose-containing solutions. *N Engl J Med.* 1968;279:176–181

14. Pierce NF, Sack RB, Mitra RC, et al. Replacement of water and electrolyte losses in cholera by an oral glucose-electrolyte solution. *Ann Intern Med.* 1969;70:1173–1181

15. Santosham M, Daum RS, Dillman L, et al. Oral rehydration therapy of infantile diarrhea: a controlled study of well-nourished children hospitalized in the United States and Panama. *N Engl J Med.* 1982;306:1070–1076

16. Tamer AM, Friedman LB, Maxwell SR, Cynamon HA, Perez HN, Cleveland WW. Oral rehydration of infants in a large urban US medical center. *J Pediatr.* 1985;107:14–19

17. Listernick R, Zieserl E, Davis AT. Outpatient oral rehydration in the United States. *Am J Dis Child.* 1986;140:211–215

18. Vesikari T, Isolauri E, Baer M. A comparative trial of rapid oral and intravenous rehydration in acute diarrhoea. *Acta Paediatr Scand.* 1987;76:300–305

19. MacKenzie A, Barnes G. Randomized controlled trial comparing oral and intravenous rehydration therapy in children with diarrhoea. *Br Med J.* 1991;303:393–396

20. Santosham M, Burns B, Nadkami V, et al. Oral rehydration therapy for acute diarrhea in ambulatory children in the United States: a double-blind comparison of four different solutions. *Pediatrics.* 1985;76:159–166

21. Carpenter CC, Greenough WB, Pierce NF. Oral rehydration therapy: the role of polymeric substrates. *N Engl J Med.* 1988;319:1346–1348

22. Gore SM, Fontaine O, Pierce NF. Impact of rice based oral rehydration solution of stool output and duration of diarrhoea: meta-analysis of 13 clinical trials. *Br Med J.* 1992;304:287–291

23. Pizarro D, Posada G, Sandi L, Moran JR. Rice-based oral electrolyte solutions for the management of infantile diarrhea. *N Engl J Med.* 1991;324:517–521

24. Santosham M, Fayad I, Hashem M, et al. A comparison of rice-based oral rehydration solution and "early feeding" for the treatment of acute diarrhea in infants. *J Pediatr.* 1990;116:868–875

25. Fayad IM, Hashem M, Duggan C, Refat M, Bakir M, Fontaine O. Comparative efficacy of rice-based and glucose-based oral rehydration salts plus early reintroduction of food. *Lancet.* 1993;342:772–775

26. Khin MU, Nyunt-Nyunt W, Myokhin AJ, et al. Effect of clinical outcome of breast feeding during acute diarrhoea. *Br Med J.* 1985;290:587–589

27. Margolis PA, Litteer T. Effects of unrestricted diet on mild infantile diarrhea: a practice-based study. *Am J Dis Child.* 1990;144:162–164

28. Gazala E, Weitzman S, Weitzman Z, et al. Early versus late refeeding in acute infantile diarrhea. *Isr J Med Sci.* 1988;24:175–179

29. Fox R, Leen CL. Acute gastroenteritis in infants under 6 months old. *Arch Dis Child.* 1990;65:936–938

30. Rees L, Brook CGD. Gradual reintroduction of full-strength milk after acute gastroenteritis in children. *Lancet.* 1979;1:770–771

31. Placzek M, Walker-Smith JA. Comparison of two feeding regimens following acute gastroenteritis in infancy. *J Pediatr Gastroenterol Nutr.* 1984;3:245–248

32. Santosham M, Foster S, Reid R, et al. Role of soy-based, lactose-free formula during treatment of acute diarrhea. *Pediatrics.* 1985;76:292–298

33. Brown KH, Gastanaduy AS, Saaverdra JM, et al. Effect of continued oral feeding on clinical and nutritional outcomes of acute diarrhea in children. *J Pediatr.* 1988;112:191–200

34. Hjelt K, Paerregaard A, Petersen W, Christiansen L, Krasilnikoff PA. Rapid versus gradual refeeding in acute gastroenteritis in childhood: energy intake and weight gain. *J Pediatr Gastroenterol Nutr.* 1989;8:75–80

35. Isolauri E, Vesikari T. Oral rehydration, rapid refeeding and cholestyramine for treatment of acute diarrhoea. *J Pediatr Gastroenterol Nutr.* 1985;4:366–374

36. Brown KH, Perez F, Gastanaduy AS. Clinical trial of modified whole milk, lactose-hydrolyzed whole milk, or cereal-milk mixtures for the dietary management of acute childhood diarrhea. *J Pediatr Gastroenterol Nutr.* 1991;12:340–350

37. Alarcon P, Montoya R, Perez F, Dongo JW, Peerson JM, Brown KH. Clinical trial of home available, mixed diets versus a lactose-free, soy-protein formula for the dietary management of acute childhood diarrhea. *J Pediatr Gastroenterol Nutr.* 1991;12:224–232

38. Brown KH, Peerson JM, Fontaine O. Use of nonhuman milks in the dietary management of young children with acute diarrhea: a meta-analysis of clinical trials. *Pediatrics.* 1994;93:17–27

39. Sunshine P, Kretchmer N. Studies of small intestine during development, III: infantile diarrhea associated with intolerance to disaccharides. *Pediatrics.* 1964;34:38–50

40. American Academy of Pediatrics, Committee on Nutrition. Use of oral fluid therapy and post-treatment feeding following enteritis in children in a developed country. *Pediatrics.* 1985;75:358–361

41. Saavedra JM, Harris GD, Li S, Finberg L. Capillary refilling (skin turgor) in the assessment of dehydration. *Am J Dis Child*. 1991;145:296–298

42. Schriger DL, Baraff L. Defining normal capillary refill: variation with age, sex, and temperature. *Ann Emerg Med*. 1988;17:932–935

43. Shaw KN. Dehydration. In: Fleisher GR, Ludwig R, eds. *Textbook of Pediatric Emergency Medicine*. 3rd ed. Baltimore, MD: Williams & Wilkins; 1993:147–151

44. Silverman BK, ed. *Advanced Pediatric Life Support*. 2nd ed. Elk Grove Village, IL: American Academy of Pediatrics, American College of Emergency Physicians; 1993

45. Chameides L, ed. *Textbook of Pediatric Advanced Life Support*. Dallas: American Heart Association, American Academy of Pediatrics; 1990

46. Schiller LR, Santa Ana CA, Morawski SG, Fordtran JS. Mechanism of the antidiarrheal effect of loperamide. *Gastroenterology*. 1984;85:1475–1483

47. Diarrhoeal Diseases Study Group (UK). Loperamide in acute diarrhoea in childhood: results of a double-blind, placebo controlled multicentre clinical trial. *Br Med J*. 1984;289:1263–1267

48. Motala C, Hill ID. Effect of loperamide on stool output and duration of acute infectious diarrhea. *J Pediatr*. 1990;117:467–471

49. Prakash P, Saxena S, Sareen DK. Loperamide versus diphenoxylate in the diarrhea of infants and children. *Indian J Pediatr*. 1980;47:303–306

50. World Health Organization. *The Rational Use of Drugs in the Management of Acute Diarrhoea in Children*. Geneva: World Health Organization; 1990

51. Bhutta TI, Tahir KI. Loperamide poisoning in children. *Lancet*. 1990;335:363

52. Chow CB, Li SH, Leung NK. Loperamide associated necrotizing enterocolitis. *Acta Pediatr Scand*. 1986;75:1034–1036

53. Minton NA, Smith PGD. Loperamide toxicity in a child after a single dose. *Br Med J*. 1987;294:1383

54. Herranz J, Luzuriaga C, Sarralle R, Florez J. Neurological symptoms precipitated by loperamide. *Anales Espanoles Pediatr*. 1980;13:1117–1120

55. Schwartz RH, Rodriguez WJ. Toxic delirium possibly caused by loperamide. *J Pediatr*. 1991;118:656–657

56. Ginsberg CM. Lomotil (diphenoxylate and atropine) intoxication. *Am J Dis Child*. 1973;125:241–242

57. Rumack BH, Temple AP. Lomotil poisoning. *Pediatrics*. 1974;53:495–500

58. Curtis JAQ, Goel KM. Lomotil poisoning in children. *Arch Dis Child*. 1979;54:222–225

59. Bala K, Khandpur S, Gujral V. Evaluation of efficacy and safety of lomotil in acute diarrheas in children. *Indian Pediatr*. 1979;16:903–907

60. DuPont HL, Hornick RB. Adverse effect of lomotil therapy in shigellosis. *JAMA*. 1973;226:1525–1528

61. Novak E, Lee JG, Seckman CE, Phillips JP, Disanto AR. Unfavorable effect of atropine-diphenoxylate (Lomotil) therapy in linomycin-caused diarrhea. *JAMA*. 1976;235:1451–1454

62. Pickering LK, Obrig TG, Stapleton FB. Hemolytic uremic syndrome and enterohemorrhagic *E coli*. *Pediatr Infect Dis J*. 1994;13:459–475

63. Reves R, Bass P, DuPont HL, Sullivan P, Mendiola J. Failure to demonstrate effectiveness of an anticholinergic drug in the symptomatic treatment of acute traveler's diarrhea. *J Clin Gastroenterol*. 1983;5:223–227

64. US Pharmacopeia. *Anticholinergic/Antispasmodics System*. Rockville, MD: US Pharmacopeia Dispensing Information; 1992;1:312

65. Ericsson CD, Evans DG, DuPont HL, Evans DJ Jr, Pickering LK. Bismuth subsalicylate inhibits activity of crude toxins of *Escherichia coli* and *Vibrio cholerae*. *J Infect Dis*. 1977;136:693–696

66. DuPont HL, Ericsson CD, Johnson PG, et al. Prevention of traveler's diarrhea by the tablet formulation of bismuth subsalicylate. *JAMA*. 1987;257:1347–1350

67. Steinhoff MC, Douglas RG Jr, Greenberg HB, Callahan DR. Bismuth subsalicylate therapy of viral gastroenteritis. *Gastroenterology*. 1980;78:1495–1499

68. Soriano-Brucher H, Avendano P, O'Ryan M, et al. Bismuth subsalicylate in the treatment of acute diarrhea in children: a clinical study. *Pediatrics*. 1991;87:18–27

69. Figueroa-Quintanilla D, Salazar-Lindo E, Sack RB, et al. A controlled trial of bismuth subsalicylate in infants with acute watery diarrheal disease. *N Engl J Med*. 1993;328:1653–1658

70. Feldman S, Chen SL, Pickering LK, Cleary TG, Ericsson CD, Hulse M. Salicylate absorption from a bismuth subsalicylate preparation. *Clin Pharmacol Ther*. 1981;29:788–792

71. Pickering LK, Feldman S, Ericsson CD, Cleary TG. Absorption of salicylate and bismuth from a bismuth subsalicylate-containing compound (Pepto-Bismol). *J Pediatr*. 1981;99:654–656

72. Mendelowitz PC, Hoffman RS, Weber S. Bismuth absorption and myoclonic encephalopathy during bismuth subsalicylate therapy. *Ann Intern Med*. 1990;112:140–141

73. Parpia SH, Nix DE, Hejmanowski LG, Goldstein HR, Wilton JH, Schentag JJ. Sucralfate reduces the gastrointestinal absorption of norfloxacin. *Antimicrob Agents Chemother*. 1989;33:99–102

74. Lidbeck A, Nord CE. Lactobacilli and the normal human anaerobic microflora. *Clin Infect Dis*. 1993;16(suppl 4):S181–S187

75. Ramakrishna BS, Mathan VI. Colonic dysfunction in acute diarrhoea: the role of luminal short chain fatty acids. *Gut*. 1993;34:1215–1218

76. Clements ML, Levine MM, Black RE, et al. *Lactobacillus* prophylaxis for diarrhea due to enterotoxigenic *Escherichia coli*. *Antimicrob Agents Chemother*. 1981;20:104–108

77. Reid G, Bruce AW, McGroorty JA, et al. Is there a role for lactobacilli in prevention of urogenital and intestinal infections? *Clin Microbiol Rev*. 1993;3:335–344

78. Saavedra JM, Bauman NA, Oung I, Perman JA, Yolken RH. Feeding *Bifidobacterium bifidum* and *Streptococcus thermophilus* to infants in hospital for prevention of diarrhoea and shedding of rotavirus. *Lancet*. 1994;334:1046–1049

79. Isolauri E, Juntunen M, Rautanen T, Sillanaukee P, Koivula T. A human *Lactobacillus* strain (*Lactobacillus casei*, sp strain GG) promotes recovery from acute diarrhea in children. *Pediatrics*. 1991;88:90–97

80. Kaila M, Isolauri E, Soppi E, Virtanen E, Laine S, Arvilommi H. Enhancement of the circulating antibody secreting cell response in human diarrhea by a human *Lactobacillus* strain. *Pediatr Res*. 1992;32:141–144

81. Donowitz M, Levine S, Watson A. New drug treatments for diarrhoea. *J Intern Med Suppl*. 1990;228:155–163

82. Schiller LR, Santa Ana CA, Morawski SG, Fordtran JS. Studies of the antidiarrheal action of clonidine: effects on motility and intestinal absorption. *Gastroenterology*. 1985;89:982–988

83. Bridges RJ, Worrell RT, Frizzell RA, Benos DJ. Stilbene disulfonate blockade of colonic secretory Cl-channels in planar lipid bilayers. *Am J Physiol*. 1989;256:907–912

84. DuPont HL, Ericsson CD, Mathewson JJ, Marani S, Knellwolf-Cousin AL, Martinez-Sandoval FG. Zalaride maleate, an intestinal calmodulin inhibitor, in the therapy of traveler's diarrhea. *Gastroenterology.* 1993;104:709–715

85. Cook DJ, Kelton JG, Stanisz AM, Collins SM. Somatostatin treatment for cryptosporidial diarrhea in a patient with the acquired immunodeficiency syndrome (AIDS). *Ann Intern Med.* 1988;108:708–709

General References

Duggan C, Santosham M, Glass RI. The management of acute diarrhea in children: oral rehydration, maintenance, and nutritional therapy. *MMWR.* 1992;41(RR-16):1–20

Pickering LK, Cleary TG. Approach to patients with gastrointestinal tract infections and food poisoning. In: Feigin RD, Cherry JC, eds. *Textbook of Pediatric Infectious Disease.* 3rd ed. Philadelphia: WB Saunders; 1992:565–596

Cohen MB, Balistreri WF. Diagnosing and treating diarrhea. *Contemp Pediatr.* 1989;6:89–114

Grisanti KA, Jaffe DM. Dehydration syndromes: oral rehydration and fluid replacement. *Emerg Med Clin North Am.* 1991;9:565–588

Management of acute diarrheal disease. Proceedings of a symposium, 1990. *J Pediatr.* 1991;118:S25–S138

Guerrant RL, Bobak DA. Bacterial and protozoal gastroenteritis. *N Engl J Med.* 1991;325:327–340

Pickering LK, Matson DO. Therapy for diarrheal illness in children. In: Blaser MJ, Smith PD, Ravdin JI, Greenburg HB, Guerrant RL, eds. *Infections of the Gastrointestinal Tract.* New York: Raven Press; 1995

Northrup RS, Flanigan TP. Gastroenteritis. *Pediatr Rev.* 1994;15:461–472

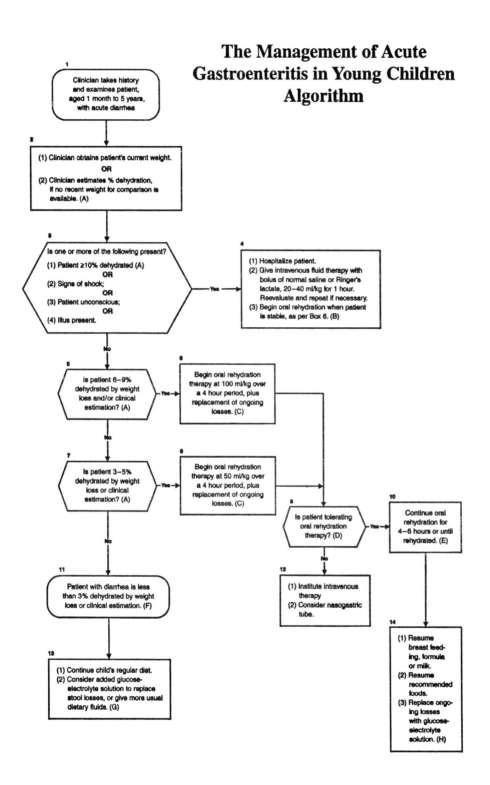

The Management of Acute Gastroenteritis in Young Children Algorithm

1
Clinician takes history and examines patient, aged 1 month to 5 years, with acute diarrhea

2
(1) Clinician obtains patient's current weight.
OR
(2) Clinician estimates % dehydration, if no recent weight for comparison is available. (A)

3
Is one or more of the following present?
(1) Patient ≥10% dehydrated (A)
OR
(2) Signs of shock;
OR
(3) Patient unconscious;
OR
(4) Ilius present.

4
(1) Hospitalize patient.
(2) Give intravenous fluid therapy with bolus of normal saline or Ringer's lactate, 20–40 ml/kg for 1 hour. Reevaluate and repeat if necessary.
(3) Begin oral rehydration when patient is stable, as per Box 6. (B)

— Yes →

5
Is patient 6–9% dehydrated by weight loss and/or clinical estimation? (A)

— Yes →

6
Begin oral rehydration therapy at 100 ml/kg over a 4 hour period, plus replacement of ongoing losses. (C)

7
Is patient 3–5% dehydrated by weight loss or clinical estimation? (A)

— Yes →

8
Begin oral rehydration therapy at 50 ml/kg over a 4 hour period, plus replacement of ongoing losses. (C)

9
Is patient tolerating oral rehydration therapy? (D)

— Yes →

10
Continue oral rehydration for 4–6 hours or until rehydrated. (E)

11
Patient with diarrhea is less than 3% dehydrated by weight loss or clinical estimation. (F)

12
(1) Institute intravenous therapy
(2) Consider nasogastric tube.

13
(1) Continue child's regular diet.
(2) Consider added glucose-electrolyte solution to replace stool losses, or give more usual dietary fluids. (G)

14
(1) Resume breast feeding, formula or milk.
(2) Resume recommended foods.
(3) Replace ongoing losses with glucose-electrolyte solution. (H)

– 231 –

Annotations for the Management of Acute Gastroenteritis in Young Children

Rehydration and Refeeding Algorithm

A. See Table 3 for guidance in the assessment of the degree of dehydration.

B. Restoration of cardiovascular stability is critical and is accomplished by giving bolus IV therapy with normal saline or Ringer's lactate solution (see text). In the patient who does not respond, consider the possibility of an underlying disorder, such as myocarditis, myocardiopathy, pericarditis, septic shock, or toxic shock syndrome. When the patient is in stable condition and has achieved satisfactory mental status, ORT can be used according to the ORT guidelines.

C. Solutions containing 45 to 90 mmol/L sodium should be given in a volume of 100 mL/kg for moderate dehydration and 50 mL/kg for mild dehydration. Giving the child these volumes requires patience and persistence, and progress must be monitored frequently.

D. Intractable, severe vomiting, unconsciousness, and ileus are contraindications to ORT. Persistent refusal to drink may require a trial of IV therapy.

E. The rehydration phase usually can be completed in 4 hours; reevaluation should occur every 1 to 2 hours. See text for guidance to decide when rehydration has been achieved.

F. The type and intensity of therapy will vary with the individual clinical situation.

G. Often, a child has diarrhea but remains adequately hydrated. The parent can be reassured but should be taught to assess hydration and to identify a worsening condition. If the stool output remains modest, ORT might not be required if early, age-appropriate feeding is instituted and increased consumption of usual dietary fluids is encouraged. More significant stool losses can be replaced with an oral rehydrating solution at the rate of 10 mL/kg for each stool.

H. Breastfeeding should be resumed. Nonlactose formula, milk-based formula, or milk may be given, although a small percentage of children will not tolerate lactose-containing fluids. Lactose-containing solutions seem to be tolerated better when combined with complex carbohydrates in weaned children. Children who are eating foods may resume eating, although certain foods are tolerated better than others. Recommended foods include complex carbohydrates (rice, wheat, potatoes, bread, and cereals), lean meats, yogurt, fruits, and vegetables. Avoid fatty foods and foods high in simple sugars (including juices and soft drinks). Supplement feeding with an oral electrolyte solution, 10 mL/kg for each diarrheal stool and the estimated amount vomited for each emesis.

Technical Report Summary:
Acute Gastroenteritis

Authors:

Gail Brown, MD, MPH
Peter Margolis, MD, PhD

The University of North Carolina at Chapel Hill

Epidemiologic Consultants to the Subcommittee on Gastroenteritis

American Academy of Pediatrics
PO Box 927, 141 Northwest Point Blvd
Elk Grove Village, IL 60009-0927

Subcommittee on Acute Gastroenteritis
1992 – 1995

Lawrence F. Nazarian, MD, Chairman

James H. Berman, MD

Gail Brown, MD, MPH

Peter A. Margolis, MD, PhD

David O. Matson, MD, PhD

Juhling McClung, MD

Larry K. Pickering, MD

John D. Snyder, MD

Provisional Committee on Quality Improvement
1993 – 1995

David A. Bergman, MD, Chairman

Richard D. Baltz, MD

James R. Cooley, MD

John B. Coombs, MD

Lawrence F. Nazarian, MD

Thomas A. Riemenschneider, MD

Kenneth B. Roberts, MD

Daniel W. Shea, MD

Liaison Representatives:

Michael J. Goldberg, MD
   Section Liaison
Charles J. Homer, MD, MPH
   Section on Epidemiology
Thomas F. Tonniges, MD
   AAP Board of Directors

Introduction

The practice parameter on acute gastroenteritis is intended to present current knowledge about optimal treatment of children with diarrhea. This technical report details the process followed in its development, and presents the evidence used to formulate the final recommendations.

Methods

The approach to developing this guideline was based on the principles for guideline development outlined by Eddy and Woolf.

Development of the Evidence Model

Definitions

In this report and in the practice parameter, acute gastroenteritis is defined as diarrheal disease of rapid onset of 10 days' duration or less. Episodes of diarrhea may or may not be accompanied by other signs and symptoms, such as vomiting, fever, or pain.

The parameter applies to children aged 1 month to 5 years who live in developed countries and who have no previously diagnosed disorders affecting major organ systems, including immunodeficiency. Not addressed are episodes of diarrhea lasting longer than 10 days, diarrhea accompanying failure to thrive, or vomiting with no accompanying diarrhea. The practice parameter is not intended to apply to chronic intestinal disorders, inflammatory bowel disease, or other previously diagnosed chronic conditions affecting major organ systems. Children with dysentery can be treated according to the principles presented here but may benefit from specific antimicrobial therapy.

Target Audience

The intended users of the practice parameter include pediatricians, family physicians, general practitioners, emergency physicians, public health nurses and nurse practitioners, physician assistants, and staff members of nutritional support groups (eg, Supplemental Feeding Program for Women, Infants, and Children [WIC]), and other individuals or organizations interested in the nutrition of children.

The practice settings targeted are the offices of private pediatricians and family physicians, hospital outpatient departments, emergency departments, acute inpatient facilities, acute care ambulatory facilities, public health clinics, and WIC programs and other nutritional support programs.

Interventions

Diagnostic interventions discussed by the subcommittee (but not necessarily included in the parameter) included tests designed to determine the severity of the patient's condition (including urinalysis), the likely cause (stool pattern and microscopic examination), and positive identification of the organism (stool culture, blood culture, sensitivities, microscopic examination for ova and parasites, and rapid identification tests). Therapeutic interventions considered included hospital vs home therapy, rehydration/restoration of electrolyte balance (oral or intravenous [IV]) adjunctive drug therapy for symptom relief or hastening of recovery, empirical antimicrobial therapy, and restoration of normal nutritional status (when to resume feeding, what foods, progression of foods, timetable of progression of foods, etc). Public health interventions considered included the primary prevention of disease through appropriate day care procedures, including hand washing, diapering, and breastfeeding.

Outcomes

The subcommittee listed the following health outcomes as potentially related to the parameter:

1. Restoration of function: return to normal functioning and state of well-being, return to normal nutritional status, and return to normal daily activities (eg, day care/school).

2. Prevention of adverse health events: hospitalization, inappropriate emergency department visits, acute complications of acute gastroenteritis (eg, shock, acute renal failure, sagittal sinus thrombosis, and seizures), severe electrolyte imbalance, cardiac arrhythmias, and death.

3. Prevention of iatrogenic complications: worsening of dehydration, electrolyte imbalance, seizures, adverse drug effects, and emergence of antibiotic-resistant organisms.

4. Avoidance of long-term complications of acute gastroenteritis: intractable diarrhea, prolonged carrier state of infectious organisms, and transmission of disease.

5. Improved patient (parental) satisfaction.

6. Cost.

Clinical outcomes used to measure improved status were expected to be state of hydration and electrolyte balance (weight, blood chemistry levels, and urine output); severity and duration of diarrhea, change in stool patterns, patient functioning (days in the hospital, and number of days out of school or day care), and the presence or absence of infectious organisms in the stool.

Although all of these outcomes were considered by the subcommittee in the initial stages of work on the parameter, not all were addressed in the parameter because of limitations in the available data.

Evidence Model

Each subcommittee member was asked to prepare a draft evidence model to help the subcommittee consider the aspects of the problem for which evidence would be required. After consideration of their models, the subcommittee chose three clinical management issues on which to focus. The three specific questions were as follows:

1. Is oral rehydration therapy (ORT) as effective as IV therapy for dehydration secondary to acute gastroenteritis?

2. For children without dehydration, or after a rehydration phase, does altering diet hasten the resolution of the disease?

3. Does drug therapy improve the course of diarrhea?

Literature Review

A literature search was conducted by staff at the American Academy of Pediatrics via the National Library of Medicine database using the terms *gastroenteritis* and *diarrhea, infantile*. The list of resulting articles was selectively reviewed by limiting studies to those involving human subjects and children older than 1 month and to the English-language literature.

For symptomatic drug therapy, staff performed a literature search using the terms *gastroenteritis* and *diarrhea*. Additional terms added to the search included *antacids, laxatives, digestants, antiemetics, bismuth, loperamide, attapulgite, diphenoxylate, scopolamine, hyoscyamine, lactobacillus, kaolin, pectin, hydroxyquinolones, toxiferine, dicyclomine, mepenzolate, donnatal, propantheline,* and *clidinium*. Addition of the term *parasympathetics* yielded no additional information. The resulting list of articles was selectively reviewed by limiting studies to those involving human subjects, and children older than 1 month, and to the English-language literature.

Additional articles were identified by subcommittee member input, bimonthly manual searches of current pediatric journals available in the American Academy of Pediatrics' library, comparison with bibliographies from other reviews, including The Public Citizen's group report to the Food and Drug Administration, *The Federal Register* notice, and the *MMWR* Recommendations and Reports on "The Management of Acute Diarrhea in Children: Oral Rehydration, Maintenance, and Nutritional Therapy." The subcommittee's literature database was compared with that in Current World Literature (sections on gastroenterology and nutrition, pathophysiology and physiology of carbohydrate absorption, and normal growth and nutrition). The two reference lists contained compatible information. This process produced no unpublished original studies.

Article Selection

Based on titles and abstract review, subcommittee members selected articles for full review. The reviewers were asked to include any article that reported outcomes of interests, specifically duration of disease, complications of therapy, parental satisfaction, and cost. Committee members were also asked to consider articles most useful if the population studied was comparable to the US population. To address the question of ORT vs IV therapy, only randomized clinical trials were considered.

A literature review form developed for this project was used by the subcommittee members to review all selected articles (Appendix). Reviewers classified articles by study type and study question. If the reviewers decided that an article did not meet the criteria listed above, it was no longer included as part of the data. If reviewers determined that an article was appropriate for inclusion, then the reviewer went on to summarize the population studied, methods, and outcomes. The form took less than an hour to complete.

The methodologists sorted the forms and articles as to clinical question and compared outcomes. Articles were incorporated into evidence tables, which formed the basis for discussion of the guidelines and also served as the background for decision making when studies could not be combined statistically.

Statistical Methods

When sufficient studies were available, the effectiveness of therapy was summarized by pooling data across studies. The difference between treatment and control groups was used as the measure of the relative benefit of one form of therapy over another. The overall impact of a therapy was calculated as the weighted average of the outcome measure across all studies (eg, mean duration and proportion of treatment failures). Pooled 95% confidence intervals (CIs) were calculated for each trial and for the combined data. The similarity of data from different studies was assessed by reviewing plots of the data and by performing a test of homogeneity. Sensitivity analyses were performed to assess the importance of individual studies on overall conclusions.

Recommendations and Level of Evidence

Recommendations are made based on the quality of scientific evidence. In the absence of high-quality scientific evidence, subcommittee consensus or a combination of evidence and consensus is used as the basis for recommendations.

Clinical Options are actions for which the subcommittee failed to find compelling evidence to support or refute. A health care provider might or might not wish to implement clinical options in the treatment of a given child.

No recommendation is made when scientific evidence is lacking and there is no compelling reason to make an expert judgment.

Results

The literature search identified 230 articles that could potentially be included in the parameter. Of these, 88 compared ORT with IV therapy for dehydration, 46 compared different refeeding strategies, and 76 reported the effects of symptomatic drug therapy. An additional 20 articles contained potentially useful general information.

ORT vs IV Therapy

Of the 88 articles initially accepted by the reviewers, five contained primary data concerning the outcomes of interest in children in developed countries. Unfortunately, these articles reported different outcomes. Outcomes reported in the studies included duration of diarrhea, weight gain, length of hospital stay, stool volume, costs, time to rehydration, stool frequency, electrolyte balance, and sodium intake. It was not possible to pool the estimates of effect across studies.

Complications of ORT and IV therapy were discussed in the five articles with original data. Two studies measured duration of illness, and two studies measured weight gain at hospital discharge. One of these studies found a statistically significant reduction in the duration of diarrhea among children receiving ORT. The other study of duration showed no difference between treatment groups. Neither study showed a significant difference in weight gain.

Although it was not possible to combine statistically the results of the five studies with original data, the tables were presented to all of the subcommittee members. These summaries, as well as data in the articles themselves, provided the basis for the recommendations. Based on an evaluation of the randomized trials documenting the effectiveness of ORT, the subcommittee recommended the use of ORT as the preferred treatment of fluid and electrolyte losses due to diarrhea in children with mild to moderate dehydration.

Refeeding

Of the 46 articles reviewed that dealt with early refeeding, 10 were combined into an evidence table. The other articles had outcomes that were not comparable or did not present original data. Four of the studies were conducted in developing countries, and six were conducted in developed countries. The studies used a variety of early refeeding regimens, including: breastfeeding, dilute soy, cow's milk formula, and rice-based formula. Because all of the studies compared dilute formula with undiluted formula and gradual reintroduction of feeding with reinstitution of normal feedings upon rehydration and used a comparable outcome measurement (duration of diarrhea), the results of the 10 studies were pooled. Data were insufficient to combine other outcomes, such as weight gain, stool output, or length of hospital stay.

The difference in the duration of diarrhea between dilute and undiluted feeding was used as the measure of effectiveness of the therapy. Combined data from all

10 studies revealed that in children who received full-strength feedings, diarrhea lasted 0.3 days (95% CI, –0.53, –0.07) less than in those in whom feedings were gradually reintroduced. However, a test of homogeneity yielded significant results (P=.011), indicating that the effectiveness of the therapy was not uniform among studies. A plot of the data from the studies suggested that studies from developing countries were associated with less of an effect of early refeeding than studies from developed countries. The plot also suggested that the study by Santosham et al might be influencing the results substantially.

Sensitivity analyses were performed to examine the impact in different studies on the duration of diarrhea. When studies from developing countries were excluded from the analysis, early refeeding was associated with 0.67 fewer days of diarrhea (95% CI, –0.96, –0.38) compared with gradual refeeding. However, the results of a test for homogeneity remained significant (P<.001). When the study by Santosham et al was excluded, the duration of diarrhea was 0.43 days less (95% CI, –0.74, –0.12), and the results of a test for homogeneity were not significant (P=.14). Exclusion of the study by Santosham et al from the original group of studies also resulted in nonsignificant results of a test of homogeneity. However, the observed reduction in the number of days of diarrhea also became nonsignificant.

In summary, these results suggest that early refeeding may be associated with a small reduction in the duration of diarrhea when studies from developed and developing countries are combined. When studies from only developed countries are considered, there is a reduction in the duration of diarrhea of about half a day. There is no evidence that early refeeding prolongs diarrhea over gradual refeeding. Based on this statistical analysis, the subcommittee observed that early refeeding appears to be associated with a clinically meaningful reduction in the duration of diarrhea and recommended the return to full-strength formula or normal feeding during an episode of diarrhea as soon as rehydration has been achieved.

Pharmacologic Therapy for Diarrhea

The literature search identified 76 articles that considered drug therapy for diarrhea. The search was not limited to studies performed in developed countries.

Four clinical trials of loperamide contained primary data and were compared in a table. The complications of these four trials were considered by the subcommittee. In addition, the four trials were combined in an evidence table that compared the duration of diarrhea in the study vs control groups. The subcommittee was impressed with the number of reports of toxic effects, especially in infants, and decided that the risks of adverse effects outweighed the limited benefits of loperamide, thus recommending that it not be used in children.

Four trials considered diphenoxylate in the treatment of acute diarrhea, but various outcomes, including duration of diarrhea, the proportion of patients responding, stool frequency, and water content of stools, were measured. Only two studies, which were summarized in an evidence table, reported duration of diarrhea. Complications reported in two studies ranged from sedation to poisoning. In light of the evidence, the subcommittee decided not to recommend the use of opiates in the management of acute diarrhea in childhood.

Two trials measured the effectiveness of bismuth subsalicylate in diarrheal disease in children. Both studies showed a decrease in duration of diarrhea in the treatment groups. However, the subcommittee observed that the benefit of bismuth subsalicylate would be minimal in most children and that there were no data about potential toxic effects. The subcommittee did not recommend the routine use of bismuth subsalicylate but recognized that future studies may demonstrate a role for this agent.

The remaining studies dealt with other pharmacologic agents or case reports of the agents mentioned above. There was not enough information on any one agent to recommend its routine use in children with diarrhea.

Discussion

The parameter contains the following subcommittee recommendations:

1. Oral rehydration therapy is recommended as the preferred treatment of fluid and electrolyte losses due to diarrhea in children with mild to moderate dehydration.

2. Appropriate diets are recommended during an episode of diarrhea as soon as rehydration has been achieved.

3. Pharmacologic agents are not recommended to treat acute childhood diarrhea.

Oral rehydration therapy was studied in-depth, but variation in measured outcomes prevented pooling of results across studies. Refeeding was covered by enough comparable studies to perform a meta-analysis and to use these data in forming recommendations. Insufficient data were available on specific drugs to demonstrate their efficacy.

The step-by-step method followed in the development of the practice parameter outlined in this technical report helped to define the questions to be addressed and to arrive at consensus opinion. Ultimately, only the question of refeeding lent itself to meta-analysis. However, the systematic evaluation of the evidence for the remaining questions points to areas needing more research. In particular, the usefulness of drug therapy for acute gastroenteritis and the use of oral rehydration in developed countries need to be examined more closely.

The Management of Hyperbilirubinemia in the Healthy Term Newborn

- *Clinical Practice Guideline*
- *Technical Report Summary*

Readers of this clinical practice guideline are urged to review the technical report to enhance the evidence-based decision-making process. For a copy of the technical report, call Carla Herrerias, MPH, at the Academy, at 800/433-9016, ext 4317.

Clinical Practice Guideline: Management of Hyperbilirubinemia in the Healthy Term Newborn

Author:

American Academy of Pediatrics
Subcommittee on Hyperbilirubinemia
Provisional Committee on Quality Improvement

American Academy of Pediatrics
PO Box 927, 141 Northwest Point Blvd
Elk Grove Village, IL 60009-0927

Subcommittee on Hyperbilirubinemia
1992–1994

William O. Robertson, MD, Chairman

Jon R. Almquist, MD
Irwin J. Light, MD
M. Jeffrey Maisels, MD

Thomas B. Newman, MD,
  MPH, Consultant
Ronald W. Poland, MD

Consultants:

Gerald B. Merenstein, MD
James A. Lemons, MD
Lawrence M. Gartner, MD
Lois Johnson, MD

Audrey K. Brown, MD
David K. Stevenson, MD
Avroy Fanaroff, MD
James Cooley, MD,
  Clinical Algorithm

Provisional Committee on Quality Improvement
1993–1994

David A. Bergman, MD, Chairman

James R. Cooley, MD
John B. Coombs, MD
Michael J. Goldberg, MD,
  Sections Liaison
Charles J. Homer, MD,
  Section on Epidemiology
  Liaison
Lawrence F. Nazarian, MD

Thomas A. Riemenschneider, MD
Kenneth B. Roberts, MD
Daniel W. Shea, MD
Thomas F. Tonniges, MD, AAP
  Board of Directors
  Liaison

Acknowledgments

The practice parameter, "Management of Hyperbilirubinemia in the Healthy Term Newborn," was reviewed by the appropriate committees and sections of the American Academy of Pediatrics (AAP), including the Chapter Review Group, a focus group of office-based pediatricians representing each AAP District: Gene R. Adams, MD; Robert M. Corwin, MD; Lawrence C. Pakula, MD; Barbara M. Harley, MD; Howard B. Weinblatt, MD; Thomas J. Herr, MD; Kenneth E. Mathews, MD; Diane Fuquay, MD; Robert D. Mines, MD; and Delosa A. Young, MD. The clinical algorithm was developed by Carmie Margolis, MD; Agnatha Golan, MD; Professor Michael Karplus, Ben Gurion University of Negev, Beer Sheva, Israel; and James R. Cooley, MD, Harvard Community Health Plan.

The American Medical Association (AMA) Specialty Society Practice Parameter Partnership reviewed the neonatal hyperbilirubinemia practice parameter and found it to be in conformance with AMA attributes for practice parameter development.

Abstract

The American Academy of Pediatrics and its Provisional Committee on Quality Improvement in collaboration with experts from the Section on Perinatal Pediatrics, general pediatricians, and research methodologists developed this practice parameter. This parameter provides recommendations for the evaluation and treatment of neonatal hyperbilirubinemia in an otherwise healthy, nonisoimmunized infant of at least 37 completed weeks of gestation. The parameter is based on the accompanying technical report developed in 1993 by the Emergency Care Research Institute (ECRI) and, in part, on the data analyses contained in a 1990 report by Newman and Maisels on jaundice in healthy newborn infants. The recommendations derive from both expert consensus and a review of the literature. A comprehensive literature review can be found in the technical report that is available from the Publications Department, American Academy of Pediatrics.

This parameter is not intended to stand alone in the treatment of neonatal hyperbilirubinemia in the healthy term newborn. It is designed to assist pediatricians by providing an analytic framework for the evaluation and treatment of this condition. It is not intended to replace clinical judgment (*Pediatrics*. 1994;94[4]:558–565).

Each year approximately 60% of the 4 million newborns in the United States become clinically jaundiced. Many receive various forms of evaluation and treatment. Few issues in neonatal medicine have generated such long-standing controversy as the possible adverse consequences of neonatal jaundice and when to begin treatment. Questions regarding potentially detrimental neurologic effects from elevated serum bilirubin levels prompt continuing concern and debate, particularly with regard to the management of the otherwise healthy term newborn without risk factors for hemolysis.[1-16] Although most data are based on infants with birth weights ≥2500 g, "term" is hereafter defined as 37 completed weeks of gestation.

Under certain circumstances, bilirubin may be toxic to the central nervous system and may cause neurologic impairment even in healthy term newborns. Most studies, however, have failed to substantiate significant associations between a specific level of total serum bilirubin (TSB) during nonhemolytic hyperbilirubinemia in term newborns and subsequent IQ or serious neurologic abnormality (including hearing impairment).[3-5] Other studies have detected subtle differences in outcomes associated with TSB levels, particularly when used in conjunction with albumin binding tests and/or duration of exposure.[5,15,17,18] In almost all published studies, the TSB concentration has been used as a predictor variable for outcome determinations.

Factors influencing bilirubin toxicity to the brain cells of newborn infants are complex and incompletely understood; they include those that affect the serum albumin concentration and those that affect the binding of bilirubin to albumin, the penetration of bilirubin into the brain, and the vulnerability of brain cells to the toxic effects of bilirubin. It is not known at what bilirubin concentration or under what circumstances significant risk of brain damage occurs or when the risk of damage exceeds the risk of treatment. Concentrations considered harmful may vary in different ethnic groups or geographic locations and may be lower outside North America or northern Europe. Reasons for apparent geographic differences in risk for kernicterus are not clear; the following practice parameter may not apply worldwide.

There are no simple solutions to the management of jaundiced neonates. Continuing uncertainties about the relationship between serum bilirubin levels and brain damage as well as differences in patient populations and practice settings contribute to variations in the management of hyperbilirubinemia. Early postpartum discharge from the hospital further complicates the management of jaundiced newborns, because it places additional responsibilities on parents or guardians to recognize and respond to developing jaundice or clinical symptoms.

Some conditions significantly increase the risk of hyperbilirubinemia, including history of a previous sibling with hyperbilirubinemia, decreasing gestational age, breast-feeding, and large weight loss after birth. Although newborns of 37 weeks' gestation and above are considered "term," infants 37 to 38 weeks of gestation may not nurse as well as more mature infants, and there is a strong correlation between decreasing gestational age and risk for hyper-bilirubinemia. Infants born at 37 weeks' gestation are much more likely to develop a serum bilirubin level of 13 mg/dL or higher than are those born at 40 weeks' gestation.[19-22]

Methodology

The Task Force on Quality Assurance (now designated the Provisional Committee on Quality Improvement) selected the management of hyper-bilirubinemia as a topic for practice parameter development and appointed a subcommittee that performed a comprehensive literature review. Two inde-pendent MEDLINE searches identified primarily retrospective epidemiologic data derived almost exclusively from North American and European litera-ture. The subcommittee also relied heavily on both the data and analyses con-tained in a 1990 report by Newman and Maisels.[3] Moreover, the total experience analyzed involved a relatively limited number of healthy term infants with bilirubin levels in excess of 25 mg/dL (428μmol/L) making it difficult to draw firm conclusions from the published data. The recommendations that fol-low stem from careful consideration of currently available information, as analyzed and interpreted by subcommittee members and consultants, and are based on evidence when appropriate data exist and derived from consensus when data are lacking. The subcommittee's recommendations are supported by a technical report containing a world literature search and analysis, and updated literature review. The technical report is available from the American Academy of Pediatrics.

Recommendations

The following recommendations were developed by the AAP to aid in the eval-uation and treatment of the healthy term infant with hyperbilirubinemia. Important in the development of these guidelines is the general belief that ther-apeutic interventions for hyperbilirubinemia in the healthy term infant may carry significant risk relative to the uncertain risk of hyperbilirubinemia in this population. In these guidelines, the AAP has attempted to describe a range of acceptable practices, recognizing that adequate data are not avail-able from the scientific literature to provide more precise recommendations.

Evaluation

1. Maternal prenatal testing should include ABO and Rh(D) typing and a serum screen for unusual isoimmune antibodies.[23]
2. A direct Coombs' test, a blood type, and an Rh(D) type on the infant's (cord) blood are recommended when the mother has not had prenatal blood grouping or is Rh-negative.
3. Institutions are encouraged to save cord blood for future testing, particu-larly when the mother's blood type is group O. Appropriate testing may then be performed as needed.

Table 1. Factors To Be Considered When Assessing a Jaundiced Infant*

Factors that suggest the possibility of hemolytic disease
    Family history of significant hemolytic disease
    Onset of jaundice before age 24 h
    A rise in serum bilirubin levels of more than 0.5 mg/dL/h
    Pallor, hepatosplenomegaly
    Rapid increase in the TSB level after 24–48 h (consider G6PD deficiency)
    Ethnicity suggestive of inherited disease (G6PD deficiency, etc)
    Failure of phototherapy to lower the TSB level
Clinical signs suggesting the possibility of other diseases such as sepsis or galactosemia in which jaundice may be one manifestation of the disease
    Vomiting
    Lethargy
    Poor feeding
    Hepatosplenomegaly
    Excessive weight loss
    Apnea
    Temperature instability
    Tachypnea
Signs of cholestatic jaundice suggesting the need to rule out biliary atresia or other causes of cholestasis
    Dark urine or urine positive for bilirubin
    Light-colored stools
    Persistent jaundice for >3 wk

* TSB indicates total serum bilirubin; G6PD, glucose-6-phosphate dehydrogenase.

4. When family history, ethnic or geographic origin, or the timing of the appearance of jaundice suggests the possibility of glucose-6-phosphate dehydrogenase deficiency or some other cause of hemolytic disease, appropriate laboratory assessment of the infant should be performed.

5. A TSB level needs to be determined in infants noted to be jaundiced in the first 24 hours of life.

6. In newborn infants, jaundice can be detected by blanching the skin with digital pressure, revealing the underlying color of the skin and subcutaneous tissue. The clinical assessment of jaundice must be done in a well-lighted room. Dermal icterus is seen first in the face and progresses caudally to the trunk and extremities. As the TSB level rises, the extent of cephalocaudad progression may be helpful in quantifying the degree of jaundice; use of an icterometer or transcutaneous jaundice meter may also be helpful.[24-26]

7. Evaluation of newborn infants who develop abnormal signs such as feeding difficulty, behavior changes, apnea, or temperature instability is recommended—regardless of whether jaundice has been detected—to rule out underlying illness (Table 1).

8. Follow-up should be provided to all neonates discharged less than 48 hours after birth by a health care professional in an office, clinic, or at home within 2 to 3 days of discharge.[23]

9. Approximately one third of healthy breast-fed infants have persistent jaundice after 2 weeks of age.[27] A report of dark urine or light stools should prompt a measurement of direct serum bilirubin. If the history (particularly the appearance of the urine and stool) and physical examination results are normal, continued observation is appropriate. If jaundice persists beyond 3 weeks, a urine sample should be tested for bilirubin, and a measurement of total and direct serum bilirubin obtained.

Table 2. Management of Hyperbilirubinemia in the Healthy Term Newborn*

Age, hours	TSB Level, mg/dL (μmol/L)			
	Consider Phototherapy[†]	Phototherapy	Exchange Transfusion if Intensive Phototherapy Fails[‡]	Exchange Transfusion and Intensive Phototherapy
≤24§	...	...	...	...
25–48	≥12 (205)	≥15 (260)	≥20 (340)	≥25 (430)
49–72	≥15 (260)	≥18 (310)	≥25 (430)	≥30 (510)
>72	≥17 (290)	≥20 (340)	≥25 (430)	≥30 (510)

*TSB indicates total serum bilirubin.
† Phototherapy at these TSB levels is a clinical option, meaning that the intervention is available and may be used *on the basis of individual clinical judgment.* For a more detailed description of phototherapy, see the Appendix.
‡ Intensive phototherapy (Appendix) should produce a decline of TSB of 1 to 2 mg/dL within 4 to 6 hours and the TSB level should continue to fall and remain below the threshold level for exchange transfusion. If this does not occur, it is considered a failure of phototherapy.
§ Term infants who are clinically jaundiced at ≤24 hours old are not considered healthy and require further evaluation (see text).

Treatment

Decisions about therapeutic intervention are tempered by clinical judgment based on the infant's history, course, and physical findings and are balanced by comparing the potential benefits with the risks. As appropriate, physicians are encouraged to discuss management options and their recommendations with parents or other guardians. The guidelines in Table 2 are recommended for infants initially seen with elevated TSB levels, as well as for infants who have been followed up for clinical jaundice. Similar guidelines have been used in Great Britain.[28,29] Direct bilirubin measurements vary substantially as a function of individual laboratories and their instrumentation. For the purposes of the otherwise healthy appearing jaundiced newborn, it is recommended that the direct bilirubin measurement not be subtracted from the TSB level and that the TSB level be relied on as the relevant criterion.

Determination of the rate of rise of TSB and the infant's age may help determine how often to monitor bilirubin levels and whether to begin phototherapy. Continued observation may be an appropriate alternative to repeated TSB testing and phototherapy.

There is continuing uncertainty about what specific TSB levels warrant exchange transfusion. Intensive phototherapy (Appendix) is recommended in infants initially seen with a TSB concentration in the exchange transfusion range (Table 2) while preparations are being made for exchange transfusion. Intensive phototherapy should produce a decline in the TSB level of 1 to 2 mg/dL within 4 to 6 hours, and the decline should continue thereafter. If the TSB level does not decline but persists above the level recommended for exchange transfusion, most experts recommend exchange transfusion (Table 2). Exchange transfusion is also indicated in infants whose TSB levels rise to exchange transfusion levels in spite of intensive phototherapy. In any of the above situations, failure of intensive phototherapy to lower the TSB level strongly suggests the presence of hemolytic disease or some other pathologic process and warrants further investigation.

These guidelines apply to infants without signs of illness or apparent hemolytic disease. It may be difficult to rule out ABO hemolytic disease as well as rarer causes of hemolysis.

The evaluation and treatment of hyperbilirubinemia in the healthy term infant is presented in the clinical Algorithm.[30]

Management of Hyperbilirubinemia in the Healthy Term Newborn by Age (in Hours)

1. Infants ≤24 hours old are excluded from Table 2, because jaundice occurring before age 24 hours is generally considered "pathologic" and requires further evaluation. Although some healthy infants appear slightly jaundiced by 24 hours, the presence of jaundice before 24 hours requires (at least) a serum bilirubin measurement and, if indicated, further evaluation for possible hemolytic disease, or other diagnoses. Phototherapy and/or exchange transfusion may be indicated for rapidly rising TSB levels in the first 24 hours of life.
2. For the treatment of the 25- to 48-hour-old infant, phototherapy may be considered (see Table 2 for definition) when the TSB level is ≥12 mg/dL (205 µmol/L). Phototherapy should be implemented when the TSB level is ≥15 mg/dL (260 µmol/L). If intensive phototherapy fails to lower a TSB level of ≥20 mg/dL (340 µmol/L), exchange transfusion is recommended. If the TSB level is ≥25 mg/dL (430 µmol/L) when the infant is first seen, inten-

sive phototherapy is recommended while preparations are made for an exchange transfusion. If intensive phototherapy fails to lower the TSB level, exchange transfusion is recommended. *The higher TSB levels in a 25- to 48-hour-old infant suggest that the infant may not be healthy and indicate the need for investigation into the cause of hyperbilirubinemia, such as hemolytic disease.*

3. Phototherapy may be considered for the 49- to 72-hour-old jaundiced infant when the TSB level is ≥15 mg/dL (260 µmol/L). Phototherapy is recommended when the TSB level reaches 18 mg/dL (310 µmol/L). If intensive phototherapy fails to lower the TSB level when it reaches or is predicted to reach 25 mg/dL (430 µmol/L), an exchange transfusion is recommended. If the TSB level is ≥30 mg/dL (510 µmol/L) when the infant is first seen, intensive phototherapy is recommended while preparations are made for exchange transfusion. If intensive phototherapy fails to lower the TSB level, an exchange transfusion is recommended.

4. For the infant >72 hours old, phototherapy may be considered if the TSB level reaches 17 mg/dL (290 µmol/L). Phototherapy needs to be implemented at a TSB level of ≥20 mg/dL (340 µmol/L). If intensive phototherapy fails to lower a TSB level of ≥25 mg/dL (430 µmol/L), exchange transfusion is recommended. If the TSB level is ≥30 mg/dL (510 µmol/L) when the infant is first seen, intensive phototherapy is recommended while preparations are made for an exchange transfusion. If intensive phototherapy fails to lower the TSB level, an exchange transfusion is recommended.

In all of the above situations, intensive phototherapy (Appendix) should be used if the TSB level does not decline under conventional phototherapy. Intensive phototherapy should produce a steady decline in the concentration of TSB. If this does not occur, the presence of hemolytic disease or some other pathologic process is suggested and warrants further investigation.

Treatment of Jaundice Associated With Breast-feeding in the Healthy Term Newborn

The AAP discourages the interruption of breast-feeding in healthy term newborns and encourages continued and frequent breast-feeding (at least eight to ten times every 24 hours). Supplementing nursing with water or dextrose water does not lower the bilirubin level in jaundiced, healthy, breast-feeding infants.[31] Depending on the mother's preference and the physician's judgment, however, a variety of options are presented in Table 3 for possible implementation beyond observation, including supplementation of breast-feeding with formula or the temporary interruption of breast-feeding and substitution with formula, either of which can be accompanied by phototherapy.

Table 3. Treatment Options for Jaundiced Breast-fed Infants

Observe
Continue breast-feeding; administer phototherapy
Supplement breast-feeding with formula with or without phototherapy
Interrupt breast-feeding; substitute formula
Interrupt breast-feeding; substitute formula; administer phototherapy

Documentation

This practice parameter is designed to assist the pediatrician and other health care providers by providing a framework for the management of hyperbilirubinemia in the healthy term newborn. It is not intended to replace the physician's clinical judgment or to establish a single protocol applicable to all such newborns with hyperbilirubinemia. It is understood that some clinical problems may not be adequately addressed by the practice parameter, which cannot be considered to represent an exclusive standard of care. Physicians are urged to document their management strategies, including any significant deviation from these or other guidelines and the rationale for the course of action taken.

Finally, all physicians and other health care providers caring for jaundiced newborns are encouraged to continue appraising and incorporating into their practices new scientific and technical advances as clinical evidence of their effectiveness becomes established.

References

1. Behrman RE, ed. *Nelson's Textbook of Pediatrics.* 14th ed. Philadelphia: WB Saunders; 1992, pp 476–481
2. Watchko JF, Oski FA. Bilirubin 20 mg/dL=vigintiphobia. *Pediatrics.* 1983;71:660–663
3. Newman TB, Maisels MJ. Does hyperbilirubinemia damage the brain of healthy newborn infants? *Clin Perinatol.* 1990;17:331–358
4. Newman TB, Maisels MJ. Evaluation and treatment of jaundice in the term infant: a kinder, gentler approach. *Pediatrics.* 1992;89:809–818
5. Newman TB, Klebanoff M. Peak serum bilirubin in normal-sized infants and neurodevelopmental outcome at age 7: a closer look at the collaborative perinatal study. *Pediatrics.* 1993;92:651–657
6. Valaes T. Bilirubin toxicity: the problem was solved a generation ago. *Pediatrics.* 1992;89:819–820
7. Wennberg RP. Bilirubin recommendations present problems: new guidelines simplistic and untested. *Pediatrics.* 1992;89:821–822
8. Merenstein GB. "New" bilirubin recommendations questioned. *Pediatrics.* 1992;89:822–823
9. Poland RL. In search of a "gold standard" for bilirubin toxicity. *Pediatrics.* 1992;89:823–824

10. Cashore WJ. Hyperbilirubinemia: should we adopt a new standard of care? *Pediatrics*. 1992;89:824–826

11. Gartner LM. Management of jaundice in the well baby. *Pediatrics*. 1992;89:826–827

12. Brown AK, Seidman DS, Stevenson DK. Jaundice in healthy term neonates: do we need new action levels or new approaches? *Pediatrics*. 1992;89:827–828

13. Johnson L. Yet another expert opinion on bilirubin toxicity! *Pediatrics*. 1992;89:829–830

14. Newman TB, Maisels MJ. Response to commentaries re: evaluation and treatment of jaundice in the term newborn: a kinder, gentler approach. *Pediatrics*. 1992;89:831–833

15. Seidman DS, Paz I, Stevenson DK, et al. Neonatal hyperbilirubinemia and physical and cognitive performances at 17 years of age. *Pediatrics*. 1991;88:828–833

16. Martinez JC, Maisels MJ, Otheguy L, et al. Hyperbilirubinemia in the breast-fed newborn: controlled trial of four interventions. *Pediatrics*. 1993;91:470–473

17. Johnson LH, Boggs TR. Bilirubin-dependent brain damage: incidence indications for treatment. In: O'Dell GB, Schaffer R, Simopoulous AP, eds. *Phototherapy in the Newborn: An Overview*. Washington, DC: National Academy of Sciences; 1974; 122–149

18. Johnson LH. Hyperbilirubinemia in the term infant: when to worry, when to treat. *NY State J Med*. 1991;91:483–489

19. Gale R, Seidman DS, Dollberg S, Stevenson DK. Epidemiology of neonatal jaundice in the Jerusalem population. *J Pediatr Gastroenterol Nutr*. 1990;10:82–86

20. Friedman L, Lewis PJ, Clifton P, et al. Factors influencing the incidence of neonatal jaundice. *Br Med J*. 1978;1:1235–1237

21. Linn S, Schoenbaum SC, Monson RR, et al. Epidemiology of neonatal hyperbilirubinemia. *Pediatrics*. 1985;75:770–774

22. Maisels MJ, Gifford KL, Antle CE, Lieb GR. Jaundice in the healthy newborn infant: a new approach to an old problem. *Pediatrics*. 1988;81:505–511

23. American Academy of Pediatrics, American College of Obstetricians and Gynecologists. *Guidelines for Perinatal Care*. 3rd ed. Elk Grove Village, IL: American Academy of Pediatrics; 1992

24. Kramer LI. Advancement of dermal icterus in the jaundiced newborn. *AJDC*. 1969; 118:454

25. Ebbesen F. The relationship between the cephalopedal progress of clinical icterus and the serum bilirubin concentration in newborn infants without blood type sensitization. *Obstet Gynecol Scand*. 1975;54:329–332

26. Schumacher RE. Noninvasive measurements of bilirubin in the newborn. *Clin Perinatol*. 1990;17:417–435

27. Alonso EM, Whitington PF, Whitington SH, Rivard WA, Given G. Enterohepatic circulation of non-conjugated bilirubin in rats fed with human milk. *J Pediatr*. 1991;118:425–430

28. Dodd KL. Neonatal jaundice—a lighter touch. *Arch Dis Child*. 1993;68:529–533

29. Finlay HVL, Tucker SM. Neonatal plasma bilirubin chart. *Arch Dis Child*. 1978;53:90–91

30. Pearson SD, Margolis CZ, Davis S, Schreier LK, Gottlieb LK. The clinical algorithm nosology: a method for comparing algorithmic guidelines. *Med Decision Making*. 1992; 12:123–131

31. Nicoll A, Ginsburg R, Tripp, JH. Supplementary feeding and jaundice in newborns. *Acta Pediatr Scand*. 1982;71:759–761

Algorithm

Management of Hyperbilirubinemia in the Healthy Term Newborn

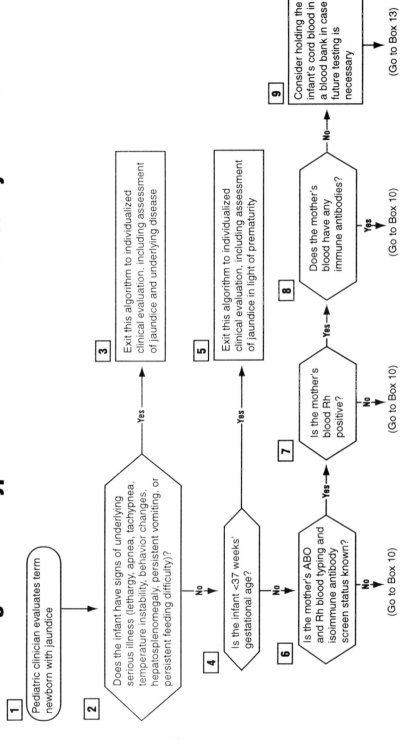

1 Pediatric clinician evaluates term newborn with jaundice

2 Does the infant have signs of underlying serious illness (lethargy, apnea, tachypnea, temperature instability, behavior changes, hepatosplenomegaly, persistent vomiting, or persistent feeding difficulty)?

3 Exit this algorithm to individualized clinical evaluation, including assessment of jaundice and underlying disease — Yes

No

4 Is the infant <37 weeks' gestational age?

5 Exit this algorithm to individualized clinical evaluation, including assessment of jaundice in light of prematurity — Yes

No

6 Is the mother's ABO and Rh blood typing and isoimmune antibody screen status known?

No (Go to Box 10)

Yes

7 Is the mother's blood Rh positive?

No (Go to Box 10)

Yes

8 Does the mother's blood have any immune antibodies?

Yes (Go to Box 10)

No

9 Consider holding the infant's cord blood in a blood bank in case future testing is necessary

(Go to Box 13)

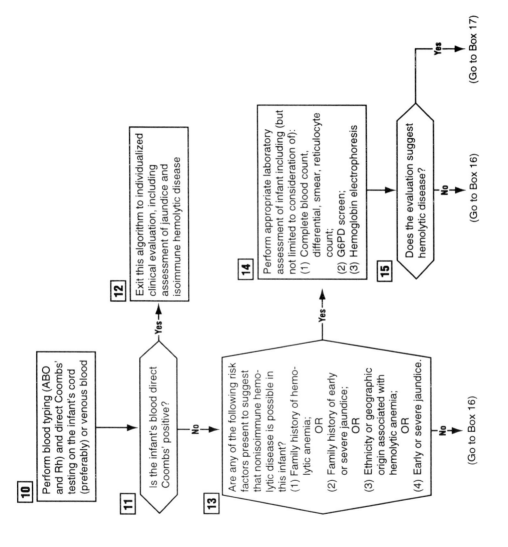

10

Perform blood typing (ABO and Rh) and direct Coombs' testing on the infant's cord (preferably) or venous blood

11

Is the infant's blood direct Coombs' positive?

Yes →

12

Exit this algorithm to individualized clinical evaluation, including assessment of jaundice and isoimmune hemolytic disease

No
↓

13

Are any of the following risk factors present to suggest that nonisoimmune hemolytic disease is possible in this infant?
(1) Family history of hemolytic anemia;
OR
(2) Family history of early or severe jaundice;
OR
(3) Ethnicity or geographic origin associated with hemolytic anemia;
OR
(4) Early or severe jaundice.

No → (Go to Box 16)

Yes →

14

Perform appropriate laboratory assessment of infant including (but not limited to consideration of):
(1) Complete blood count, differential, smear, reticulocyte count;
(2) G6PD screen;
(3) Hemoglobin electrophoresis

↓

15

Does the evaluation suggest hemolytic disease?

No → (Go to Box 16)

Yes → (Go to Box 17)

– 263 –

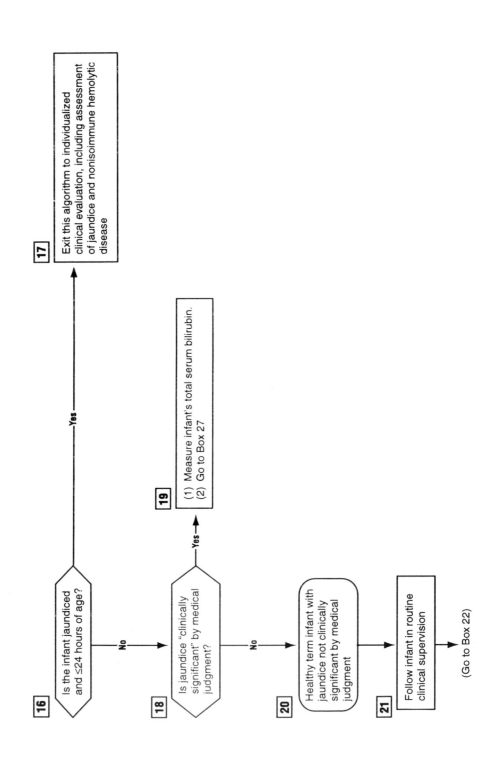

16 Is the infant jaundiced and ≤24 hours of age?

Yes →

17 Exit this algorithm to individualized clinical evaluation, including assessment of jaundice and nonisoimmune hemolytic disease

No →

18 Is jaundice "clinically significant" by medical judgment?

Yes →

19
(1) Measure infant's total serum bilirubin.
(2) Go to Box 27

No →

20 Healthy term infant with jaundice not clinically significant by medical judgment

21 Follow infant in routine clinical supervision

(Go to Box 22)

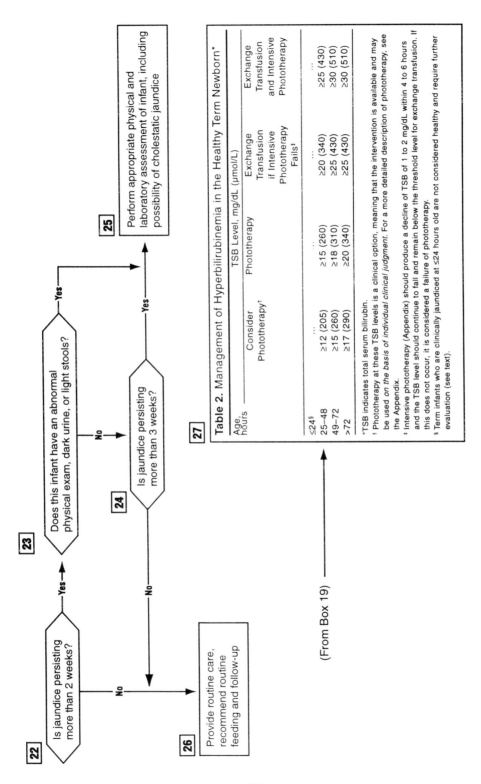

22 Is jaundice persisting more than 2 weeks?

No → **26** Provide routine care, recommend routine feeding and follow-up

Yes → **23** Does this infant have an abnormal physical exam, dark urine, or light stools?

23 No → **24** Is jaundice persisting more than 3 weeks?

24 No → **26**

24 Yes → **25**

23 Yes → **25** Perform appropriate physical and laboratory assessment of infant, including possibility of cholestatic jaundice

(From Box 19)

27

Table 2. Management of Hyperbilirubinemia in the Healthy Term Newborn*

Age, hours	TSB Level, mg/dL (µmol/L)			
	Consider Phototherapy†	Phototherapy	Exchange Transfusion if Intensive Phototherapy Fails‡	Exchange Transfusion and Intensive Phototherapy
≤24§	...	...	...	...
25–48	≥12 (205)	≥15 (260)	≥20 (340)	≥25 (430)
49–72	≥15 (260)	≥18 (310)	≥25 (430)	≥30 (510)
>72	≥17 (290)	≥20 (340)	≥25 (430)	≥30 (510)

*TSB indicates total serum bilirubin.

† Phototherapy at these TSB levels is a clinical option, meaning that the intervention is available and may be used *on the basis of individual clinical judgment*. For a more detailed description of phototherapy, see the Appendix.

‡ Intensive phototherapy (Appendix) should produce a decline of TSB of 1 to 2 mg/dL within 4 to 6 hours and the TSB level should continue to fall and remain below the threshold level for exchange transfusion. If this does not occur, it is considered a failure of phototherapy.

§ Term infants who are clinically jaundiced at ≤24 hours old are not considered healthy and require further evaluation (see text).

– 265 –

Appendix

Phototherapy

There is no standardized method for delivering phototherapy. Phototherapy units vary widely, as do the types of lamps used in these units. The following factors strongly influence the efficacy of phototherapy:

> The energy output (or irradiance) of the phototherapy light in the blue spectrum, measured in $\mu W/cm^2$;

> The spectrum of light delivered by the phototherapy unit, determined by the type of light source.

> The surface area of the infant exposed to phototherapy.

Commonly used phototherapy units contain a number of daylight, cool white, blue, or "special blue" fluorescent tubes. Other units use tungsten-halogen lamps in different configurations, either free-standing or as part of a radiant warming device. Most recently, fiberoptic systems have been developed that deliver light from a high-intensity lamp to a fiberoptic blanket. Most of these devices deliver enough output in the blue-green region of the visible spectrum to be effective for standard phototherapy use. When bilirubin levels approach the range at which exchange transfusion might be indicated, maximal efficacy should be sought. This can be achieved in the following manner.

The use of special blue tubes in standard fluorescent phototherapy units. Note that special blue (narrow spectrum) tubes carry the designation F20 T12/BB are not the same as blue tubes (F20 T12/B).[1] Special blue lights have the disadvantage of making the infant look blue, but in healthy newborns this is generally not a concern during the relatively brief period that phototherapy is necessary. To mitigate this effect, four special blue tubes may be used in the central portion of a standard phototherapy unit and two daylight fluorescent tubes may be used on either side.[2]

Regardless of the type of light used, its maximum irradiance should be employed. Standard fluorescent lamps accomplish this by bringing the light as close to the baby as possible. In the full-term nursery, this is most easily achieved by placing the infant in a bassinet (not an incubator) and lowering the lamps to within 15 to 20 cm of the infant. If this treatment causes slight warming of the infant, the lamps need to be elevated slightly. With halogen phototherapy lamps, however, there are no data to indicate how close to the baby the lamp can be positioned without incurring the risk of a burn. When halogen lamps are used, manufacturers' recommendations should be followed. The reflectors, light source, and transparent light filters (if any) should be kept clean.

The third way to improve phototherapy efficiency is to increase the surface area of the infant exposed to the lights. This is done, most simply, by placing the infant on a fiberoptic blanket while using a standard phototherapy system described above.[3] If fiberoptic units are not available, several phototherapy lamps can be placed around the infant. When a single phototherapy unit is used, the area of exposure can be increased by placing a white reflecting surface (such as a sheet) around the bassinet so that light is reflected onto the baby's skin. Removing diapers will also increase the exposed surface area.

Intermittent Versus Continuous Phototherapy

Clinical studies comparing intermittent with continuous phototherapy have produced conflicting results.[4-6] Because all light exposure increases bilirubin excretion (compared with darkness), no plausible scientific rationale exists for using intermittent phototherapy. In the majority of circumstances, however, phototherapy does not need to be continuous. Phototherapy may be interrupted during feeding or brief parental visits. Individual judgment should be exercised. If the infant is admitted to the hospital with a bilirubin level ≥25 mg/dL (428 μmol/L), intensive phototherapy should be administered continuously until a satisfactory decline in the serum bilirubin level occurs or exchange transfusion is initiated.

Intensity of Phototherapy

The intensity of phototherapy (number of lights, distance from infant, and use of double phototherapy, use of special lights) should also be tailored to the infant's needs. In many circumstances intensive phototherapy is not necessary. However, if the serum bilirubin level is rising in spite of conventional phototherapy or the infant is admitted with a serum bilirubin concentration within the exchange transfusion range, the necessary steps should be taken to increase the intensity of phototherapy during preparation for exchange transfusion. With the light sources commonly used, it is impossible to overdose the patient.

Hydration

To our knowledge, no evidence exists that excess fluid administration affects the serum bilirubin concentration. Some infants who are admitted with high bilirubin levels are also mildly dehydrated, however, may need supplemental fluid intake to correct their dehydration. As these infants are almost always breast-fed, the best fluid to use in these circumstances is a milk-based formula, because it inhibits the enterohepatic circulation of bilirubin and helps lower the serum bilirubin level. Because the photoproducts responsible for the decline in serum bilirubin are excreted in both urine and bile, maintaining adequate hydration and good urine output should help improve the efficacy of phototherapy.[7] Routine supplementation (with dextrose water) of infants receiving phototherapy is not indicated.

When Should Phototherapy Be Stopped?

A recent study found that, in infants who do not have hemolytic disease, the average bilirubin rebound after phototherapy is less than 1 mg/dL (17 µmol/L).[8] Phototherapy may be discontinued when the serum bilirubin level falls below 14 to 15 mg/dL. Discharge from the hospital need not be delayed in order to observe the infant for rebound and, in most cases, no further measurement of bilirubin is necessary. If phototherapy is initiated early and discontinued before the infant is 3 to 4 days old, additional outpatient follow-up may be necessary.

Appendix References

1. Ennever JF. Blue light, green light, white light, more light: treatment of neonatal jaundice. *Clin Perinatol.* 1990;17:407–478
2. Hammerman C, Eidelman A, Lee K-S, et al. Comparative measurements of phototherapy: a practical guide. *Pediatrics.* 1981;67:368–372
3. Holtrop PC, Ruedisueli K, Maisels MJ. Double versus single phototherapy in low birthweight infants. *Pediatrics.* 1992;90:674–677
4. Maurer HM, Shumway C, Draper DA, et al. Controlled trial comparing agar, intermittent phototherapy, and continuous phototherapy for reducing neonatal hyperbilirubinemia. *J Pediatr.* 1973;82:73–76
5. Rubaltelli FF, Zanardo V, Granati B. Effect of various phototherapy regimens on bilirubin decrement. *Pediatrics.* 1978;61:838–841
6. Lau SP, Fung KP. Serum bilirubin kinetics in intermittent phototherapy of physiological jaundice. *Arch Dis Child.* 1984;59:892–894
7. Wu PYK, Hodgman JE, Kirkpatrick BV, et al. Metabolic aspects of phototherapy. *Pediatrics.* 1985;75:427–433
8. Lazar L, Litwin A, Nerlob P. Phototherapy for neonatal nonhemolytic hyperbilirubinemia. Analysis of rebound and indications for discontinuing phototherapy. *Clin Pediatr.* 1993;32:264–267

Technical Report Summary

**Management of
Hyperbilirubinemia
in Healthy Newborns**

Author:
Zaid Smith, PhD

American Academy of Pediatrics
PO Box 927, 141 Northwest Point Blvd
Elk Grove Village, IL 60009-0927

1.0 Introduction

In May 1993, Emergency Care Research Institute (ECRI) was asked by the American Academy of Pediatrics (AAP) to participate in the formation of a new practice parameter for the treatment of hyperbilirubinemia in otherwise healthy newborns.

ECRI is the leading independent organization committed to the assessment, evaluation, and continued improvement of health care technology. ECRI's mission is to improve the safety, efficacy, and cost-effectiveness of health technology, and broadly encompasses devices, drugs, procedures, facilities, and related standards and guidelines. The results of ECRI's research and experience are made available through publications, information systems, laboratory services, seminars, and technical assistance and management programs. The Institute has more than 25 years' experience. Its 200-member staff includes physicians, doctoral life scientists, epidemiologists, and bio-statisticians; biomedical, electrical, chemical, and mechanical engineers; nurses; hospital planners; attorneys; and specialists in hospital administration, financial and policy analysis, risk management, and medical research data-bases. ECRI's strict enforcement of conflict-of-interest guidelines guarantees an unbiased approach to all projects. ECRI strives to maintain an environment that encourages maximum objectivity and integrity of process. Neither ECRI nor any of its staff members has a financial interest in the sale of any medical technology, and no form of remuneration from pharmaceutical or device manufacturers is permitted.

ECRI was asked to write the technical report, a supplement to the practice parameter for the treatment of hyperbilirubinemia in newborns. To accomplish this task, ECRI independently assessed the scientific data upon which the Scientific Committee based its decisions as well as the assumptions upon which the scientific and clinical literature was based. The first part of the report (Section 2) presents evidence pertaining to the incidence of brain damage caused by hyperbilirubinemia in healthy term neonates. Specific topics in the practice parameter are amplified in Section 3. The appendix in the full technical report provides a detailed review of recent literature pertaining to hyperbilirubinemia in healthy term infants along with the search strategy employed to generate a database of more than 3400 articles on neonatal jaundice. This database has been turned over to the AAP.

ECRI findings indicate that the changes in the treatment of hyperbilirubinemia proposed in the new practice parameter appear not to pose any added risk of adverse outcome in jaundiced infants. Evidence also indicates that for many infants, less intervention is beneficial. Significant gaps exist, however, in our knowledge of the association between hyperbilirubinemia and brain damage. Efforts should be made to gather information on the impact of this new standard on patient outcome.

2.0 The Current Status of the Evidence for Bilirubin Toxicity in Healthy Full-Term Newborns

Literature from the past 3 decades pertaining to hyperbilirubinemia's effects on the mental and physical development of healthy term infants has been reviewed critically. For the most part, data from studies on the following groups were not included: isoimmunized infants, those with genetic predispositions to jaundice (eg, glucose-6-phosphate dehydrogenase [G6PD] deficiency), and neonates with birth weights less than 2500 g or gestational ages of less than 37 weeks. Infants with these characteristics who were studied in the Collaborative Perinatal Project (CPP) were not excluded, however, because of their size and importance. The study population consisted primarily of full-term, healthy newborns; often the data on preterm and isoimmunized infants were not singled out for separate analysis.

This literature has also been examined in detail elsewhere by Newman and Maisels and Newman and Klebanoff. Our general conclusion, after careful statistical analyses of the studies on which these reviews are based, is that for full-term (over 37 weeks' gestation), full-weight (over 2500 g) infants who do not have isoimmunization, genetic predisposition (eg, G6PD), or sepsis, there appears to be little, if any, risk of toxicity from serum bilirubin levels up to 20 mg/dL (342 µmol/L). This does not mean that levels above 20 mg/dL are dangerous, but rather that the data are less determinate for this group because of the small number of infants with these bilirubin concentrations. Although no risk of toxicity has been proven for these infants, bilirubin at these levels has not been proven to be harmless.

The most important epidemiological data linking bilirubin to brain damage in the healthy population came from the CPP, a massive, inclusive study of newborns that was designed originally to elucidate the perinatal correlates of cerebral palsy. The study was not designed explicitly to test the hypothesis that high bilirubin levels cause brain damage (or, more precisely, are a close correlate). One result showed that the number of bilirubin measurements made varied among the infants, depending on their birth weight or the results of their previous bilirubin test. Infants were not tested consistently over time, and only the peak level of bilirubin was recorded. Extrapolations of the duration of exposure to a given bilirubin level have been made based on the data, but these are tenuous.

Another result of the CPP (which was designed to examine bilirubin as a correlate to brain damage *per se*), in addition to the inadequate data gathered on the predictor variable, showed that the data had a post-hoc element. Because the possible confounding effects of bilirubin (eg, isoimmunization, maternal diabetes, G6PD deficiency) were not factored into the design of the study, researchers were left with the task of parsing out the potential (negative) effects of this pigment statistically. Although this approach is not without validity, it is limited by the quality and types of data gathered initially.

Successive analyses of the data (or subsets thereof) have been progressively more sophisticated, and yet progressively less effective, culminating in the recent reanalysis by Newman and Klebanoff, which basically found that elevated levels of bilirubin have no adverse effects.

Historically, the CPP has had a great impact on the treatment of hyperbilirubinemia—in part because the study was so large and in part because its early results suggested that any level of bilirubin was toxic. Flaws in its design—most notably, its inability to address the effects of high bilirubin levels—have led to its eventual decay, however, as a cynosure study. Even if these results are taken at face value, the effects of bilirubin on the target population are quite modest, if detectable at all. Newman and Maisels had the same findings essentially. The results of their review were expressed in millipoints of IQ decrement per milligrams per deciliter of bilirubin, however, which could suggest that bilirubin, like lead, generally has a depressive effect on brain functioning. This has not been established.

Studies other than those associated with the CPP and designed more explicitly to examine the effects of hyperbilirubinemia on brain functioning have been less supportive of a deleterious effect of bilirubin on the healthy infant population. In general, little consistent evidence of bilirubin affecting IQ or cognitive functions has been forthcoming, at least for the healthy, full-term infant. The evidence that hyperbilirubinemia is associated with hearing loss or motor dysfunctions is more ambiguous, with some researchers finding an association, while others do not. Sometimes these opposing results are from studies on the same (or similar) populations. As discussed later, there is reason to suspect that all forms of hyperbilirubinemia are not equally relevant to nervous system damage.

There is no solid evidence that a particular value of bilirubin is the threshold level for toxic effects. Newman and Klebanoff, in their reanalysis of the CPP data, searched explicitly for a threshold value but found none. Seidman and colleagues suggested a possible toxicity threshold of 20 mg/dL; their analysis neither ruled it out nor confirmed this theory. Thus, the thresholds for treatment of hyperbilirubinemia described in the practice parameter are those that were deemed prudent despite the considerable ambiguity in the clinical literature.

3.0 Comments and Recommendations on the Proposed Practice Parameter

3.1 Possible Impact of the Proposed Parameter

On the basis of ECRI's analysis of the current literature pertaining to hyperbilirubinemia in healthy newborns and literature analyzed by Newman and Maisels, it appears that the proposed changes in the treatment of hyperbilirubinemia in healthy newborns entail minimal risk. The evidence supports the view that the new practice parameter will not increase the risk of deleterious outcomes in jaundiced infants and may markedly decrease the amount of intervention required.

Who will be affected by this practice parameter? Data from the United States on the distribution of peak serum bilirubin levels indicate that 2% or fewer untreated infants will have peak bilirubin levels greater than 20 mg/dL (>342 μmol/L); European data suggest that as many as 6% will have these levels. Because comparatively few infants have jaundice of this magnitude, these percentages are not entirely reliable, and vary depending on the frequency of breastfeeding, ethnicity of the hospital's population, method of bilirubin measurement, and other factors. When phototherapy is administered, however, the number of infants who have serum bilirubin levels above 20 mg/dL appears to be about 0.2%.

Because the practice parameter model has established bilirubin's toxicity to be greatest when the serum levels are high, the children who are of most interest are those with the highest bilirubin levels. The population of infants who currently have bilirubin levels reaching 20 mg/dL or greater is likely to remain constant, since this group has presumably received phototherapy before their bilirubin reached this level. This group probably comprises 2% of all newborns. It follows that 98% of neonates will not receive phototherapy if the trigger point is moved to 20 mg/dL. The exact number of infants currently receiving phototherapy is unknown, but if a threshold for initiation of therapy at 15 mg/dL (257 μmol/L) is being used, 5% of all infants are probably treated. Thus about 3% of all the newborns (about 120 000 per year) who may be receiving phototherapy might be spared the trouble of undergoing this treatment.

Although the percentage of infants currently receiving phototherapy who are treated at home is unknown, this number is presumably increasing as hospitals discharge infants earlier. For the sake of discussion, we assume it is 60%. Published costs for hospital phototherapy range from $125 to $600 per day, while home phototherapy may cost $40 to $125 daily. ECRI has observed, however, that many companies administering home phototherapy charge a flat rate, often around $600, on the assumption that phototherapy will last less than 4 days. If the latter figure, and the average hospital cost is $1200, the total national savings is roughly $ 100 million a year. If the costs of phototherapy are higher, or if the percentage of patients being treated at home is lower, the savings is even greater, a figure of $140 million is certainly possible. ECRI does not believe that potential savings should be a basis for adopting the proposed practice parameter, however.

Will changing the thresholds for initiation of phototherapy increase the number of neonates who receive exchange transfusions? Probably not, since in most infants, serum bilirubin levels increase fairly slowly and decrease rapidly in response to phototherapy. Moreover, there is evidence that delaying the onset of phototherapy until bilirubin levels reach 18.7 mg/dL (320 μmol/L) has no adverse effects compared with initiating therapy at 14.6 mg/dL (250 μmol/L). Thus the population of infants with bilirubin levels that reach 30 mg/dL (513 μmol/L) is not likely to increase, even if phototherapy is not initiated until the infant's bilirubin level reaches 20 mg/dL. In fact, administering phototherapy at greater intensities will probably decrease this population. The issue of exchange transfusions may need further consideration, however. The risk of mortality from exchange transfusion is estimated to be between 0.2% and 2%, with a morbidity risk of around 5%; however, the data on the risks of this procedure probably are somewhat out of date.

Since the advent of phototherapy, exchange transfusions have become rarer events, and the number of hospital personnel familiar with the procedure has probably become smaller, making the risks higher than before. The present risk of kernicterus is unknown—0.3% or 0.003%, but it is low enough to pose the question of where the balance of risk between exchange transfusions and kernicterus should lie. Determining the criteria for performing exchange transfusions has not been easy.

There is widespread variability in the manner in which hyperbilirubinemia is treated. Some have argued that the "kinder, gentler" guidelines that have been proposed would change nothing, because they are being practiced already. Others have argued correctly that changing the current recommendations for treatment could mean subjecting society to an enormous experiment. ECRI has encountered some physicians treating hyperbilirubinemia in healthy newborns with bilirubin levels of 7 mg/dL, and others waiting until levels reach 20 or 25 mg/dL; apparently such variability is common. Thus the experiment is being conducted already—but no one is gathering the results. Actual widespread treatment practices cannot be assumed to be the same as those published by neonatologists who are particularly involved with bilirubin. ECRI recommends that the AAP gather more information on the variations in current treatment practices and outcomes. Acquiring such data is essential to determining whether changing the treatment of hyperbilirubinemia has any effect, positive or negative.

3.2 Comments on the Aspects of the Practice Parameter

Clinicians should remember that measurements of bilirubin are not particularly accurate nor precise. Measurements of direct bilirubin are subject to wide variations and should not be used. Direct bilirubin has only a loose relationship with unconjugated bilirubin. Because of its photosensitivity and insolubility, bilirubin is difficult to measure accurately. Although high-pressure liquid chromatography is the most effective method of measuring bilirubin, it is not usually clinically practical. The Kodak Ektachem test is probably the second most effective method; it is somewhat superior to the more widely used diazo and spectrophotometric methods. Measurements of total serum bilirubin have always varied widely between laboratories. The coefficient of variation (CV) of bilirubin testing is approximately 20%, and nearly the same whether the test is automated or not. (For comparison, the CV of albumin testing is 7%, and of cholesterol testing, 8%.) These uncertainties associated with bilirubin measurement are not new, but are worth mentioning in light of the renewed context of decisions based on them. Practitioners should be informed of the methods and reliability of bilirubin testing conducted in the clinics, and regard the action levels in the practice parameter as relative guides, rather than absolutes.

Although icterometers or transcutaneous bilirubinometers may be useful for taking rough measurements of bilirubin in serum, they are neither accurate nor reliable enough to be used for critical determinations.

In a large randomized trial, the safety of phototherapy was demonstrated to be comparable to having no treatment; it follows then that receiving no treatment is as safe as phototherapy. Given that phototherapy will be administered, however, the guidelines for its application are reasonable. Intensive phototherapy has been used in Europe, America, and elsewhere. Variations exist in the expressions of light intensity and in the bulbs used. The Phillips TL20W/52 is used in foreign studies as opposed to the F20 T12/BB mentioned in the practice parameter. Both bulbs are reported to have a narrow spectrum of output, near the bilirubin absorbance spectrum. If it is assumed that the lamps have equal outputs, levels as high as 30 $\mu W/cm^2/nm$ may be use. For comparison, we measured the illumination intensity of the sun in the blue wavelengths used for phototherapy on a rainy day to be about 18 $\mu W/cm^2/nm$ (40°N latitude on the solstice at 2 pm), while on a cloudless day, the intensity was reported to be over 100 $\mu W/cm^2/nm$. It is possible that infants are quite tolerant of the irradiance levels of intensive phototherapy.

As an aside, in the United Kingdom phototherapy is sometimes given intermittently, reportedly with equal effectiveness.

Phototherapy is reputed to be effective in preventing kernicterus. (This has not been proven, however; the one study that examined this issue is inconclusive because the sample size was too small.) The diagnosis of hyperbilirubinemia and the subsequent therapy does impose a psychological cost on the mother-child relationship. It is hoped that a less invasive means of treating jaundice will be developed, and that efforts will be made to keep mothers from being alarmed over this common occurrence.

Breast-feeding infants are likely to have higher bilirubin levels than those who are formula-fed. The manner in which breast milk augments bilirubin levels is not known. Because breast milk is the natural food of the human neonate, the levels of jaundice seen in breast-fed infants should be considered the biological norm, which has been artificially depressed in infants fed formula. Mothers should not be led to believe that some substance in their milk is adversely affecting their infant. In the United States, breast-feeding may not result in a substantially higher number of infants with hyperbilirubinemia, at bilirubin levels of 16 mg/dL (274 μmol/L) or greater. The continuation of breast-feeding while administering phototherapy is practically as effective as suspending breastfeeding; interruption of breast-feeding is unnecessary.

Home phototherapy may be more conducive to breast-feeding than is hospitalization. A possible alternative to phototherapy, or to the cessation of breast-feeding in some cases, may be supplementation of breast milk with formula, which would provide the child access to the bilirubin-inhibiting factor in cow's milk.

3.3 Questions for Further Study

There are many outstanding questions about hyperbilirubinemia. Some of those questions pertaining to the biologic action of bilirubin have been discussed previously, but more can be addressed.

The precise relationship between serum bilirubin levels and brain damage is elusive; this could be due to secular and population changes in the nature of the disease, or to the confounding of several different conditions, which results in similar symptoms. Using current methods (including current standards for experimental design), we need to obtain a better understanding of the nature of the disease we are attempting to prevent. The free bilirubin hypothesis may provide an elegant theoretic explanation of how bilirubin toxicity could occur, but the postulated interrelatedness of albumin, age, pH, and bilirubin levels has not been translated into workable clinical measurements.

We need to know what the incidence of kernicterus is in the present population. Who are the infants who get the disease? How many are there? Cases of the kernicterus occur despite our efforts to prevent it, which tells us one thing, if nothing else—that we don't understand the cause(s).

It may be unknown whether bilirubin actually enters the brain, and if so, how. The only way to be certain that bilirubin has or has not entered the brain is to perform autoradiography, followed by recovery of the labeled substance to ensure it is still bilirubin. Studies in which radiolabeled bilirubin has been infused, followed by flushing of the vasculature and scintillation counting of the brain tissue, may have shown only that bilirubin is absorbed on the surface of endothelial cells, or is taken up by them, without entering the brain.

We know very little about the circumstances that allow albumin to release bilirubin. If, as it now appears, specific albumin receptors on the liver are nonexistent, albumin could be releasing bilirubin to cells of other tissues as well. Albumin may be thought of more usefully as a transport protein, rather than as an "end sink" for bilirubin.

The development of the blood-brain barrier in humans, and the factors that may lead to its opening need to be better.

The enterohepatic circulation of bilirubin may still provide an alternative means for interdiction of hyperbilirubinemia. Should an effective absorber of bilirubin be found (possibly a purified agar), hyperbilirubinemia could be treatable at home at very little cost or inconvenience.

Because our perception and knowledge of hyperbilirubinemia will certainly change in the coming years, it is possible that these issues will require revisiting in the future. Currently, the best available data indicate that the proposed practice parameter is a safe step in the right direction.

The Management of Minor Closed Head Injury in Children

- *Clinical Practice Guideline*
- *Technical Report Summary*

Readers of this clinical practice guideline are urged to review the technical report to enhance the evidence-based decision-making process. The report is available on the Pediatrics electronic pages Web site at the following URL: http://www.pediatrics.org/cgi/content/full/104/6/e78.

Clinical Practice Guideline:
The Management of Minor Closed Head Injury in Children

Author:

Subcommittee on Minor Head Trauma

American Academy of Pediatrics
Committee on Quality Improvement
American Academy of Family Physicians
Commission on Clinical Policies and Research

American Academy of Pediatrics
PO Box 927, 141 Northwest Point Blvd
Elk Grove Village, IL 60009-0927

Subcommittee on Management of Minor Head Injury

John B. Coombs, MD, Chairperson

Hannan Bell, PhD, AAFP,
   Methodologic Consultant
Robert L. Davis, MD, MPH,
   AAP, Consultant
Theodore G. Ganiats, MD, AAFP
Michael D. Hagen, MD, AAFP,
   1992–1993
Jack Haller, MD, AAP, Consultant
Charles J. Homer, MD, MPH,
   AAP, Subcommittee
   Methodologist

David M. Jaffee, MD,
   AAP Section on Emergency
   Medicine Liaison
Hector James, MD, AAP
Larry Kleinman, MD, AAP,
   Consultant 1992–1994
Jane Knapp, MD, AAP
J. Michael Dean, MD, AAP
Patricia Nobel, MD, AAP
Sanford Schneider, MD, AAP

AAP Committee on Quality Improvement
1992–1997

David A. Bergman, MD, Chairperson

Richard D. Baltz, MD
James R. Cooley, MD
John B. Coombs, MD
Michael J. Goldberg, MD
   Sections Liaison
Charles J. Homer, MD, MPH,
   Section on Epidemiology
   Liaison

Paul V. Miles, MD
Lawrence F. Nazarian, MD, 1992–1994
Thomas A. Riemenschneider, MD
   1992–1995
Kenneth B. Roberts, MD
Daniel W. Shea, MD, 1992–1995
William M. Zurhellen, MD

AAFP Commission on Clinical Policies and Research
1996–1997

Joseph E. Scherger, MD, Chairperson, 1997
Richard G. Roberts, MD, JD, Chairperson, 1996

Roman M. Hendrickson, MD
William J. Hueston, MD, 1996
Stephen J. Spann, MD
Thomas Gilbert, MD, MPH, 1997
Theodore G. Ganiats, MD
William R. Phillips, MD, MPH
Richard K. Zimmerman, MD, MPH
Lee A. Green, MD, MPH
Jonathan E. Rodnick, MD
Barbara P. Yawn, MD, MSc
Linda L. Barrett, MD, Resident
   Representative, 1997
Enrico G. Jones, MD, Resident
   Representative, 1996

Theresa-Ann Clark, Student
   Representative
Ross R. Black, MD, Liaison,
   Commission on Quality and
   Scope of Practice
Leah Raye Mabry, MD, Liaison,
   Commission on Public Health
Herbert F. Young, MD, MA,
   Staff Executive
Hanan S. Bell, PhD,
   Assistant Staff Executive

Abstract

The American Academy of Pediatrics (AAP) and its Committee on Quality Improvement in collaboration with the American Academy of Family Physicians (AAFP) and its Commission on Clinical Policies and Research, and in conjunction with experts in neurology, emergency medicine and critical care, research methodologists, and practicing physicians have developed this practice parameter. This parameter provides recommendations for the management of a previously neurologically healthy child with a minor closed head injury who, at the time of injury, may have experienced temporary loss of consciousness, experienced an impact seizure, vomited, or experienced other signs and symptoms. These recommendations derive from a thorough review of the literature and expert consensus. The methods and results of the literature review and data analyses including evidence tables can be found in the technical report. This practice parameter is not intended as a sole source of guidance for the management of children with minor closed head injuries. Rather, it is designed to assist physicians by providing an analytic framework for the evaluation and management of this condition. It is not intended to replace clinical judgment or establish a protocol for all patients with a minor head injury, and rarely will provide the only appropriate approach to the problem.

The practice parameter, "The Management of Minor Closed Head Injury in Children," was reviewed by the AAFP Commission on Clinical Policies and Research and individuals appointed by the AAFP and appropriate committees and sections of the AAP including the Chapter Review Group, a focus group of office-based pediatricians representing each AAP District: Gene R. Adams, MD; Robert M. Corwin, MD; Diane Fuquay, MD; Barbara M. Harley, MD; Thomas J. Herr, MD, Chair; Kenneth E. Mathews, MD; Robert D. Mines, MD; Lawrence C. Pakula, MD; Howard B. Weinblatt, MD; and Delosa A. Young, MD.

The supporting data are contained in a technical report available at http://www.pediatrics.org/cgi/content/full/104/6/e78.

Minor closed head injury is one of the most frequent reasons for visits to a physician.[1] Although >95 000 children experience a traumatic brain injury each year in the United States,[2] consensus is lacking about the acute care of children with minor closed head injury. The evaluation and management of injured children may be influenced by local practice customs, settings where children are evaluated, the type and extent of financial coverage, and the availability of technology and medical staffing.

Because of the magnitude of the problem and the potential seriousness of closed head injury among children, the AAP and the American Academy of Family Physicians (AAFP) undertook the development of an evidence-based parameter for health care professionals who care for children with minor closed head injury. In this document, the term Subcommittee is used to denote the Subcommittee on Minor Closed Head Injury, which reports to the AAP Committee on Quality Improvement, and the AAFP Commission on Clinical Policies, Research, and Scientific Affairs.

While developing this practice parameter, the Subcommittee attempted to find evidence of benefits resulting from 1 or more patient management options. However, at many points, adequate data were not available from the medical literature to provide guidance for the management of children with mild head injury. When such data were unavailable, we did not make specific recommendations for physicians and other professionals but instead we presented a range of practice options deemed acceptable by the Subcommittee.

An algorithm at the end of this parameter presents recommendations and options in the context of direct patient care. Management is discussed for the initial evaluation of a child with minor closed head injury, and the disposition after evaluation. These recommendations and options may be modified to fit the needs of individual patients.

Purpose and Scope

This practice parameter is specifically intended for previously neurologically healthy children of either sex 2 through 20 years of age, with isolated minor closed head injury.

The parameter defines children with minor closed head injury as those who have normal mental status at the initial examination, who have no abnormal or focal findings on neurologic (including fundoscopic) examination, and who have no physical evidence of skull fracture (such as hemotympanum, Battle's sign, or palpable bone depression).

This parameter also is intended to address children who may have experienced temporary loss of consciousness (duration <1 minute) with injury, may have had a seizure immediately after injury, may have vomited after injury, or may have exhibited signs and symptoms such as headache and lethargy. The treatment of these children is addressed by this parameter, provided that they seem to be normal as described in the preceding paragraph at the time of evaluation.

This parameter is not intended for victims of multiple trauma, for children with unobserved loss of consciousness, or for patients with known or suspected cervical spine injury. Children who may otherwise fulfill the criteria for minor closed head injury, but for whom this parameter is not intended include patients with a history of bleeding diatheses or neurologic disorders potentially aggravated by trauma (such as arteriovenous malformations or shunts), patients with suspected intentional head trauma (eg, suspected child abuse), or patients with a language barrier.

The term brief loss of consciousness in this parameter refers to a duration of loss of consciousness of 1 minute or less. This parameter does not make any inference that the risk for intracranial injury changes with any specific length of unconsciousness lasting <1 minute. The treatment of children with loss of consciousness of longer duration is not addressed by this parameter.

Finally, this parameter refers only to the management of children evaluated by a health care professional immediately or shortly after (within 24 hours) injury. This parameter is not intended for the management of children who are initially evaluated >24 hours after injury.

Methods for Parameter Development

The literature review encompassed original research on minor closed head trauma in children, including studies on the prevalence of intracranial injury, the sensitivity and specificity of different imaging modalities, the utility of early diagnosis of intracranial injury, the effectiveness of various patient management strategies, and the impact of minor closed head injury on subsequent child health. Research was included if it had data exclusively on children or identifiable child-specific data, if cases were comparable with the case definition in the parameter, and if the data were published in a peer-reviewed journal. Review articles and articles based solely on expert opinion were excluded.

An initial search was performed on several computerized databases including Medline (1966–1993) using the terms head trauma and head injury. The search was restricted to infants, children, and adolescents, and to English-language articles published after 1966. A total of 422 articles were identified. Titles and abstracts were reviewed by the Subcommittee and articles were reviewed if any reviewer considered the title relevant. This process identified 168 articles that were sent to Subcommittee members with a literature review form to categorize study design, identify study questions, and abstract pertinent data. In addition, reference lists in the articles were reviewed for additional sources, and 125 additional articles were identified. After excluding review articles and other studies not meeting entry criteria, a total of 64 articles were included for review. All articles were reabstracted by the methodologists and the data summarized on evidence tables. Differences in case definition, outcome definition, and study samples precluded pooling of data among studies.

The published data proved extremely limited for a number of study questions, and direct queries were placed to several authors for child-specific data. Because these data have not been formally published, the Subcommittee does not rest strong conclusions on them; however, they are included in the Technical Report. The Technical Report produced along with this practice parameter contains supporting scientific data and analysis including evidence tables and is available at http://www.pediatrics.org/cgi/content/full/104/6/e78.

Summary

Initial Evaluation and Management of the Child With
Minor Closed Head Injury and No Loss of Consciousness

Observation

For children with minor closed head injury and no loss of consciousness, a thorough history and appropriate physical and neurologic examination should be performed. Observation in the clinic, office, emergency department, or at home, under the care of a competent caregiver is recommended for children with minor closed head injury and no loss of consciousness. Observation implies regular monitoring by a competent adult who would be able to recognize abnormalities and to seek appropriate assistance. The use of cranial computed tomography (CT) scan, skull radiograph, or magnetic resonance imaging (MRI) is not recommended for the initial evaluation and management of the child with minor closed head injury and no loss of consciousness.

Initial Evaluation of the Child With Minor Closed
Head Injury With Brief Loss of Consciousness

Observation or Cranial CT Scan

For children with minor closed head injury and brief loss of consciousness (<1 minute), a thorough history and an appropriate physical and neurologic examination should be performed. Observation, in the office, clinic, emergency department, hospital, or home under the care of a competent caregiver, may be used to evaluate children with minor closed head injury with brief loss of consciousness. Cranial CT scanning may also be used, in addition to observation, in the initial evaluation and management of children with minor closed head injury with loss of consciousness.

The use of skull radiographs or MRI in the initial management of children with minor closed head injury and loss of consciousness is not recommended. However, there are limited situations in which MRI and skull radiography are options (see sections on skull radiographs and on MRI).

Patient Management Considerations

Many factors may influence how management strategies influence outcomes for children with minor closed head injury. These factors include: 1) the prevalence of intracranial injury, 2) the percentage of intracranial injuries that need medical or neurosurgical intervention (ie, the percentage of these injuries that, if left undiagnosed or untreated, leads to disability or death), 3) the relative accuracy of clinical examination, skull radiographs, and CT scans as diagnostic tools to detect such intracranial injuries that benefit from medical or neurosurgical intervention, 4) the efficacy of treatment for intracranial injuries, and 5) the detrimental effect on outcome, if any, of delay from the time of injury to the time of diagnosis and intervention.

This last factor, delay of diagnosis and intervention, is particularly relevant when trying to decide between a clinical strategy of immediate CT scanning of all patients as opposed to a strategy that relies primarily on patient observation, with CT scanning reserved for rare patients whose conditions change. To our knowledge, no published studies were available for review that compared clinically meaningful outcomes (ie, morbidity or mortality) between children receiving different management regimens such as immediate neuroimaging, or observation. Although some studies were able to demonstrate the presence of intracranial abnormalities on CT scans or MRIs among children with minor head injury, no known evidence suggested that immediate neuroimaging of asymptomatic children improved outcomes for these children, compared with the outcomes for children managed primarily with examination and observation.

Initial Management of the Child With Minor Closed Head Injury and No Loss of Consciousness

Minor closed head injury without loss of consciousness is a common occurrence in childhood. Available data suggest that the risk of intracranial injury is negligible in this situation. Population-based studies have found that fewer than 1 in 5000 patients with minor closed head injury and no loss of consciousness have intracranial injuries that require medical or neurosurgical intervention. In 1 study of 5252 low-risk patients, mostly adults, none were found to have an intracranial injury after minor head injury.[3] Comparably sized studies do not exist for children. In 2 much smaller studies of children with minor head injury, among those with normal neurologic examination findings and no loss of consciousness, amnesia, vomiting, headache, or mental status abnormalities, no children had abnormal CT scan findings.[4,5]

Observation

Among children with minor closed head injury and no loss of consciousness, a thorough history and appropriate physical and neurologic examination should be performed. Subcommittee consensus was that observation, in the clinic, office, emergency department, or home under the care of a competent observer, be used as the primary management strategy. If on examination the patient's condition appears normal (as outlined earlier), no additional tests are needed and the child can be safely discharged to the care of a responsible caregiver. The recommended duration of observation is discussed in the section titled "Disposition of the Child With Minor Head Injury."

CT Scan/MRI

With such a low prevalence of intracranial injury, the Subcommittee believed that the marginal benefits of early detection of intracranial injury afforded by routine brain imaging studies such as CT or MRI were outweighed by considerations of cost, inconvenience, resource allocation, and possible side effects attributable to sedation or inappropriate interventions (eg, medical, surgical, or other interventions based on incidental CT findings in asymptomatic children).

Skull Radiographs

Skull radiographs have only a very limited role in the evaluation of children with minor closed head injury, no loss of consciousness, and no signs of skull fracture (ie, no palpable depression, hemotympanum, or Battle's sign). The substantial rate of false-positive results provided by skull radiographs (ie, a skull fracture detected on skull radiographs in the absence of intracranial injury) along with the low prevalence of intracranial injury among this specific subset of patients, leads to a low predictive value of skull radiographs. Most children with abnormal skull radiographs will not harbor significant intracranial lesions and conversely intracranial injury occurs in the absence of a skull fracture detected on skull radiographs.

There may be some clinical scenarios in which a practitioner desires imaging such as the case of a child with a scalp hematoma over the course of the meningeal artery. In situations such as these, the Subcommittee believes that clinical judgment should prevail. However, given the relatively low predictive value of skull radiographs, the Subcommittee believes that, if imaging is desired, cranial CT scan is the more satisfactory imaging modality.

Initial Management of the Child With Minor Closed Head Injury and Brief Loss of Consciousness

Among children with minor closed head injury, loss of consciousness is uncommon but is associated with an increased risk for intracranial injury. Studies performed since the advent of CT scanning suggest that children with loss of consciousness, or who demonstrate amnesia at the time of evaluation, or who have headache or vomiting at the time of evaluation, have a prevalence of intracranial injury detectable on CT that ranges from 0% to 7%.[5-8] Although most of these intracranial lesions will remain clinically insignificant, a substantial proportion of children, between 2% and 5% of those with minor head injury and loss of consciousness, may require neurosurgical intervention.[6-8] The differences in findings among studies are likely attributable to differences in selection criteria, along with random variation among studies with limited sample size. Although these findings might have been biased somewhat if more seriously injured patients were preferentially selected for CT scans, even studies in which patients were explicitly stated to be neurologically normal and asymptomatic found children with clinically significant injuries that required intervention.[6]

In past studies of children with minor head injury, patient selection may have led to overestimates of the prevalence of intracranial injury. Many of these studies looked at patients referred to emergency departments or trauma centers, patients brought to emergency departments after examination in the field by emergency personnel, or patients for whom the reason for obtaining CT scans was not clearly stated. These factors may have led to the selection of a patient population at higher risk for intracranial injury than the patients specifically addressed in this practice parameter.

As evidence of this, population-based studies before the widespread availability of CT scanning found the prevalence of clinically significant intracranial injury after minor closed head injury to be far less than estimated by the aforementioned studies. One study found a prevalence of intracranial injury that required neurosurgery to be as low as .02%.[9] This discrepancy is consistent also with the fact that many lesions currently identified with cranial CT were not recognized before the availability of this technology. Because most of these lesions do not progress or require neurosurgical intervention, most would not have been diagnosed in studies before the availability of CT scan.

Observation

As discussed earlier, the Subcommittee did not find evidence to show that immediate neuroimaging of asymptomatic children produced demonstrable benefits compared with a management strategy of initial observation alone. In light of these considerations, there was Subcommittee consensus based on limited evidence that for children who are neurologically normal after minor closed head injury with loss of consciousness, patient observation was an acceptable management option.

If the health care practitioner chooses observation alone, it may be performed in the clinic, office, emergency department, hospital, or at home under the care of a competent observer, typically a parent or suitable guardian. If the observer seems unable to follow or comply with the instructions for home observation, observation under the supervision of a health care practitioner is to be considered.

CT Scan

Data that support the routine use of CT scanning of children with minor head injury and loss of consciousness indicate that children with intracranial lesions after minor closed head injury are not easily distinguishable clinically from the large majority with no intracranial injury.[10,11] Children with nonspecific signs such as headache, vomiting, or lethargy after minor closed head injury may be more likely to have intracranial injury than children without such signs. However, these clinical signs are of limited predictive value, and most children with headache, lethargy, or vomiting after minor closed head injury do not have demonstrable intracranial injury. In addition, some children with intracranial injury do not have any signs or symptoms. Because of these findings, many investigators have concluded that the physical and neurologic examination are inadequate predictors of intracranial injury, and that cranial CT is more sensitive than physical and neurologic examinations for the diagnosis of intracranial injury.

The most accurate and rapid means of detecting intracranial injury would be with a clinical protocol that routinely obtained intracranial imaging for all children after head injury. Rapid diagnosis and treatment of subdural hematomas was found in 1 study to significantly reduce morbidity and mortality among severely injured adults.[12] However, this result was not replicated in other studies of subdural or epidural hematomas[13–15] and similar studies have not addressed less severely head injured children, or children with minor closed head injury.

CT itself is a safe procedure. However, some healthy children require sedation or anesthesia, and the benefits gained from cranial CT should be carefully weighed against the possible harm of sedating and/or anesthetizing a large number of children. In addition, CT scans obtained for asymptomatic children may show incidental findings that lead to subsequent unnecessary medical or surgical interventions. To our knowledge, no data are available that demonstrate that children who undergo CT scanning early after minor closed head injury with loss of consciousness have different outcomes compared with children who receive observation alone after injury. A clinical trial comparing the risks and benefits of immediate CT scanning with simple monitored observation for children with minor closed head injury has not been performed, primarily because intracranial injury after minor closed head injury is so rare that the cost and logistics of such a study would be prohibitive. As a result, the risk-benefit ratio for the evaluation and management modalities of CT scanning or observation is unknown.

Simple observation by a reliable parent or guardian is the management option with the least initial costs, while CT scans typically cost less than observation performed in the hospital. A study that compares costs of CT and observation strategies would need data on the cost of following up children with positive CT scans, as well as the potential costs associated with late detection and emergency therapy among those managed by observation alone.

Because of these considerations, there was Subcommittee consensus based on limited evidence that for children who are neurologically normal after minor closed head injury with loss of consciousness, cranial CT scanning along with observation was also an acceptable management option.

Skull Radiographs

Before the availability of CT imaging, skull radiographs were a common means to evaluate children with head injury. Skull radiographs may identify skull fractures, but they do not directly show brain injury or other intracranial trauma. Although intracranial injury is more common in the presence of a skull fracture, many studies have demonstrated that intracranial lesions are not always associated with skull fractures and that skull fractures do not always indicate an underlying intracranial lesion.[7,8,16]

Large studies of children and adults have shown that the sensitivity of skull radiographs for identifying intracranial injury in children is quite low (~25% in some studies). More recent studies limited to children have reported sensitivities between 50% and 100%, with the latter higher figure reported from studies of adolescent patients.[7,8,15,16] The specificity of skull radiographs for intracranial injury (the proportion of patients without intracranial injury who have normal radiographs) has been reported as between 53% and 97% in these same studies. Given the limited specificity of skull radiographs and the low prevalence of intracranial injury, the skull radiographs would likely be interpreted as abnormal for a substantial proportion of patients without intracranial injury. Furthermore, the low sensitivity of the radiographs will result in the interpretation of skull radiographs as normal for some patients with intracranial injury.

The Subcommittee consensus was that skull radiographs have only a limited role in the management of the child with loss of consciousness. If imaging is desired by the health care practitioner and if CT and skull radiographs are available, the Subcommittee believes that CT scanning is the imaging modality of choice, based on the increased sensitivity and specificity of CT scans. When CT scanning is not readily available, skull radiographs may assist the practitioner to define the extent of injury and risk for intracranial injury. In this situation, there was Subcommittee consensus that, for a child who has suffered minor closed head injury with loss of consciousness, skull radiographs are an acceptable management option. However, as noted, skull fractures may be detected on skull radiographs in the absence of intracranial injury, and intracranial injury may be present when no skull fracture is detected on skull radiographs. These limitations should be considered carefully by physicians who elect to use skull radiographs. Regardless of findings on skull films (should the physician elect to obtain them) close observation, as described previously, remains a cornerstone of patient management.

MRI

MRI is another available modality for neuroimaging. Although MRI has been shown to be more sensitive than cranial CT in detecting certain types of intracranial abnormalities, CT is more sensitive for hyperacute and acute intracranial hemorrhage (especially subarachnoid hemorrhage). CT is more quickly and easily performed than MRI, and costs for CT scans generally are less than those for MRI. The consensus of the Subcommittee was that cranial CT offered substantial advantages over MRI in the acute care of children with minor closed head injury.

As is the case with skull radiographs, there may be situations in which CT scanning is not readily available and the health care professional desires to obtain imaging studies. There was Subcommittee consensus that, for a child who has experienced minor closed head injury with loss of consciousness, MRI to evaluate the intracranial status of the child was an acceptable management option.

Disposition of Children With Minor Closed Head Injury

Children Managed by Observation Alone

Children who appear neurologically normal after minor closed head injury are at very low risk for subsequent deterioration in their condition and are unlikely to require medical intervention. Therefore, although observation is recommended for patients after the initial evaluation is completed, such observation may take place in many different settings. The strategy chosen by the health care practitioner may depend on the resources available for observation. Other factors, such as the distance and time it would take to reach appropriate care if the patient's clinical status worsened, may influence where observation occurs.

Historically, when hospitalization has been used to observe children after head injury, the length of stay averaged 12 to 48 hours. This practice was based on the reasoning that most life-threatening complications occur within 24 hours after head injury. The Subcommittee believes that a prudent duration of observation would extend at least 24 hours, and could be accomplished in any combination of locations, including the emergency department, hospital, clinic, office, or home. However, it is important for physicians, parents, and other guardians to have a high index of suspicion about any change in the patient's clinical status for several days after the injury. Parents or guardians require careful instruction to seek medical attention if the patient's condition worsens at any time during the first several days after injury.

In all cases, the health care professional is to make a careful assessment of the parent or guardian's anticipated compliance with the instructions to monitor the patient. If the caregiver is incompetent, unavailable, intoxicated, or otherwise incapacitated, other provisions must be made to ensure adequate observation of the child. These provisions may differ based on the characteristics of each case.

The physician has an important role in educating the parents or guardians of children with minor closed head injury. Understandable, printed instructions should be given to the parent or guardian detailing how to monitor the patient and including information on how and when to seek medical attention if necessary. All children discharged should be released to the care of a reliable parent or guardian who has adequate transportation and who has the capability to seek medical attention if the child's condition worsens.

Children Evaluated by Cranial CT

Neurologically normal patients with normal cranial CT scans are at extremely low risk for subsequent problems. Although there are many reports of patients with head injuries in whom extradural or intracerebral bleeding developed after an initial stable clinical period,[18-22] there are only a few reports of patients in whom extradural or intracerebral bleeding developed after a postinjury CT scan was interpreted as normal.[23-25] Most often when such cases have been described, the patients had sustained a more severe initial head injury than the patient for whom this parameter is intended, and the neurologic status of the patients was not intact at the initial examination following the injury. A number of studies have demonstrated the safety of using cranial CT as a triage instrument for neurologically normal and clinically stable patients after minor closed head injury.[26-31]

Patients may be discharged from the hospital for observation by a reliable observer if the postinjury CT scan is interpreted as normal. The length of observation should be similar to that described in the preceding section. If the cranial CT reveals abnormalities, proper disposition depends on a thorough consideration of the abnormalities and, when warranted, consultations with appropriate subspecialists.

Research Issues

Classification of Head Injury in Children and Prognostic Features

Much remains to be learned about minor closed head injury in children. The implications of clinical events such as loss of consciousness and signs or symptoms such as seizures, nausea, vomiting, and headache remain unclear. Data on patients with low-risk head injuries but with loss of consciousness, such as the data provided on a primarily adult population, are not available for children. Moreover, this practice parameter deals with clinically normal patients who did not lose consciousness at the time of injury and with patients who did lose consciousness with injury. Children with minor head injury, who have experienced loss of consciousness, vomiting or seizures have been found to have a prevalence of intracranial injury ranging from 2% to 5%. Questions remain about the selection of patients for many of these studies, and there is considerable uncertainty about the generalizability of these results to patients within this parameter.

Future studies on minor closed head injury should assess the relationship between characteristics such as these and the risk for intracranial injury among children who are clinically asymptomatic. Specifically, studies should address the question of whether such a history of loss of consciousness is associated with an increased risk for clinically significant intracranial abnormalities. Such studies should not be limited to patients seen in referral settings, but instead should cover patients from a wide range of settings, including those managed in clinics and offices, and if possible, those managed over the phone.

These studies should also address the independent prognostic value of other signs and symptoms for which the clinical significance in children is uncertain. In particular, practitioners are often faced with managing patients who are asymptomatic except for episodes of repeated vomiting or moderate to severe headache. The Subcommittee did not find evidence in the literature that helped differentiate the risk status of children with such symptoms from children without such symptoms. If studies are performed on this population, information should be collected on the presence of signs or symptoms including posttraumatic seizures, nausea with or without vomiting, posttraumatic amnesia, scalp lacerations and hematomas, headache, and dizziness, and their relationship to intracranial injury.

The Benefit of Early Detection of, and Intervention for, Intracranial Lesions in Asymptomatic Children

The outcome for asymptomatic patients found to have intracranial hematomas is of particular interest. Additional studies are needed to determine whether a strategy of immediate CT scan provides measurably improved outcomes for children with minor closed head injury compared with a strategy of observation followed by CT scan for children whose clinical status changes. Although rapid detection and neurosurgical intervention for intracranial injuries such as subdural hematomas has been shown to improve outcome in some studies of patients with more serious head injuries, it is unclear whether the same benefit would accrue to asymptomatic neurologically normal children.

A randomized, controlled trial would provide the most direct information on the risks and benefits of each management strategy. However, such a study would be extremely difficult and expensive to perform because of the rarity of adverse outcomes. Retrospective observational studies among children with minor head injury could be performed more easily and at less cost. However, correct characterization of the patient's clinical status before any treatment strategy or diagnostic procedure would be essential to eliminate bias in the evaluation of the comparison groups.

Finally, if such studies are performed to compare different diagnostic and management strategies, the outcomes should include not only mortality and short-term morbidity, but also long-term outcomes such as persistent psychological problems or learning disorders.

The Management of the Asymptomatic Patient With Intracranial Hemorrhage

The optimal management and prognosis for asymptomatic patients with intracranial hemorrhage is unknown. Because surgery is not always indicated or beneficial, some neurosurgeons and neurologists now advocate an expectant approach of close observation for small intracranial and extradural hematomas, considering hematoma size, shift of intracranial structures, and other factors.

If all asymptomatic children with minor head injury undergo cranial CT scanning, a substantial number of patients with an abnormal result on CT may undergo surgery that is unnecessary or even harmful. Additional research is needed to determine the proper management of asymptomatic children with intracranial hemorrhage. Outcome measures should include mortality and morbidity outcomes such as seizures, learning disabilities, and behavioral disabilities.

Research Into Other Imaging Modalities

As newer modalities for neuroimaging are developed and disseminated, careful evaluation of their relative utility is necessary before they are used for patients with minor closed head injury. Although such new modalities frequently provide new and different types of information to the health care professional, it is important that they be submitted to scientific study to assess their effect on patient outcome.

Algorithm

The notes below are integral to the algorithm. The letters in parentheses correspond to the algorithm.

A. This parameter addresses the management of previously neurologically healthy children with minor closed head injury who have normal mental status on presentation, no abnormal or focal findings on neurologic (including fundoscopic) examination, and no physical evidence of skull fracture (such as hemotympanum, Battle's sign, or palpable depression).

B. Observation in the clinic, office, emergency department, or home, under the care of a competent caregiver is recommended for children with minor closed head injury and no loss of consciousness.

C. Observation in the office, clinic, emergency department, hospital, or home under the care of a competent caregiver may be used to manage children with minor closed head injury with loss of consciousness.

D. Cranial CT scanning along with observation may also be used in the initial evaluation and management of children with minor closed head injury with brief loss of consciousness.

E. If imaging is desired by the health care practitioner and if both CT and skull radiography are available, CT scanning is the imaging modality of choice, because of its increased sensitivity and specificity. When CT scanning is not readily available, skull radiographs may assist the practitioner to define the risk for intracranial injury. However skull fractures may be detected on skull radiographs in the absence of intracranial injury, and occasionally intracra-

Evaluation and Triage of Children and Adolescents With Minor Head Trauma

Algorithm

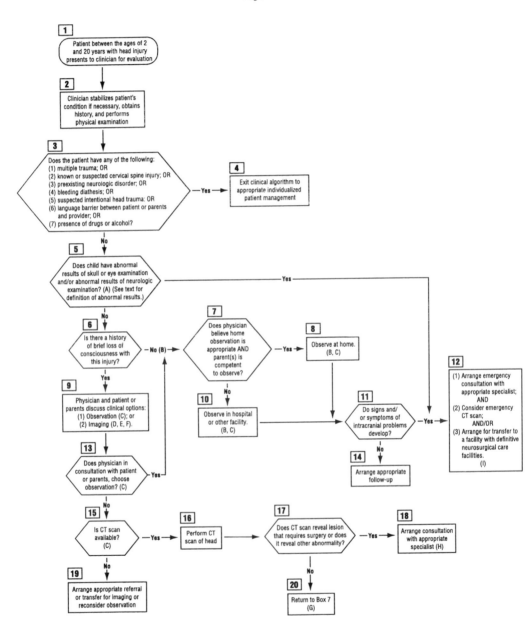

nial injury is present despite the absence of a skull fracture detected on skull radiographs. These limitations should be considered by physicians who elect to use skull radiographs. Whether the changed probabilities for harboring an intracranial injury based on the results of the skull radiographs is sufficient to alter the management strategy may depend on the preferences of the family and physician.

F. In some studies MRI has been shown to be more sensitive than CT in diagnosing certain intracranial lesions. However, there is currently no appreciable difference between CT and MRI in the diagnosis of clinically significant acute intracranial injury and bleeding that requires neurosurgical intervention. CT is more quickly and easily performed than MRI, and the costs for CT scans generally are less than those for MRI. Because of this, the consensus among the Subcommittee was that cranial CT offered advantages over MRI in the acute care of children with minor closed head injury.

G. Neurologically normal patients with a normal cranial CT scan are at very low risk for subsequent deterioration. Patients may be discharged from the hospital for observation by a reliable observer if the postinjury CT scan is normal. The decision to observe at home takes into consideration the delay that would ensue if the child had to return to the hospital as well as the reliability of the parents or other caregivers. Otherwise, depending on the preferences of the patient and physician, observation also may take place in the office, clinic, emergency department, or hospital.

H. If the cranial CT reveals abnormalities, proper disposition depends on a thorough consideration of the abnormalities and, when warranted, consultation with appropriate subspecialists.

I. If the child's neurologic condition worsens during observation, a thorough neurologic examination is to be performed, along with immediate cranial CT after the patient's condition is stabilized. If a repeat CT scan shows new intracranial pathologic abnormalities, consultation with the appropriate subspecialist is warranted.

References

1. Levin HS, Mattis S, Ruff RM, et al. Neurobehavioral outcome following minor head injury: a three-center study. *J Neurosurg.* 1987;66:234–243
2. Krauss JF, Black MA, Hessol N, et al. The incidence of acute brain injury and serious impairment in a defined population. *Am J Epidemiol.* 1984;119:186–201
3. Masters SJ, McClean PM, Arcarese JS, et al. Skull radiograph examinations after head trauma: recommendations by a multidisciplinary panel and validation study. *N Engl J Med.* 1987;316:84–91
4. Hennes H, Lee M, Smith D, Sty JR, Losek J. Clinical predictors of severe head trauma in children. *Am J Dis Child.* 1988;142:1045–1047
5. Dietrich AM, Bowman MJ, Ginn-Pease ME, Kusnick E, King DR. Pediatric head injuries: can clinical factors reliably predict an abnormality on computed tomography? *Ann Emerg Med.* 1993;22:1535–1540

6. Dacey RG Jr, Alves WM, Rimel RW, Winn HR, Jane JA. Neurosurgical complications after apparently minor head injury: assessment of risk in a series of 610 patients. *J Neurosurg.* 1986;65:203–210

7. Hahn YS, McLone DG. Risk factors in the outcome of children with minor head injury. *Pediatr Neurosurg.* 1993;19:135–142

8. Rosenthal BW, Bergman I. Intracranial injury after moderate head trauma in children. *J Pediatr.* 1989;115:346–350

9. Teasdale GM, Murray G, Anderson E, et al. Risks of acute traumatic intracranial complications in hematoma in children and adults: implications for head injuries. *Br Med J.* 1990;300:363–367

10. Rivara F, Taniguchi D, Parish RA, et al. Poor prediction of positive computed tomographic scans by clinical criteria in symptomatic pediatric head trauma. *Pediatrics.* 1987;80:579–584

11. Davis RL, Mullen N, Makela M, Taylor JA, Cohen W, Rivara FP. Cranial computed tomography scans in children after minimal head injury with loss of consciousness. *Ann Emerg Med.* 1994;24:640–645

12. Seelig JM, Becker DP, Miller JD, Greenberg RP, Ward JD, Choi SC. Traumatic acute subdural hematoma: major mortality reduction in comatose patients treated within four hours. *N Engl J Med.* 1981;304:1511–1518

13. Chen TY, Wong CW, Chang CN, et al. The expectant treatment of asymptomatic supratentorial epidural hematomas. *Neurosurgery.* 1993;32:176–179

14. Hatashita S, Koga N, Hosaka Y, Takagi S. Acute subdural hematoma: severity of injury, surgical intervention, and mortality. *Neurol Med Chir (Tokyo).* 1993;33:13–18

15. Lobato RD, Rivas JJ, Gomez PA, et al. Head injured patients who talk and deteriorate into coma. *J Neurosurg.* 1991;75:256–261

16. Zimmerman RA, Bilaniuk LT, Gennarelli T, Bruce D, Dolinskas C, Uzzell B. Cranial computed tomography in diagnosis and management of acute head trauma. *AJR Am J Roentgenol.* 1978;131:27–34

17. Borovich B, Braun J, Guilburd JN, et al. Delayed onset of traumatic extradural hematoma. *J Neurosurg.* 1985;63:30–34

18. Miller JD, Murray LS, Teasdale GM. Development of a traumatic intracranial hematoma after a "minor" head injury. *Neurosurgery.* 1990;27:669–673

19. Rosenthal BW, Bergman I. Intracranial injury after moderate head trauma in children. *J Pediatr.* 1989;115:346–350

20. Dacey RG, Alves WM, Rimel RW, Winn HR, Jane JA. Neurosurgical complications after apparently minor head injury. *J Neurosurg.* 1986;65:203–210

21. Deitch D, Kirshner HS. Subdural hematoma after normal CT. *Neurology.* 1989;39:985–987

22. Poon WS, Rehman SU, Poon CY, Li AK. Traumatic extradural hematoma of delayed onset is not a rarity. *Neurosurgery.* 1992;30:681–686

23. Brown FD, Mullan S, Duda EE. Delayed traumatic intracerebral hematomas. *J Neurosurg.* 1978;48:1019–1022

24. Lipper MH, Kishore PR, Girevendulis AK, Miller JD, Becker DP. Delayed intracranial hematoma in patients with severe head injury. *Radiology.* 1979;133:645–649

25. Diaz FG, Yock DH Jr, Larson D, Rockswold GL. Early diagnosis of delayed posttraumatic intracerebral hematomas. *J Neurosurg.* 1979;50:217–223

26. Stein SC, Ross SE. The value of computed tomographic scans in patients with low-risk head injuries. *Neurosurgery.* 1990;29:638–640

27. Stein SC, Ross SE. Mild head injury: a plea for routine early CT scanning. *J Trauma.* 1992;33:11–13

28. Harad FT, Kerstein MD. Inadequacy of bedside clinical indicators in identifying significant intracranial injury in trauma patients. *J Trauma.* 1992;32:359–363

29. Livingston DH, Loder PA, Koziol J, Hunt CD. The use of CT scanning to triage patients requiring admission following minimal head injury. *J Trauma.* 1991;31:483–489

30. Feurman T, Wackym PA, Gade GF, Becker DP. Value of skull radiography, head computed tomographic scanning, and admission for observation in cases of minor head injury. *Neurosurgery.* 1988;22:449–453

31. Livingston DH, Loder PA, Hunt CD. Minimal head injury: is admission necessary? *Am Surg.* 1991;57:14–17

**Technical Report Summary:
Minor Head Injury in Children**

Author:

Charles J. Homer, MD, MPH, and
Lawrence Kleinman. MD, MPH

American Academy of Pediatrics
PO Box 927, 141 Northwest Point Blvd
Elk Grove Village, IL 60009-0927

Abstract

Minor head trauma affecting children is a common reason for medical consultation and evaluation. In order to provide evidence on which to base a clinical practice guideline for the American Academy of Pediatrics, we undertook a systematic review of the literature on minor head trauma in children.

Methods. Medline and Health databases were searched for articles published between 1966 and 1993 on head trauma or head injury, limited to infants, children, and adolescents. Abstracts were reviewed for relevance to mild head trauma consistent with the index case defined by the AAP subcommittee. Relevant articles were identified, reviewed, and abstracted. Additional citations were identified by review of references and expert suggestions. Unpublished data were also identified through contact with authors highlighting child-specific information. Abstracted data were summarized in evidence tables. The process was repeated in 1998, updating the review for articles published between 1993 and 1997.

Results. A total of 108 articles were abstracted from 1033 abstracts and articles identified through the various search strategies. Variation in definitions precluded any pooling of data from different studies. Prevalence of intracranial injury in children with mild head trauma varied from 0% to 7%. Children with no clinical risk characteristics are at lower risk than are children with such characteristics; the magnitude of increased risk was inconsistent across studies. Computed tomography scan is most sensitive and specific for detection of intracranial abnormalities; sensitivity and specificity of skull radiographs ranged from 21% to 100% and 53% to 97%, respectively. No high quality studies tested alternative strategies for management of such children. Outcome studies are inconclusive as to the impact of minor head trauma on long-term cognitive function.

Conclusions. The literature on mild head trauma does not provide a sufficient scientific basis for evidence-based recommendations about most of the key issues in clinical management. More consistent definitions and multisite assessments are needed to clarify this field. Pediatrics 1999;104(6). URL: http://www.pediatrics.org/ cgi/content/full/104/6/e78. *Keywords: head trauma, imaging, literature review.*

Minor head trauma affecting a child is a common reason for medical consultation and evaluation. No consensus exists concerning the appropriate diagnostic assessment of such children. Previous surveys of physicians indicated significant variation in practice, and examination of hospitalization rates shows substantial regional variation for this condition. The American Academy of Pediatrics, in coordination with the American Academy of Family Physicians, launched an initiative to develop a clinical practice guideline to reduce variation and improve the quality of care of children with minor head trauma.

This report provides the technical information on the literature concerning minor head trauma in children that was used by the American Academy of Pediatrics/American Academy of Family Physicians' subcommittee in formulating this guideline.

Methods

The literature review included the following salient aspects of minor head trauma in children:

- Prevalence of intracranial injury
- Sensitivity and specificity of different imaging modalities in detecting intracranial injury, including skull radiography, computed tomography (CT), and magnetic resonance imaging (MRI)
- Utility of early diagnosis of intracranial injury
- Effectiveness of alternative management strategies, and
- Impact of minor head injury on subsequent child health.

The data included for review met the following criteria:

1. publication in a peer-reviewed journal,
2. data related exclusively to children or was identifiable as being specifically related to children, and
3. assurance that cases described in the article were comparable with the case described in the practice guideline. Review articles and expert opinion were excluded.

A medical librarian undertook an initial search of several computerized databases, including Medline (1966–1993) and Health, searching terms of head trauma and head injury, restricted to infancy, children, and adolescents. Four hundred twenty-two articles were identified. Titles and abstracts were reviewed by 4 initial reviewers, including the subcommittee chairperson, American Academy of Pediatrics staff, and methodologic consultants, and articles were obtained when reviewers considered the title to be relevant. Through this process, 168 articles were identified.

Articles were sent to subcommittee members with an article review form, which asked reviewers to categorize the study design, identify the study question, and abstract the data to enable data pooling and meta-analysis. In addition, reviewers were asked to check the article references to see whether additional sources could be found.

Of the initial 168 articles sent out, reviewers excluded 134 papers and included 34 papers in their reviews.

An additional 125 references were identified through bibliography tracing, of which 30 were included for review by the epidemiologist/pediatrician consultants.

All articles included were then abstracted again by the epidemiologist/pediatrician consultants, and the data were compiled using summary tables and evidence tables. Differences in case definition, outcome definition, and study samples precluded pooling of data to arrive at common estimates.

Because the published data proved extremely limited for a number of study questions, direct queries were given to several authors for child-specific data. Because these data have not been formally published, we did not rest strong conclusions on them; when available, however, they are presented with this report.

Because of the lengthy period between the initial review of the literature and final approval of the guideline, a second literature review was performed to assure that the literature review was current. This literature review used the same search headings and targeted the period between January 1, 1993, and July 1, 1997. For this review, only an electronic search was performed. The review identified an additional 486 abstracts, of which 44 were selected for detailed review by the epidemiologist and 11 included in the evidence tables.

Results

In general, interpretation of clinical studies of head trauma was complicated by several characteristics of the literature. Specifically, the head trauma literature suffers by the nonstandardized ways of categorizing head injury, clinical examinations, radiologic outcomes, and clinical outcomes, and by the inconsistent reporting of the subjects included in a study population.

The results of the literature review are presented by each area for which evidence was sought.

Risk of Intracranial Injury

Ten published articles were identified that provided estimates of the prevalence of intracranial injury in children with mild head injury, with CT scans used as the "gold standard". Among these articles, however, 3 included patients with more severe symptoms or findings than specified by the guideline case description (including Glasgow coma scale [GCS] scores as low as 13), and 1 included trivial abnormalities on CT as the principal outcome measure. Among those studies restricting their subjects to GCS scores of 15, and considering abnormal findings to be subdural, extradural, or intracerebral hematomas, ranges of the prevalence of intracranial injury ranged from 0% to 7%. The high estimate of 7% comes from a study in which both initial and delayed (24-hour) CT scans were obtained for most patients; how many patients were referred for care at this institution because of clinical deterioration was not noted.

Three unpublished studies provided prevalence estimates of intracranial injuries ranging from 4% to 10% among patients with a GCS score of 15, without focal neurologic findings, but with either a history of (brief) loss of consciousness or amnesia (J. Finkelstein, 1994; S. C. Stein, 1994; S. C. Stein, 1994).

We sought to determine within these articles whether any clinical characteristics were associated with the presence or absence of significant CT scan abnormalities. Two studies indicated that among patients with a GCS score of 15, normal neurologic examinations, no history of loss of consciousness or amnesia, no vomiting, headache, or subtle changes in mental status, there were no abnormal CT scan findings. One additional case series (49 children) found that no child with a GCS of 15, a completely normal neurologic examination, and no trauma aside from the head injury experienced an intracranial lesion, even with a history of loss of consciousness or amnesia. The upper limits for the 95% confidene interval for this estimate is 6%, and the analysis that identified this group of predictors is exploratory; no confirmatory analyses were undertaken in a second dataset.

One pediatric study used surgery for intracranial bleeding as an indicator of intracranial injury. This study found that .017% of cases with a GCS score of 15 required surgery.

We conclude from these data that:

- the true prevalence of intracranial injury following mild head injury is not clearly known;
- the population as defined by the head trauma task force is likely heterogeneous in its risk;
- children with clinically trivial head injury—no loss of consciousness or amnesia, normal examinations, no vomiting, headache, and a GCS score of 15—are at substantially <1% risk of having an intracranial abnormality of immediate clinical significance;
- children with mild head injury but who have experienced loss of consciousness, amnesia, vomiting, or seizures are at higher risk of having an intracranial injury detected using CT, likely in the 1% to 5% range, with a significantly lower amount requiring any intervention (see below).

We extended this section of the literature review to examine the significance of the abnormalities detected by CT scanning in such patients No studies randomly assigned patients with abnormal CT scans to receive or not receive surgery. Rather, several reports on the management decisions among those children found to have abnormal CT scans. These studies, and the unpublished data provided to us, indicated that between 20% and 80% of children with abnormal CT scans underwent a neurosurgical procedure, a proportion of which was intracranial pressure monitoring only.

Imaging Modalities

Through the 1970s and early 1980s, controversy raged concerning the role of skull radiography in the assessment of acute head trauma. Although fewer articles are now being written on this topic, the lack of access to CT scanners in some practice settings prompted review of this literature.

We identified 5 studies that examined the sensitivity and specificity of skull radiographs for the detection of intracranial injury, using intracranial abnormality or bleeding as determined by CT scanning as the gold standard. (Table 3). These studies found that the sensitivity of skull films varied from 50% to 100%; 1 of the studies showing 100% sensitivity was restricted to adolescents. The specificity of skull films for intracranial injury (ie, the proportion of patients without intracranial injury who have normal films) has been reported to be between 53% and 97%. Thus, a substantial proportion of patients without intracranial injury will have abnormal skull films.

A few studies have examined the role of MRI in head trauma. These studies indicate that although subtle forms of neural injury can be better detected by MRI, and that isodense subdural collections (as may be found in chronic subdural injuries in adults) also may be more readily identified, in acute settings with children MRI offers no advantage in detecting lesions of clinical concern.

We conclude from this literature that 1) although an abnormal skull film increases the likelihood of a significant intracranial lesion, the test is not of sufficient sensitivity or specificity to be clinically useful in most settings, and 2) CT is sufficiently sensitive and specific as the imaging modality of choice at this time; in most cases, a normal CT scan in a child who meets the case definition provides assurance that subsequent adverse outcomes are very unlikely. A cohort of 399 such children (GCS .12 and normal CT scan) found 3 patients who were readmitted within 1 month, 1 of whom had an intercranial contusion, but none required neurosurgical intervention. Rarely, cases are reported in the literature of children with normal CT scans who subsequently develop "flash edema," or, even more rarely, intracranial (especially epidural) hematomas.

Utility of Early Diagnosis

In the course of the literature review, because the reviewers identified several papers and unpublished reports that noted a higher frequency of intracranial abnormalities than the subcommittee members had anticipated, the subcommittee requested that literature examining the utility of the early diagnosis of these abnormalities be examined. Little child-specific data are available that relate to this question, ie, "Are children with apparently mild head trauma who are discovered to have an intracranial injury better off if the discovery is made sooner rather than later?" Although a classic and often cited study of comatose adults with subdural hematoma showed a dramatic benefit associated with rapid diagnosis and treatment, subsequent study has not replicated that report for either subdural or epidural bleeding. Small case series have similarly not found a correlation between delay in diagnosis of intracranial bleeding and outcome in children. The extreme limitations of these reports in their sample size, and the appropriately nonrandom allocation of time to diagnosis and treatment make any inferences from this work extremely limited.

Effectiveness of Alternative Management Strategies

An ideal study seeking to determine the relative effectiveness of alternative management strategies would initially define a homogeneous population of children with mild head trauma, and randomly assign such children to 1 of 2 or more potential approaches. Such approaches might include inpatient observation for a defined period of time without initial imaging, outpatient observation without imaging, or CT scanning followed by outpatient observation if scans are normal. No such study has been identified in the pediatric literature. The rarity of adverse outcomes would make such a study difficult to perform, and would require careful collaboration across multiple institutions.

One decision analysis has been published that assesses the cost-effectiveness of a particular strategy for the evaluation of head trauma. This analysis, although not limited to children, utilized much pediatric data in developing the probabilities required for the analysis. The authors recommend immediate CT scanning for patients with abnormal clinical signs; for patients who are otherwise normal, these authors recommend skull radiography, with CT if radiographs are abnormal. If such a strategy were followed for 10 000 persons presenting with mild head trauma, of 10 000 individuals with head injuries, the 9900 additional skull films and 250 CT scans would identify 6 or 7 additional cases of early intracranial hemorrhage.

Outcome of Mild Head Trauma

In an idealized decision analytic framework, the "utilities" to patients of the various clinical outcomes are incorporated in assessing the value of each potential treatment arm. We sought to identify through the literature the long-term outcome for the index case, assuming no significant intracranial abnormalities were identified.

Several studies did not specifically report on outcomes for pediatric patients, although authors typically commented that outcomes for children were better than those for adults. Four studies, however, did specifically examine outcomes for children. One large cohort study of children with "minimal" (or "trivial") head injury, ie, excluding children with skull fracture, loss of consciousness, or having been admitted to an inpatient unit, found physical health 1 month after injury to be identical to that of a normal population, but that role limitations, eg, school absenteeism, was substantially increased. Unfortunately, this study could not distinguish whether this effect was the result of the head injury, or associated either with the use of the emergency department or with whatever factors led to the injury. A smaller study of children with mild injury including "concussion" found a slight increase in teacher-reported hyperactivity (activity and inattentiveness) 10 years after the injury, with no other differences in school performance, cognitive ability, or behavioral symptoms. In this relatively small cohort, no differences in these outcomes between those patients who had been observed in inpatient or out-patient settings were identified. Two more recent studies also suggested some possible long-term impact of head injury. Comparing a cohort of 95 children followed up 1 year after hospitalization for head trauma of varying degree with population norms, investigators found that the children with head injuries had higher levels of physical and behavioral impairment; this investigation did not control for preexisting morbidity leading to the injury. Only patients at the most severe end of the spectrum (Abbreviated Injury Scale level 5) had demonstrably worse outcomes than those with milder injuries (Abbreviated Injury Scale level 2). A more compelling study from New Zealand compared children ages 2½ to 3½ years of age with mild head trauma (evaluated in an emergency department but not admitted to the hospital) with injury date-matched children with other forms of mild trauma 1, 6, and 12 months after the injury and when the children were 6½ years of age. The investigators found specific deficits in solving visual puzzles beginning 6 months after injury and persisting throughout the observation; these children were also more likely to have reading disabilities. We conclude from these investigations that children who present with head injuries or other types of injuries are different from the general population and more likely to have some functional impairment unrelated to the injury per se; at the same time, children with mild or minimal head injury may be more likely to experience subtle abnormalities in specific cognitive functions.

Conclusion

The literature on mild head trauma does not provide a sufficient scientific basis on which clinical management decisions can be made with certainty. The field remains burdened by inconsistent definitions of case severity, inadequate specification of the population base, and varied and incomplete definition of outcome. Nonetheless, the published data do indicate that 1) a small proportion of children with minimal and mild head injury will have significant intracranial injury; 2) the presence of either loss of consciousness or amnesia increases the probability that an injury is present in many, but not all studies; 3) CT scanning is the most sensitive, specific, and clinically safe mode of identifying such injury, whereas plain radiographs in this pediatric age group have neither sufficient sensitivity nor specificity to recommend their general use; 4) extremely rare children with normal examinations and CT scans will experience delayed bleeding or edema; and 5) long-term outcomes for children with minimal or mild head injury, in the absence of significant intracranial hemorrhage, are generally very good, with a suggestion of a small increase in risk for subtle specific deficits in particular cognitive skills.

The confusion in this field mandates that multicenter, collaborative investigations be performed that will begin to address the limited information base on which such a large volume of clinical care rests.

Otitis Media with Effusion in Young Children

• *Quick Reference Guide for Clinicians*

Managing Otitis Media with Effusion in Young Children
Quick Reference Guide for Clinicians

- **Diagnosis and Hearing Evaluation**

- **Environmental Risk Factors**

- **Therapeutic Intervention**

- **Algorithm**

Author:

U.S. Department of Health and Human Services
Public Health Service
Agency for Health Care Policy and Research

The *Quick Reference Guide for Clinicians, Managing Otitis Media with Effusion in Young Children,* was developed by the American Academy of Pediatrics under contract with the Agency for Health Care Policy and Research (AHCPR) and in consortium with the American Academy of Family Physicians and the American Academy of Otolaryngology–Head and Neck Surgery (the "Consortium"). With AHCPR approval, the Consortium convened an interdisciplinary, non-Federal panel comprising health care professionals and a consumer representative. Panel members were:

Sylvan E. Stool, MD *(Co-chair)*	Janice A. Goertz, RN, BS, CPNP
Alfred O. Berg, MD, MPH *(Co-chair)*	Allan J. Goldstein, MD
Stephen Berman, MD	Kenneth M. Grundfast, MD
Cynthia J. Carney	Douglas G. Long, MD
James R. Cooley, MD	Loretta L. Macconi, RN, MSN,
Larry Culpepper, MD, MPH	CRNP
Roland D. Eavey, MD	LoBirtha Melton, RN, BSN, MPA
Lynne V. Feagans, PhD	Joanne Erwick Roberts, PhD,
Terese Finitzo, PhD, CCC/A	CCC-SLP & AUD
Ellen Friedman, MD	Jessie L. Sherrod, MD, MPH
	Jane E. Sisk, PhD

For a description of the guideline development process and information about the sponsoring agency (AHCPR), see the *Clinical Practice Guideline, Otitis Media with Effusion in Young Children* (AHCPR Publication No. 94-0622). To receive copies of the *Clinical Practice Guideline,* call toll free 800-358-9295 or write the AHCPR Publications Clearinghouse, P.O. Box 8547, Silver Spring, MD 20907.

AHCPR invites comments and suggestions from users for consideration in development and updating of future guidelines. Please send written comments to Director, Office of the Forum for Quality and Effectiveness in Health Care, AHCPR, Willco Building, Suite 310, 6000 Executive Boulevard, Rockville, MD 20852.

Note: This *Quick Reference Guide for Clinicians* presents summary points from the *Clinical Practice Guideline.* The *Clinical Practice Guideline* provides more detailed analysis and discussion of the available research, health care decisionmaking, critical evaluation of the assumptions and knowledge of the field, considerations for patients with special needs, and references. Decisions to adopt any particular recommendation from any publication must be made by practitioners in light of available resources and circumstances presented by individual patients.

Abstract

This *Quick Reference Guide for Clinicians* contains highlights from the *Clinical Practice Guideline, Otitis Media with Effusion in Young Children.* The Otitis Media Guideline Panel, a private-sector panel of health care providers, developed the *Guideline* after comprehensively analyzing the research literature and current scientific knowledge of the development, diagnosis, and treatment of otitis media with effusion in young children.

Specific recommendations are given for the management of otitis media with effusion in young children age 1 through 3 years with no craniofacial or neurologic abnormalities or sensory deficits. The natural history of otitis media with effusion, the functional impairments that may result from otitis media with effusion, and the difficulty of measuring the effects of medical and surgical interventions on long-term outcomes are included. The medical interventions studied involve antibiotic therapy, steroid therapy, and antihistamine/decongestant therapy. The surgical interventions studied involve myringotomy with insertion of tympanostomy tubes, adenoidectomy, and tonsillectomy. Short-term outcomes addressed are resolution of effusion and restoration of hearing.

Stool SE, Berg AO, Berman S, Carney CJ, Cooley JR, Culpepper L, Eavey RD, Feagans LV, Finitzo T, Friedman E, et al. *Managing Otitis Media with Effusion in Young Children. Quick Reference Guide for Clinicians*. AHCPR Publication No. 94-0623. Rockville, MD: Agency for Health Care Policy and Research, Public Health Service, U.S. Department of Health and Human Services. July 1994.

Managing Otitis Media with Effusion in Young Children

Purpose and Scope

Otitis media (inflammation of the middle ear) is the most frequent primary diagnosis at visits to U.S. physician offices by children younger than 15 years. Otitis media particularly affects infants and preschoolers: almost all children experience one or more episodes of otitis media before age 6.

The American Academy of Pediatrics, the American Academy of Family Physicians, and the American Academy of Otolaryngology–Head and Neck Surgery, with the review and approval of the Agency for Health Care Policy and Research of the U.S. Department of Health and Human Services, convened a panel of experts to develop a guideline on otitis media for providers and consumers of health care for young children. Providers include primary care and specialist physicians, professional nurses and nurse practitioners, physician assistants, audiologists, speech-language pathologists, and child development specialists. Because the term otitis media encompasses a range of diseases, from acute to chronic and with or without symptoms, the Otitis Media Guideline Panel narrowed the topic. Two types of otitis media often encountered by clinicians were considered:

- **Acute otitis media**—fluid in the middle ear accompanied by signs or symptoms of ear infection (bulging eardrum usually accompanied by pain; or perforated eardrum, often with drainage of purulent material).
- **Otitis media with effusion**—fluid in the middle ear without signs or symptoms of ear infection.

The *Clinical Practice Guideline, Otitis Media with Effusion in Young Children,* and this *Quick Reference Guide for Clinicians, Managing Otitis Media with Effusion in Young Children*, based on the *Guideline*, discuss only otitis media with effusion. Further, the *Guideline* and this *Quick Reference Guide* narrow their discussion of the identification and management of otitis media with effusion to a very specific "target patient":

- A child age 1 through 3 years.
- With no craniofacial or neurologic abnormalities or sensory deficits.
- Who is healthy except for otitis media with effusion.

When the scientific evidence for management permitted, Guideline recommendations were broadened to include older children.

Highlights of Patient Management

Congenital or early onset hearing impairment is widely accepted as a risk factor for impaired speech and language development. In general, the earlier the hearing problem begins and the more severe it is, the worse its effects on speech and language development. Because otitis media with effusion is often associated with a mild to moderate hearing loss, most clinicians have been eager to treat the condition to restore hearing to normal and thus prevent any long-term problems.

Studies of the effects of otitis media with effusion on hearing have varied in design and have examined several aspects of hearing and communication skills. Because of these differences, the results cannot be combined to provide a clear picture of the relationship between otitis media with effusion and hearing. Also, it is uncertain whether changes in hearing due to middle ear fluid have any long-term effects on development. Evidence of dysfunctions mediated by otitis media with effusion that have persisted into later childhood, despite resolution of the middle ear fluid and a return to normal hearing, would provide a compelling argument for early, decisive intervention. There is, however, no consistent, reliable evidence that otitis media with effusion has such long-term effects on language or learning.

The following recommendations for managing otitis media with effusion are tempered by the failure to find rigorous, methodologically sound research to support the theory that untreated otitis media with effusion results in speech/language delays or deficits.

Recommendations and options were developed for the diagnosis and management of otitis media with effusion in otherwise healthy young children. The following steps parallel the management algorithm provided at the end of this booklet.

Diagnosis and Hearing Evaluation

1. Suspect otitis media with effusion in young children.
Most children have at least one episode of otitis media with effusion before entering school. Otitis media with effusion may be identified following an acute episode of otitis media, or it may be an incidental finding. Symptoms may include discomfort or behavior changes.

2. Use pneumatic otoscopy to assess middle ear status.
Pneumatic otoscopy is recommended for assessment of the middle ear because it combines visualization of the tympanic membrane (otoscopy) with a test of membrane mobility (pneumatic otoscopy). When pneumatic otoscopy is performed by an experienced examiner, the accuracy for diagnosis of otitis media with effusion may be between 70 and 79 percent.

3. **Tympanometry may be performed to confirm suspected otitis media with effusion.**

Tympanometry provides an indirect measure of tympanic membrane compliance and an estimate of middle ear air pressure. The positive predictive value of an abnormal (type B, flat) tympanogram is between 49 and 99 percent; that is, as few as half of ears with abnormal tympanograms may have otitis media with effusion. The negative predictive value of this test is better—the majority of middle ears with normal tympanograms will in fact be normal. Because the strengths of tympanometry (it provides a quantitative measure of tympanic membrane mobility) and pneumatic otoscopy (many abnormalities of the eardrum and ear canal that can skew the results of tympanometry are visualized) offset the weaknesses of each, using the two tests together improves the accuracy of diagnosis.

- **Acoustic reflectometry** has not been studied well enough for a recommendation to be made for or against its use to diagnose otitis media with effusion.
- **Tuning fork tests:** No recommendation is made regarding the use of tuning fork tests to screen for or diagnose otitis media with effusion, except to note that they are inappropriate in the youngest children.

4. **A child who has had fluid in both middle ears for a total of 3 months should undergo hearing evaluation. Before 3 months of effusion, hearing evaluation is an option.**

A change in hearing threshold is both a clinical outcome and a possible indicator of the presence of otitis media with effusion. Methods used to determine a child's hearing acuity will vary depending on the resources available and the child's willingness and ability to participate in testing. Optimally, air- and bone-conduction thresholds can be established for 500, 1,000, 2,000, and 4,000 Hz, and an air-conduction pure tone average can be calculated. This result should be verified by obtaining a measure of speech sensitivity. Determinations of speech reception threshold or speech awareness threshold alone may be used if the child cannot cooperate for pure tone testing. If none of the test techniques is available or tolerated by the child, the examiner should use his/her best judgment as to adequacy of hearing. In these cases, the health care provider should be aware of whether the child is achieving the appropriate developmental milestones for verbal communication.

Although hearing evaluation may be difficult to perform in young children, evaluation is recommended after otitis media with effusion has been present bilaterally for 3 months, because of the strong belief that surgery is not indicated unless otitis media with effusion is causing hearing impairment (defined as equal to or worse than 20 decibels hearing threshold level in the better-hearing ear).

Natural History

Longitudinal studies of otitis media with effusion show spontaneous resolution of the condition in more than half of children within 3 months from development of the effusion. After 3 months the rate of spontaneous resolution remains constant, so that only a small percentage of children experience otitis media with effusion lasting a year or longer. In most children, episodes of otitis media with effusion do not persist beyond early childhood. The likelihood that middle ear fluid will resolve by itself underlies the recommendations made for management of otitis media with effusion.

Environmental Risk Factors

Scientific evidence showed that the following environmental factors may increase potential risks of getting acute otitis media or otitis media with effusion:

- Bottle-feeding rather than breast-feeding infants.
- Passive smoking.
- Group child-care facility attendance.

Because the target child for Guideline recommendations is beyond the age when the choice of breast-feeding versus bottle-feeding is an issue, this risk factor was not considered at length.

Passive smoking (exposure to another's cigarette smoke) is associated with higher risk of otitis media with effusion. Although there is no proof that stopping passive smoking will help prevent middle ear fluid, there are many health reasons for not exposing persons of any age to tobacco smoke. Therefore, clinicians should advise parents of the benefits of decreasing children's exposure to tobacco smoke.

Studies of otitis media with effusion in children cared for at home compared to those in group child-care facilities found that children in group child-care facilities have a slightly higher relative risk (less than 2.0) of getting otitis media with effusion. Research did not show whether removing the child from the group child-care facility helped prevent otitis media with effusion.

Therapeutic Interventions

5. **Observation OR antibiotic therapy are treatment options for children with effusion that has been present less than 4 to 6 months and at any time in children without a 20-decibel hearing threshold level or worse in the better-hearing ear.**
   Most cases of otitis media with effusion resolve spontaneously. Meta-analysis of controlled studies showed a 14 percent increase in the resolution rate when antibiotics were given. Length of treatment in these studies was typically 10 days.

   The most common adverse effects of antibiotic therapy are gastrointestinal. Dermatologic reactions may occur in 3 to 5 percent of cases; severe anaphylactic reactions are much rarer; severe hematologic, cardiovascular, central nervous system, endocrine, renal, hepatic, and respiratory adverse effects are rarer still. The potential for the development of microbial resistance is always present with antibiotics.

6. **For the child who has had bilateral effusion for a total of 3 months and who has a bilateral hearing deficiency (defined as a 20-decibel hearing threshold level or worse in the better-hearing ear), bilateral myringotomy with tube insertion becomes an additional treatment option. Placement of tympanostomy tubes is recommended after a total of 4 to 6 months of bilateral effusion with a bilateral hearing deficit.**
   The principal benefits of myringotomy with insertion of tympanostomy tubes are the restoration of hearing to the pre-effusion threshold and clearance of the fluid and possible feeling of pressure. While patent and in place, tubes may prevent further accumulation of fluid in the middle ear. Although there is insufficient evidence to prove that there are long-term deleterious effects of otitis media with effusion, concern about the possibility of such effects led the panel to recommend surgery, based on their expert opinion. Tubes are available in a myriad of designs, most constructed from plastic and/or metal. Data comparing outcomes with tubes of various designs are sparse, and so there were assumed to be no notable differences between available tympanostomy tubes.

   Insertion of tympanostomy tubes is performed under general anesthesia in young children. Calculation of the risks for two specific complications of myringotomy with tympanostomy tube insertion showed that tympanosclerosis might occur after this procedure in 51 percent, and postoperative otorrhea in 13 percent, of children.

A number of treatments are not recommended for treatment of otitis media with effusion in the otherwise healthy child age 1 through 3 years.

- **Steroid medications** are not recommended to treat otitis media with effusion in a child of any age because of limited scientific evidence that this treatment is effective and the opinion of many experts that the possible adverse effects (agitation, behavior change, and more serious problems such as disseminated varicella in children exposed to this virus within the month before therapy) outweighed possible benefits.
- **Antihistamine/decongestant therapy** is not recommended for treatment of otitis media with effusion in a child of any age, because review of the literature showed that these agents are not effective for this condition, either separately or together.
- **Adenoidectomy** is not an appropriate treatment for uncomplicated middle ear effusion in the child younger than age 4 years when adenoid pathology is not present (based on the lack of scientific evidence). Potential harms for children of all ages include the risks of general anesthesia and the possibility of excessive postoperative bleeding.
- **Tonsillectomy, either alone or with adenoidectomy**, has not been found effective for treatment of otitis media with effusion.
- **The association between allergy and otitis media with effusion** was not clear from available evidence. Thus, although close anatomic relationships between the nasopharynx, eustachian tube, and middle ear have led many experts to suggest a role for allergy management in treating otitis media with effusion, no recommendation was made for or against such treatment.
- **Evidence regarding other therapies for the treatment of otitis media with effusion** was sought, but no reports of chiropractic, holistic, naturopathic, traditional/indigenous, homeopathic, or other treatments contained information obtained in randomized controlled studies. Therefore, no recommendation was made regarding such other therapies for the treatment of otitis media with effusion in children.

Treatment Outcomes

The following table summarizes the benefits and harms identified for management interventions in the target child with otitis media with effusion.

Table 1. Outcomes of treating otitis media with effusion[1]

Intervention	Benefits[2]	Harms[2]
Observation	Base Case.	Base Case.
Antibiotics	Improved clearance of effusion at 1 month or less, 14.0% (95% CI [3.6%, 24.2%]). Possible reduction in future infections.	Nausea, vomiting, diarrhea (2%–32% depending on dose and antibiotic). Cutaneous reactions (≤5%). Numerous rare organ system effects, including very rare fatalities. Cost. Possible development of resistant strains of bacteria.
Antibiotics plus steroids	Possible improved clearance at 1 month, 25.1% (95% CI [-1.3%, 49.9%]).[3] Possible reduction in future infections.	See antibiotics and steroids separately.
Steroids alone	Possible improved clearance at 1 month, 4.5% (95% CI [-11.7%, 20.6%]).[3]	Possible exacerbation of varicella. Long-term complications not established for low doses. Cost.
Antihistamine/ decongestant	Same as base case.	Drowsiness and/or excitability.[4] Cost.
Myringotomy with tubes	Immediate clearance of effusion in all children. Improved hearing.	Invasive procedure. Anesthesia risk. Cost. Tympanosclerosis. Otorrhea. Possible restrictions on swimming.
Adenoidectomy	Benefits for young children have not been established.	Invasive procedure.[4] Anesthesia risk. Cost.
Tonsillectomy	Same as base case.	Invasive procedure.[4] Anesthesia risk. Cost.

1 The target patient is an otherwise healthy child age 1 through 3 years with no craniofacial or neurologic abnormalities or sensory deficits.

2 Outcomes are reported as differences from observation, which is treated as the base case. When possible, meta-analysis was performed to provide a mean and associated confidence interval (CI).

3 Difference from base case not statistically significant.

4 Risks were not examined in detail because no benefits were identified.

Algorithm

The notes below are an integral part of the algorithm that follows.

Notes to Algorithm

(A) Otitis media with effusion (OME) is defined as fluid in the middle ear without signs or symptoms of infection; OME is not to be confused with acute otitis media (inflammation of the middle ear with signs of infection). The Guideline and this algorithm apply only to the child with otitis media with effusion. This algorithm assumes followup intervals of 6 weeks.

(B) The algorithm applies only to a child age 1 through 3 years with no craniofacial or neurologic abnormalities or sensory deficits (except as noted) who is healthy except for otitis media with effusion. The Guideline recommendations and algorithm do not apply if the child has any craniofacial or neurologic abnormality (for example, cleft palate or mental retardation) or sensory deficit (for example, decreased visual acuity or pre-existing hearing deficit).

(C) The Panel found some evidence that pneumatic otoscopy is more accurate than otoscopy performed without the pneumatic test of eardrum mobility.

(D) Tympanometry may be used as confirmation of pneumatic otoscopy in the diagnosis of otitis media with effusion (OME). Hearing evaluation is recommended for the otherwise healthy child who has had bilateral OME for 3 months; before 3 months, hearing evaluation is a clinical option.

(E) In most cases, otitis media with effusion (OME) resolves spontaneously within 3 months.

(F) The antibiotic drugs studied for treatment of otitis media with effusion (OME) were amoxicillin, amoxicillin-clavulanate potassium, cefaclor, erythromycin, erythromycin-sulfisoxazole, sulfisoxazole, and trimethoprim-sulfamethoxazole.

(G) Exposure to cigarette smoke (passive smoking) has been shown to increase the risk of otitis media with effusion (OME). For bottle-feeding versus breast-feeding and for child-care facility placement, associations were found with OME, but evidence available to the Panel did not show decreased incidence of OME with breast-feeding or with removal from child-care facilities.

(H) The recommendation against tonsillectomy is based on the lack of added benefit from tonsillectomy when combined with adenoidectomy to treat otitis media with effusion in older children. Tonsillectomy and adenoidectomy may be appropriate for reasons other than otitis media with effusion.

(I) The Panel found evidence that decongestants and/or antihistamines are ineffective treatments for otitis media with effusion.

(J) Meta-analysis failed to show a significant benefit for steroid medications without antibiotic medications in treating otitis media with effusion in children.

Algorithm for managing otitis media with effusion in an otherwise healthy child age 1 through 3 years

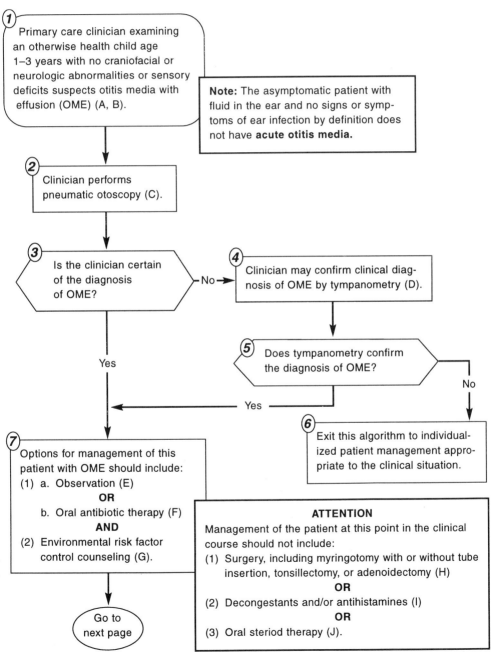

1 Primary care clinician examining an otherwise health child age 1–3 years with no craniofacial or neurologic abnormalities or sensory deficits suspects otitis media with effusion (OME) (A, B).

Note: The asymptomatic patient with fluid in the ear and no signs or symptoms of ear infection by definition does not have **acute otitis media.**

2 Clinician performs pneumatic otoscopy (C).

3 Is the clinician certain of the diagnosis of OME?

— No →

4 Clinician may confirm clinical diagnosis of OME by tympanometry (D).

5 Does tympanometry confirm the diagnosis of OME?

No

Yes

Yes

6 Exit this algorithm to individualized patient management appropriate to the clinical situation.

7 Options for management of this patient with OME should include:
(1) a. Observation (E)
   OR
   b. Oral antibiotic therapy (F)
   AND
(2) Environmental risk factor control counseling (G).

ATTENTION
Management of the patient at this point in the clinical course should not include:
(1) Surgery, including myringotomy with or without tube insertion, tonsillectomy, or adenoidectomy (H)
   OR
(2) Decongestants and/or antihistamines (I)
   OR
(3) Oral steriod therapy (J).

Go to next page

Algorithm (continued)

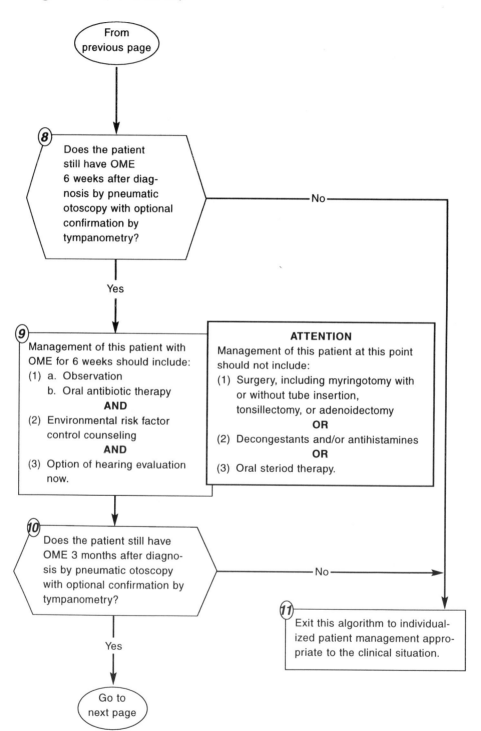

From previous page

8 Does the patient still have OME 6 weeks after diagnosis by pneumatic otoscopy with optional confirmation by tympanometry?

No →

Yes ↓

9 Management of this patient with OME for 6 weeks should include:
(1) a. Observation
   b. Oral antibiotic therapy
   AND
(2) Environmental risk factor control counseling
   AND
(3) Option of hearing evaluation now.

ATTENTION
Management of this patient at this point should not include:
(1) Surgery, including myringotomy with or without tube insertion, tonsillectomy, or adenoidectomy
   OR
(2) Decongestants and/or antihistamines
   OR
(3) Oral steriod therapy.

10 Does the patient still have OME 3 months after diagnosis by pneumatic otoscopy with optional confirmation by tympanometry?

No →

Yes ↓

11 Exit this algorithm to individualized patient management appropriate to the clinical situation.

Go to next page

Algorithm (continued)

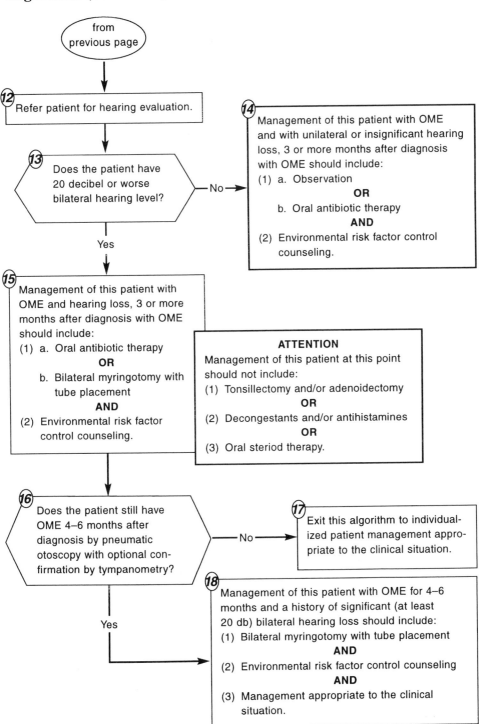

from previous page

12 Refer patient for hearing evaluation.

13 Does the patient have 20 decibel or worse bilateral hearing level?

—No→

14 Management of this patient with OME and with unilateral or insignificant hearing loss, 3 or more months after diagnosis with OME should include:
(1) a. Observation
   OR
   b. Oral antibiotic therapy
   AND
(2) Environmental risk factor control counseling.

Yes

15 Management of this patient with OME and hearing loss, 3 or more months after diagnosis with OME should include:
(1) a. Oral antibiotic therapy
   OR
   b. Bilateral myringotomy with tube placement
   AND
(2) Environmental risk factor control counseling.

ATTENTION
Management of this patient at this point should not include:
(1) Tonsillectomy and/or adenoidectomy
   OR
(2) Decongestants and/or antihistamines
   OR
(3) Oral steriod therapy.

16 Does the patient still have OME 4–6 months after diagnosis by pneumatic otoscopy with optional confirmation by tympanometry?

—No→

17 Exit this algorithm to individualized patient management appropriate to the clinical situation.

Yes

18 Management of this patient with OME for 4–6 months and a history of significant (at least 20 db) bilateral hearing loss should include:
(1) Bilateral myringotomy with tube placement
   AND
(2) Environmental risk factor control counseling
   AND
(3) Management appropriate to the clinical situation.

Selected Bibliography

Black N. The aetiology of glue ear—a case-control study. Int J Pediatr Otorhinolaryngol 1985; 9(2):121–33.

Cantekin EI, Mandel EM, Bluestone CD, Rockette HE, Paradise JL, Stool SE, Fria TJ, Rogers KD. Lack of efficacy of a decongestant-antihistamine combination for otitis media with effusion ("secretory" otitis media) in children: results of a double-blind, randomized trial. N Engl J Med 1983;308(6):297–301.

Casselbrant ML, Brostoff LM, Cantekin EI, Flaherty MR, Doyle WJ, Bluestone CD, Fria TJ. Otitis media with effusion in preschool children. Laryngoscope 1985 Apr;95:428–36.

Etzel RA, Pattishall EN, Haley NJ, Fletcher RH, Henderson FW. Passive smoking and middle ear effusion among children in day care. Pediatrics 1992 Aug;90(2):228–32.

Friel-Patti S, Finitzo T. Language learning in a prospective study of otitis media with effusion in the first two years of life. J Speech Hear Res 1990;33:188–94.

Maw AR. Development of tympanosclerosis in children with otitis media with effusion and ventilation tubes. J Laryngol Otol 1991;105(8):614–7.

Rosenfeld RM, Mandel EM, Bluestone CD. Systemic steroids for otitis media with effusion in children. Arch Otolaryngol Head Neck Surg 1991 Sept;117:984–9.

Rosenfeld RM, Post JC. Meta-analysis of antibiotics for the treatment of otitis media with effusion. Otolaryngol Head Neck Surg 1992;106:378–86.

Teele DW, Klein JO, Rosner B; the Greater Boston Otitis Media Study Group. Middle ear disease and the practice of pediatrics. Burden during the first five years of life. JAMA 1983 Feb 25;249(8):1026–9.

Teele DW, Klein JO, Rosner B; the Greater Boston Otitis Media Study Group. Otitis media with effusion during the first three years of life and development of speech and language. Pediatrics 1984;74(2):282–7.

Toner JG, Mains B. Pneumatic otoscopy and tympanometry in the detection of middle ear effusion. Clin Otolaryngol 1990;15(2):121–3.

Williams RL, Chalmers TC, Stange KC, Chalmers FT, Bowlin SJ. Use of antibiotics in preventing recurrent acute otitis media and in treating otitis media with effusion: a meta-analytic attempt to resolve the brouhaha. JAMA 1993 Sep 15; 270(11):1344–51.

Zielhuis GA, Straatman H, Rach GH, van den Broek P. Analysis and presentation of data on the natural course of otitis media with effusion in children. Int J Epidemiol 1990 Dec; 19(4):1037–44.

The Diagnosis, Treatment, and Evaluation of the Initial Urinary Tract Infection in Febrile Infants and Young Children

- *Clinical Practice Guideline*
- *Technical Report Summary*

Readers of this clinical practice guideline are urged to review the technical report to enhance the evidence-based decision-making process. The report is available on the Pediatrics electronic pages Web site at the following URL: http://www.pediatrics.org/cgi/content/full/103/4/e54.

Clinical Practice Guideline:
The Diagnosis, Treatment, and Evaluation of the Initial Urinary Tract Infection in Febrile Infants and Young Children

Author:

Subcommittee on Urinary Tract Infection
Committee on Quality Improvement

American Academy of Pediatrics
PO Box 927, 141 Northwest Point Blvd
Elk Grove Village, IL 60009-0927

Subcommittee on Urinary Tract Infection

Kenneth B. Roberts, MD, Chairperson

Stephen M. Downs, MD, MS

Stanley Hellerstein, MD

Michael J. Holmes, MD, PhD

Robert L. Lebowitz, MD

Jacob A. Lohr, MD

Linda D. Shortliffe, MD

Russell W. Steele, MD

Committee on Quality Improvement, 1999

David A. Bergman, MD, Chairperson

Richard D. Baltz, MD

James R. Cooley, MD

Gerald B. Hickson, MD

Paul V. Miles, MD

Joan E. Shook, MD

William M. Zurhellen, MD

Liaison Representatives:

Michael J. Goldberg, MD,
  Sections Liaison
Charles J. Homer, MD, MPH,
  Section on Epidemiology Liaison

Betty A. Lowe, MD, NACHRI
  Liaison

Abstract

Objective. To formulate recommendations for health care professionals about the diagnosis, treatment, and evaluation of an initial urinary tract infection (UTI) in febrile infants and young children (ages 2 months to 2 years).

Design. Comprehensive search and analysis of the medical literature, supplemented with consensus opinion of Subcommittee members.

Participants. The American Academy of Pediatrics (AAP) Committee on Quality Improvement selected a Subcommittee composed of pediatricians with expertise in the fields of epidemiology and informatics, infectious diseases, nephrology, pediatric practice, radiology, and urology to draft the parameter. The Subcommittee, the AAP Committee on Quality Improvement, a review panel of office-based practitioners, and other groups within and outside the AAP reviewed and revised the parameter.

Methods. The Subcommittee identified the population at highest risk of incurring renal damage from UTI—infants and young children with UTI and fever. A comprehensive bibliography on UTI in infants and young children was compiled. Literature was abstracted in a formal manner, and evidence tables were constructed. Decision analysis and cost-effectiveness analyses were performed to assess various strategies for diagnosis, treatment, and evaluation.

Technical Report. The overall problem of managing UTI in children between 2 months and 2 years of age was conceptualized as an evidence model. The model depicts the relationship between the steps in diagnosis and management of UTI. The steps are divided into the following four phases: 1) recognizing the child at risk for UTI, 2) making the diagnosis of UTI, 3) short-term treatment of UTI, and 4) evaluation of the child with UTI for possible urinary tract abnormality.

Phase 1 represents the recognition of the child at risk for UTI. Age and other clinical features define a prevalence or a prior probability of UTI, determining whether the diagnosis should be pursued.

Phase 2 depicts the diagnosis of UTI. Alternative diagnostic strategies may be characterized by their cost, sensitivity, and specificity. The result of testing is the division of patients into groups according to a relatively higher or lower probability of having a UTI. The probability of UTI in each of these groups depends not only on the sensitivity and specificity of the test, but also on the prior probability of the UTI among the children being tested. In this way, the usefulness of a diagnostic test depends on the prior probability of UTI established in Phase 1.

Phase 3 represents the short-term treatment of UTI. Alternatives for treatment of UTI may be compared, based on their likelihood of clearing the initial UTI.

Phase 4 depicts the imaging evaluation of infants with the diagnosis of UTI to identify those with urinary tract abnormalities such as vesicoureteral reflux (VUR). Children with VUR are believed to be at risk for ongoing renal damage with subsequent infections, resulting in hypertension and renal failure. Prophylactic antibiotic therapy or surgical procedures such as ureteral reimplantation may prevent progressive renal damage. Therefore, identifying urinary abnormalities may offer the benefit of preventing hypertension and renal failure.

Because the consequences of detection and early management of UTI are affected by subsequent evaluation and long-term management and, likewise, long-term management of patients with UTI depends on how they are detected at the outset, the Subcommittee elected to analyze the entire process from detection of UTI to the evaluation for, and consequences of, urinary tract abnormalities. The full analysis of these data can be found in the technical report. History of the literature review along with evidence-tables and a comprehensive bibliography also are available in the report. This report is published in *Pediatrics electronic pages* and can be accessed at the following URL: http://www.pediatrics.org/cgi/content/full/103/4/e54.

Results. Eleven recommendations are proposed for the diagnosis, management, and follow-up evaluation of infants and young children with unexplained fever who are later found to have a diagnosed UTI. Infants and young children are of particular concern because UTI in this age group (approximately 5%) may cause few recognizable signs or symptoms other than fever and has a higher potential for renal damage than in older children. Strategies for diagnosis and treatment depend on the clinician's assessment of the illness in the infant or young child. Diagnosis is based on the culture of a properly collected specimen of urine; urinalysis can only suggest the diagnosis. A sonogram should be performed on all infants and young children with fever and their first documented UTI; voiding cysto-urethrography or radionuclide cystography should be strongly considered.

ABBREVIATIONS: UTI, urinary tract infections; SPA, suprapubic aspiration; VUR, vesicoureteral reflux; WBC, white blood cell; TMP-SMX, trimethoprim-sulfamethoxazole; VCUG, voiding cystourethrography; RNC, radionuclide cystography.

The urinary tract is a relatively common site of infection in infants and young children. Urinary tract infections (UTIs) are important because they cause acute morbidity and may result in long-term medical problems, including hypertension and reduced renal function. Management of children with UTI involves repeated patient visits, use of antimicrobials, exposure to radiation, and cost. Accurate diagnosis is extremely important for two reasons: to permit identification, treatment, and evaluation of the children who are at risk for kidney damage and to avoid unnecessary treatment and evaluation of children who are not at risk, for whom interventions are costly and potentially harmful but provide no benefit. Infants and young children with UTI are of particular concern because the risk of renal damage is greatest in this age group and because the diagnosis is frequently challenging: the clinical presentation tends to be nonspecific and valid urine specimens cannot be obtained without invasive methods (suprapubic aspiration [SPA], transurethral catheterization).

Considerable variation in the methods of diagnosis, treatment, and evaluation of children with UTI was documented more than 2 decades ago.[1] Since then, various changes have been proposed to aid in diagnosis, treatment, and evaluation, but no data are available to suggest that such innovations have resulted in reduced variation in practice. This practice parameter focuses on the diagnosis, treatment, and evaluation of febrile infants and young children (2 months to 2 years of age). Excluded are those with obvious neurologic or anatomic abnormalities known to be associated with recurrent UTI and renal damage. Neonates and infants younger than 2 months have been excluded from consideration in this practice parameter. Children older than 2 years experiencing their first UTI also are excluded because they are more likely than younger children to have symptoms referable to the urinary tract, are less likely to have factors predisposing them to renal damage, and are at lower risk of developing renal damage.

This parameter is intended for use by clinicians who treat infants and young children in a variety of clinical settings (eg, office, emergency department, hospital).

Methods

A comprehensive literature review was conducted to provide data for evidence tables that could be used to generate a decision tree. More than 2000 titles were identified from MEDLINE and bibliographies of current review articles from 1966 to 1996, and the authors' files. Of these, 402 articles contained relevant original data that were abstracted in a formal, standardized manner. An evidence-based model was developed using quantitative outcomes derived from the literature and cost data from the University of North Carolina. Decision analysis was used to perform risk analyses and cost-effectiveness analyses of alternative strategies for the diagnosis, management, and evaluation of UTI, using hypertension and end-stage renal disease as the undesirable outcomes. The calculated probability of undesirable outcome is the product of the probabilities of several steps (diagnosis, treatment, evaluation) and therefore is an estimate, influenced by approximations at each step. Cost-effectiveness of various strategies was assessed using the methods of Rice and associates[2] in which the break-even cost to prevent a chronic condition, such as hypertension or end-stage renal disease, is considered to be $700 000, an amount based on the estimated lifetime productivity of a healthy, young adult. Once this cost is assigned to the untoward clinical outcome (ie, hypertension or end-stage renal disease), it is possible to use the threshold method of decision-making.[3] The threshold approach to decision-making involves changing the value of a variable in the decision analysis to determine the value at which one strategy of diagnosis, treatment, and evaluation exceeds the break-even cost and an alternative strategy is preferred. Based on the results of these analyses and consensus, when necessary, an Algorithm was developed representing the strategies with the greatest benefit-risk characteristics. The strength of evidence on which recommendations were based was rated by the Subcommittee methodologist as strong, good, fair, or opinion/consensus. A detailed description of the methods by which the parameter was derived is available in a technical report from the American Academy of Pediatrics.

Diagnosis

Recommendation 1

The presence of UTI should be considered in infants and young children 2 months to 2 years of age with unexplained fever (strength of evidence: strong).

The prevalence of UTI in infants and young children 2 months to 2 years of age who have no fever source evident from history or physical examination is high, ~5%.[4-8] The genders are not affected equally, however. The prevalence of UTI in febrile girls age 2 months to 2 years is more than twice that in boys (relative risk, 2.27). The prevalence of UTI in girls younger than 1 year of age is 6.5%; in boys, it is 3.3%. The prevalence of UTI in girls between 1 and 2 years of age is 8.1%; in boys it is 1.9%. The rate in circumcised boys is low, 0.2% to 0.4%.[9-13] The literature suggests that the rate in uncircumcised boys is 5 to 20 times higher than in circumcised boys.

Infants and young children are at higher risk than are older children for incurring acute renal injury with UTI. The incidence of vesicoureteral reflux (VUR) is higher in this age group than in older children (Fig 1), and the severity of VUR is greater, with the most severe form (with intrarenal reflux or pyelotubular backflow) virtually limited to infants.

Infants and young children with UTI warrant special attention because of the opportunity to prevent kidney damage. First, the UTI may bring to attention a child with an obstructive anomaly or severe VUR. Second, because infants and young children with UTI may have a febrile illness and no localizing findings, there may be a delay in diagnosis and treatment of the UTI. Clinical and experi-

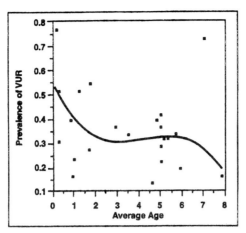

Fig. 1.
Prevalence of VUR by age. Plotted are the prevalences reported in 54 studies of urinary tract infections in children (references in Technical Report). The studies are weighted by sample size. The line is a third order polynomial fit to the data.

mental data support the concept that delay in instituting appropriate treatment of acute pyelonephritis increases the risk of kidney damage.[14,15] Third, the risk of renal damage increases as the number of recurrences increases[16] (Fig 2).

The presence of fever has long been considered a finding of special importance in infants and young children with UTI, because it has been accepted as a clinical marker of renal parenchymal involvement (pyelonephritis). The concept that otherwise unexplained fever in a child with UTI indicates that renal parenchymal involvement is based on comparison of children with high fever (≥39°C) and the clinical diagnosis of acute pyelonephritis with those with no fever (≤38°C) and a clinical diagnosis of cystitis.[17] Indirect tests for localization of the site of UTI,

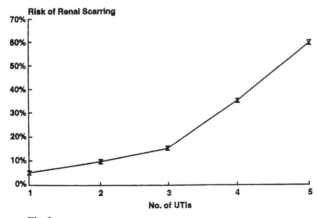

Fig. 2.
Relationship between renal scarring and number of urinary tract infections.[16]

such as the presence of a reversible defect in renal concentrating ability and high levels of antibody titer to the infecting strains of *Escherichia coli*, and nonspecific tests of inflammation, such as elevated white blood cell (WBC) count, C-reactive protein, or sedimentation rate, are encountered more frequently in children with clinical pyelonephritis than in those with clinical cystitis. However, the indirect tests for localization of the site of infection and the nonspecific indicators of inflammation do not provide confirmatory evidence that the febrile infant or young child with UTI has pyelonephritis. Cortical imaging studies using technetium 99 m Tc-dimercaptosuccinic acid (DMSA) or 99 m Tc-glucoheptonate may prove useful in determining whether the presence of high fever does identify children with pyelonephritis and distinguish them from those with cystitis; currently available studies with data that can be used to assess fever as a marker of pyelonephritis (defined by a positive scan) provide a wide range of sensitivity (53% to 84%) and specificity (44% to 92%).[18–20]

The likelihood that UTI is the cause of the fever may be increased if there is a history of crying on urination or of foul-smelling urine. An altered voiding pattern may be recognized as a symptom of UTI as early as the second year after birth in some children. Dysuria, urgency, frequency, or hesitancy may be present but are difficult to discern in this age group. Nonspecific signs and symptoms, such as irritability, vomiting, diarrhea, and failure to thrive, also may reflect the presence of UTI, but data are not available to assess the sensitivity, specificity, and predictive value of these clinical manifestations.

Decision analysis and cost-effectiveness analyses were performed, considering the different prevalences for age, gender, and circumcision status, and the prevalence of VUR by age. For girls and uncircumcised boys, it is cost-effective to pursue the diagnosis of UTI by invasive means and to perform imaging studies of the urinary tract. For circumcised boys younger than 1 year, the cost-benefit analysis is equivocal, but the Subcommittee supports the same diagnostic and evaluation measures as for girls and uncircumcised boys. Circumcised boys older than 1 year have a lower prevalence of UTI, and the prevalence of reflux is lower than that in those younger than 1 year. As a result, the cost-effectiveness analysis does not support invasive diagnostic procedures for all circumcised boys older than 1 year with unexplained fever. Analysis of a bag-collected specimen is a reasonable screening test in these boys, as long as they do not appear so ill as to warrant the initiation of antimicrobial therapy. Those who will be given antimicrobials on clinical grounds should have a specimen obtained for culture that is unlikely to be contaminated.

Recommendation 2

In infants and young children 2 months to 2 years of age with unexplained fever, the degree of toxicity, dehydration, and ability to retain oral intake must be carefully assessed (strength of evidence: strong).

In addition to seeking an explanation for fever, such as a source of infection, clinicians make a subjective assessment of the degree of illness or toxicity. Attempts have been made to objectify this assessment, using the prediction of bacteremia or serious bacterial infection as the outcome measure.[21] This clinical assessment, operationalized as whether antimicrobial therapy will be initiated, affects the diagnostic and therapeutic process regarding UTI as follows. If the clinician determines that the degree of illness warrants antimicrobial therapy, a valid urine specimen should be obtained before antimicrobials are administered, because the antimicrobials commonly prescribed in such situations will be effective against the usual urinary pathogens; invasive means are required to obtain such a specimen. If the clinician determines that the degree of illness does not require antimicrobial therapy, a urine culture is not essential immediately. In this situation, some clinicians may choose to obtain a specimen by noninvasive means (eg, in a collection bag attached to the perineum). The false-positive rate with such specimens dictates that before diagnosing UTI, all positive results be confirmed with culture of a urine specimen unlikely to be contaminated (see below).

Recommendation 3

If an infant or young child 2 months to 2 years of age with unexplained fever is assessed as being sufficiently ill to warrant immediate antimicrobial therapy, a urine specimen should be obtained by SPA or transurethral bladder catheterization; the diagnosis of UTI cannot be established by a culture of urine collected in a bag (strength of evidence: good).

Urine obtained by SPA or transurethral catheterization is unlikely to be contaminated and therefore is the preferred specimen for documenting UTI. In a clinical setting in which the physician has determined that immediate antimicrobial therapy is appropriate, the use of a bag-collected urine specimen is insufficient to document the presence of UTI.

Establishing a diagnosis of UTI requires a strategy that minimizes false-negative and false-positive results. Urine obtained by SPA is the least likely to be contaminated; urine obtained by transurethral bladder catheterization is next best. Either SPA or transurethral bladder catheterization should be used to establish the diagnosis of UTI. Cultures of urine specimens collected in a bag applied to the perineum have an unacceptably high false-positive rate; the combination of a 5% prevalence of UTI and a high rate of false-positive results (specificity, ~70%) results in a positive culture of urine collected in a bag to be a *false*-positive result 85% of the time. If antimicrobial therapy is initiated before obtaining a specimen of urine for culture that is unlikely to be contaminated, the opportunity may be lost to confirm the presence or establish the absence of UTI. Therefore, in the situation in which antimicrobial therapy will be initiated, SPA or catheterization is required to establish the diagnosis of UTI.

SPA has been considered the "gold standard" for obtaining urine for detecting bacteria in bladder urine accurately. The technique has limited risks. However, variable success rates for obtaining urine have been reported (23% to 90%),[16,22–24] technical expertise and experience are required, and many parents and physicians perceive the procedure as unacceptably invasive compared with catheterization. There may be no acceptable alternative in the boy with moderate or severe phimosis, however.

Urine obtained by transurethral catheterization of the urinary bladder for urine culture has a sensitivity of 95% and a specificity of 99% compared with that obtained by SPA.[23,25] Catheterization requires some skill and experience to obtain uncontaminated specimens, particularly in small infants, girls, and uncircumcised boys. Early studies in adults provided widely varying estimates of risk of introducing infection by a single, in-out catheterization. Turck and colleagues[26] demonstrated that the rate of bacteriuria secondary to transurethral catheterization in healthy young adults was considerably lower than that in hospitalized, older adults. Of the 200 healthy young adults studied, 100 men and 100 women, bacteriuria ultimately developed in only 1 woman—2 weeks after catheterization; bacteriuria was documented not to be present during the first 1 to 2 weeks after her catheterization. The risk of introducing infection in infants by transurethral catheterization has not been determined precisely, but it is the consensus of the Subcommittee that the risk is sufficiently low to recommend the procedure when UTI is suspected.

The techniques required for transurethral bladder catheterization and SPA are well described.[27] When SPA or transurethral catheterization is being attempted, the clinician should have a sterile container ready to collect a urine specimen voided because of the stimulus of the patient by manipulation in preparation for or during the procedure.

Recommendation 4

If an infant or young child 2 months to 2 years of age with unexplained fever is assessed as not being so ill as to require immediate antimicrobial therapy, there are two options (strength of evidence: good).

Option 1
Obtain and culture a urine specimen collected by SPA or transurethral bladder catheterization.

Option 2
Obtain a urine specimen by the most convenient means and perform a urinalysis. If the urinalysis suggests a UTI, obtain and culture a urine specimen collected by SPA or transurethral bladder catheterization; if urinalysis

does not suggest a UTI, it is reasonable to follow the clinical course without initiating antimicrobial therapy, recognizing that a negative urinalysis does not rule out a UTI.

The option with the highest sensitivity is to obtain and culture a urine specimen collected by SPA or transurethral bladder catheterization; however, this approach may be resisted by some families and clinicians. In infants and young children assessed as *not* being so ill as to require immediate antimicrobial therapy, a urinalysis may help distinguish those with higher and lower likelihood of UTI. The urinalysis can be performed on any specimen, including one collected from a bag applied to the perineum, and has the advantage of convenience. The major disadvantage of collecting a specimen in a bag is that it is unsuitable for quantitative culture. In addition, there may be a delay of 1 hour or longer for the infant or young child to void; then, if the urinalysis suggests UTI, a second specimen is required. The sensitivity of the bag method for detecting UTI is essentially 100%, but the false-positive rate of this method is also high, as demonstrated in several studies.[23,25,28] If the prevalence of UTI is 5%, 85% of positive cultures will be false-positive results; if the prevalence of UTI is 2% (febrile boys), the rate of false-positive results is 93%; if the prevalence of UTI is 0.2% (circumcised boys), the rate of false-positive results is 99%. The use of bag-collected urine specimens persists because collection of urine by this method is noninvasive and requires limited personnel time and expertise. Moreover, a negative (sterile) culture of a bag-collected urine specimen effectively eliminates the diagnosis of UTI, provided that the child is not receiving antimicrobials and that the urine is not contaminated with an antibacterial skin cleansing agent. Based on their experience, many clinicians believe that this collection technique has a low contamination rate under the following circumstances: the patient's perineum is properly cleansed and rinsed before application of the collection bag; the urine bag is removed promptly after urine is voided into the bag; and the specimen is refrigerated or processed immediately. Nevertheless, even if contamination from the perineal skin is minimized, there may be significant contamination from the vagina in girls or the prepuce in uncircumcised boys. Published results demonstrate that although a negative culture of a bag-collected specimen effectively rules out UTI, a positive culture does not document UTI. Confirmation requires culture of a specimen collected by transurethral bladder catheterization or SPA. Transurethral catheterization does not eliminate completely the possibility of contamination in girls and uncircumcised boys.

Of the components of urinalysis, the three most useful in the evaluation of possible UTI are leukocyte esterase test, nitrite test, and microscopy. A positive result on a leukocyte esterase test seems to be as sensitive as the identification of WBCs microscopically, but the sensitivity of either test is so low that the risk of missing UTI by either test alone is unacceptably high (Table 1). The nitrite test has a very high specificity and positive predictive value when urine specimens are processed promptly after collection. Using either a positive leukocyte esterase or nitrite test improves sensitivity at the expense of specificity; that

TABLE 1 Sensitivity and Specificity of Components of the Urinalysis, Alone and in Combination (References in Text)

Test	Sensitivity % (Range)	Specificity % (Range)
Leukocyte esterase	83 (67–94)	78 (64–92)
Nitrite	53 (15–82)	98 (90–100)
Leukocyte esterase *or* nitrite positive	93 (90–100)	72 (58–91)
Microscopy: WBCs	73 (32–100)	81 (45–98)
Microscopy: bacteria	81 (16–99)	83 (11–100)
Leukocyte esterase *or* nitrite *or* microscopy positive	99.8 (99–100)	70 (60–92)

is, there are many false-positive results. The wide range of reported test characteristics for microscopy indicates the difficulty in ensuring quality performance; the best results are achieved with skilled technicians processing fresh urine specimens.

The urinalysis cannot substitute for a urine culture to document the presence of UTI, but the urinalysis can be valuable in selecting individuals for prompt initiation of treatment while waiting for the results of the urine culture. Any of the following are suggestive (although not diagnostic) of UTI: positive result of a leukocyte esterase or nitrite test, more than 5 white blood cells per high-power field of a properly spun specimen, or bacteria present on an unspun Gram-stained specimen.

In circumcised boys, whose low a priori rate of UTI (0.2% to 0.4%) does not routinely justify an invasive, potentially traumatic procedure, a normal urinalysis reduces the likelihood of UTI as the cause of the fever still further, to the order of 0.1%.

Recommendation 5

Diagnosis of UTI requires a culture of the urine (strength of evidence: strong).

All urine specimens should be processed as expediently as possible. If the specimen is not processed promptly, it should be refrigerated to prevent the growth of organisms that can occur in urine at room temperature. For the same reason, specimens requiring transportation to another site for processing should be transported on ice.

The standard test for the diagnosis of UTI is a quantitative urine culture; no element of the urinalysis or combination of elements is as sensitive and specific. A properly collected urine specimen should be inoculated on culture media that will allow identification of urinary tract pathogens.

UTI is confirmed or excluded based on the number of colony-forming units that grow on the culture media. Defining significant colony counts with regard to the method of collection considers that the distal urethra is commonly colonized by

TABLE 2   Criteria for the Diagnosis of UTI[53]

Method of Collection	Colony Count (Pure Culture)	Probability of Infection (%)
SPA	Gram-negative bacilli: any number Gram-positive cocci: more than a few thousand	>99%
Transurethral catheterization	$>10^5$ 10^4–10^5 10^3–10^4 $<10^3$	95%; Infection likely suspicious; repeat infection unlikely
Clean void		
Boy	$>10^4$	Infection likely
Girl	3 Specimens $\geq 10^5$ 2 Specimens $\geq 10^5$ 1 Specimen $\geq 10^5$ 5×10^4 – 10^5 10^4 – 5×10^4 $<10^4$	95% 90% 80% Suspicious, repeat Symptomatic: suspicious, repeat Asymptomatic: infection unlikely infection unlikely

the same bacteria that may cause UTI; thus, a low colony count may be present in a specimen obtained by voiding or by transurethral catheterization when bacteria are not present in bladder urine. As noted in Table 2, what constitutes a significant colony count depends on the collection method and the clinical status of the patient; definitions of positive and negative cultures are operational and not absolute. Significance also depends on the identification of the isolated organism as a pathogen. Organisms such as *Lactobacillus* species, coagulase-negative staphylococci, and *Corynebacterium* species are not considered clinically relevant urine isolates in the otherwise healthy 2-month to 2-year-old. Alternative culture methods such as the dipslide may have a place in the office setting; sensitivity is reported in the range of 87% to 100%, and specificity, 92% to 98%.

Treatment

Recommendation 6

If the infant or young child 2 months to 2 years of age with suspected UTI is assessed as toxic, dehydrated, or unable to retain oral intake, initial antimicrobial therapy should be administered parenterally and hospitalization should be considered (strength of evidence: opinion/consensus).

The goals of treatment of acute UTI are to eliminate the acute infection, to prevent urosepsis, and to reduce the likelihood of renal damage. Patients who are toxic-appearing, dehydrated, or unable to retain oral intake (including medications) should receive an antimicrobial parenterally (Table 3) until they are improved clinically and are able to retain oral fluids and medications. The parenteral route is recommended because it ensures optimal antimicrobial levels in

TABLE 3   Some Antimicrobials for Parenteral Treatment of UTI

Antimicrobial	Daily Dosage
Ceftriaxone	75 mg/kg every 24 h
Cefotaxime	150 mg/kg/d divided every 6 h
Ceftazidime	150 mg/kg/d divided every 6 h
Cefazolin	50 mg/kg/d divided every 8 h
Gentamicin	7.5 mg/kg/d divided every 8 h
Tobramycin	5 mg/kg/d divided every 8 h
Ticarcillin	300 mg/kg/d divided every 6 h
Ampicillin	100 mg/kg/d divided every 6 h

these high-risk patients. Parenteral administration of an antimicrobial also should be considered when compliance with obtaining and/or administering an antimicrobial orally cannot be ensured. In patients with compromised renal function, the use of potentially nephrotoxic antimicrobials (eg, aminoglycosides) requires caution, and serum creatinine and peak and trough antimicrobial concentrations need to be monitored. The clinical conditions of most patients improve within 24 to 48 hours; the route of antimicrobial administration then can be changed to oral (Table 4) to complete a 7- to 14-day course of therapy.

Hospitalization is necessary if patients have clinical urosepsis or are considered likely to have bacteremia based on clinical or laboratory evaluation. These patients need careful monitoring and repeated clinical examinations.

For children who do not appear toxic but who are vomiting, or when noncompliance is a concern, options include beginning therapy in the hospital or administering an antimicrobial parenterally on an outpatient basis. The route of administration is changed to oral when the child is no longer vomiting, and compliance appears to be ensured.

Recommendation 7

In the infant or young child 2 months to 2 years of age who may not appear ill but who has a culture confirming the presence of UTI, antimicro-

TABLE 4   Some Antimicrobials for Oral Treatment of UTI

Antimicrobial	Dosage
Amoxicillin	20–40 mg/kg/d in 3 doses
Sulfonamide	
TMP in combination	6–12 mg TMP, 30–60 mg
with SMX	SMX per kg per d in 2 doses
Sulfisoxazole	120–150 mg/kg/d in 4 doses
Cephalosporin	
Cefixime	8 mg/kg/d in 2 doses
Cefpodixime	10 mg/kg/d in 2 doses
Cefprozil	30 mg/kg/d in 2 doses
Cephalexin	50–100 mg/kg/d in 4 doses
Loracarbef	15–30 mg/kg/d in 2 doses

bial therapy should be initiated, parenterally or orally (strength of evidence: good).

The usual choices for treatment of UTI orally include amoxicillin, a sulfonamide-containing antimicrobial (sulfisoxazole or trimethoprim-sulfamethoxazole [TMP-SMX]), or a cephalosporin (Table 4). Emerging resistance of *E coli* to ampicillin appears to have rendered ampicillin and amoxicillin less effective than alternative agents. Studies comparing amoxicillin with TMP-SMX have demonstrated consistently higher cure rates with TMP-SMX (4% to 42%), regardless of the duration of therapy (1 dose, 3 to 4 days, or 10 days).[29-45]

Agents that are excreted in the urine but do not achieve therapeutic concentrations in the bloodstream, such as nalidixic acid or nitrofurantoin, should not be used to treat UTI in febrile infants and young children in whom renal involvement is likely.

Recommendation 8

Infants and young children 2 months to 2 years of age with UTI who have not had the expected clinical response with 2 days of antimicrobial therapy should be reevaluated and another urine specimen should be cultured (strength of evidence: good).

Routine reculturing of the urine after 2 days of antimicrobial therapy is generally not necessary if the infant or young child has had the expected clinical response and the uropathogen is determined to be sensitive to the antimicrobial being administered. Antimicrobial sensitivity testing is determined most commonly by the application of disks containing the usual serum concentration of the antimicrobial to the culture plate. Because many antimicrobial agents are excreted in the urine in extremely high concentrations, an intermediately sensitive organism may be fully eradicated. Studies of minimal inhibitory concentration may be required to clarify the appropriateness of a given antimicrobial. If the sensitivity of the organism to the chosen antimicrobial is determined to be intermediate or resistant, or if sensitivity testing is not performed, a "proof-of-bacteriologic cure" culture should be performed after 48 hours of treatment. Data are not available to determine that clinical response alone ensures bacteriologic cure.

Recommendation 9

Infants and young children 2 months to 2 years of age, including those whose treatment initially was administered parenterally, should complete a 7- to 14-day antimicrobial course orally (strength of evidence: strong).

In 8 of 10 comparisons of long treatment duration (7 to 10 days) and short duration (1 dose or up to 3 days), results were better with long duration, with an attributable improvement in outcome of 5% to 21%.[33,38,41,44-48] Most uncomplicated UTIs are eliminated with a 7- to 10-day antimicrobial course, but many experts prefer 14 days for ill-appearing children with clinical evidence of pyelonephritis. Data comparing 10 days and 14 days are not available.

Recommendation 10

After a 7- to 14-day course of antimicrobial therapy and sterilization of the urine, infants and young children 2 months to 2 years of age with UTI should receive antimicrobials in therapeutic or prophylactic dosages until the imaging studies are completed (strength of evidence: good).

Although this practice parameter deals with the acute UTI, it is important to recognize the significance of recurrent infections. The association between recurrent bouts of febrile UTI and renal scarring follows an exponential curve[16] (Fig 2). Because the risk of recurrence is highest during the first months after UTI, children treated for UTI should continue antimicrobial treatment or prophylaxis (Table 5) until the imaging studies are completed and assessed. Additional treatment is based on the imaging findings assuming sterilization of the urine.

Evaluation: Imaging

Recommendation 11

Infants and young children, 2 months to 2 years, with UTI, who do not demonstrate the expected clinical response within 2 days of antimicrobial therapy, should undergo ultrasonography promptly. Voiding cystourethrography (VCUG) or radionuclide cystography (RNC) is strongly encouraged to be performed at the earliest convenient time. Infants and young children who have the expected response to antimicrobials should have a sonogram performed at the earliest convenient time; a VCUG or RNC is strongly encouraged (strength of evidence: fair).

UTI in young children serve as a marker for abnormalities of the urinary tract. Imaging of the urinary tract is recommended in every febrile infant or young child with a first UTI to identify those with abnormalities that predispose to

TABLE 5 Some Antimicrobials for Prophylaxis of UTI	
Antimicrobial	Dosage
TMP in combination with SMX	2 mg of TMP, 10 mg of SMX per kg as single bedtime dose *or* 5 mg of TMP, 25 mg of SMX per kg twice per week
Nitrofurantoin	1–2 mg/kg as single daily dose
Sulfisoxazole	10–20 mg/kg divided every 12 h
Nalidixic acid	30 mg/kg divided every 12 h
Methenamine mandelate	75 mg/kg divided every 12 h

renal damage. Imaging should consist of urinary tract ultrasonography to detect dilatation secondary to obstruction and a study to detect VUR.

Ultrasonography

Urinary tract ultrasonography consists of examination of the kidneys to identify hydronephrosis and examination of the bladder to identify dilatation of the distal ureters, hypertrophy of the bladder wall, and the presence of ureteroceles. Previously, excretory urography (commonly called intravenous pyelography) was used to reveal these abnormalities, but now ultrasonography shows them more safely, less invasively, and often less expensively. Ultrasonography does have limitations, however. A normal ultrasound does not exclude VUR. Ultrasonography may show signs of acute renal inflammation and established renal scars, but it is not as sensitive as other renal imaging techniques.

Usually the timing of the ultrasound is not crucial, but when the rate of clinical improvement is slower than anticipated during treatment, ultrasonography should be performed promptly to look for a cause such as obstruction or abscess.

VUR

The most common abnormality detected in imaging studies is VUR (Fig 1). The rate of VUR among children younger than 1 year of age with UTI exceeds 50%. VUR is not an all-or-none phenomenon; grades of severity are recognized, designated I to V in the International Study Classification (International Reflux Study Committee, 1981), based on the extent of the reflux and associated dilatation of the ureter and pelvis. The grading of VUR is important because the natural history differs by grade, as does the risk of renal damage. Patients with high-grade VUR are 4 to 6 times more likely to have scarring than those with low-grade VUR and 8 to 10 times more likely than those without VUR.[16,49]

VCUG; RNC

Either traditional contrast VCUG or RNC is recommended for detecting reflux. Although children may have pyelonephritis without reflux, the child with reflux is at increased risk of pyelonephritis and of scarring from UTI. With VCUG and RNC, a voiding phase is important because some reflux occurs only during voiding. If the predicted bladder capacity is not reached, the study may underestimate the presence or degree of reflux.

VCUG with fluoroscopy characterizes reflux better than does RNC. In addition, RNC does not show urethral or bladder abnormalities; for this reason, boys, whose urethra must be examined for posterior urethral valves, or girls, who have symptoms of voiding dysfunction when not infected, should have a standard fluoroscopic contrast VCUG as part of their initial studies. RNC has a lower radiation dose and therefore may be preferred in follow-up examinations of children with reflux. However, the introduction of low-dose radiographic equipment has narrowed the gap in radiation between the VCUG and RNC.[50]

There is no benefit in delaying performance of these studies as long as the child is free of infection and bladder irritability is absent. While waiting for reflux study results, the child should be receiving an antimicrobial, either as part of the initial treatment or as posttreatment prophylaxis (Table 5).

Radionuclide Renal Scans

Renal cortical scintigraphy (with 99 m Tc-DMSA or 99 m Tc-glucoheptonate) and enhanced computed tomography are very sensitive means of identifying acute changes from pyelonephritis or renal scarring. However, the role of these imaging modalities in the clinical management of the child with UTI still is unclear.

Conclusions

Eleven recommendations are proposed for the diagnosis, management, and evaluation of infants and young children with UTI and unexplained fever. Infants and children younger than 2 years of age with unexplained fever are identified for particular concern because UTI has a high prevalence in this group (~5%), may cause few recognizable signs or symptoms other than fever, and has a greater potential for renal damage than in older children. Strategies of diagnosis and treatment depend on how ill the clinician assesses the infant or young child to be, ie, whether antimicrobial therapy is warranted immediately or can be delayed safely until the results of urine culture are available. Diagnosis is based on the culture of an appropriately collected specimen of urine; urinalysis can only suggest the diagnosis. Imaging studies should be performed on all infants and young children with a documented initial UTI.

Areas for Future Research

The relationship between UTI in infants and young children and reduced renal function in adults has been established but is not well characterized in quantitative terms. The ideal prospective cohort study from birth to age 40 to 50 years has not been conducted and is unlikely to be conducted. Thus, estimates of undesirable outcomes in adulthood, such as hypertension and end-stage renal disease, are based on the mathematical product of probabilities at several steps, each of which is subject to bias and error. Other attempts at decision analysis[51] and thoughtful literature review[52] have recognized the same limitations. Until recently, imaging tools available to assess the effect of UTI have been insensitive. With the imaging techniques available now, it may be possible to follow a cohort of infants and young children who present with fever and UTI to assess the development of scars and functional impairment. Research is underway in this area.

The development of noninvasive methods of obtaining a urine specimen or of techniques that obviate the need for invasive sampling would be valuable for general use. One component of the urinalysis that merits particular attention is the assessment of WBCs in the urine. Bacteriuria can occur without pyuria, but it is not clear whether pyuria is a specific marker for renal inflammation, obviating the need for culture if WBCs are not present in the urine. Research is underway in this area under conditions that optimize the detection of WBCs in the urine by microscopy. If studies continue to demonstrate usefulness of microscopy, the general applicability of the test will need to be studied, particularly in offices without on-site laboratories or trained laboratory staff. Special attention will need to be given to specimens from girls and from uncircumcised boys, particularly infants, because transurethral catheterization may be difficult and produce a contaminated specimen. An alternative to SPA, which is not commonly performed anymore, would be welcome in clinical practice and in research to clarify such issues as the true prevalence of UTI in young uncircumcised boys.

There is consensus about the antimicrobial treatment of infants and young children with acute UTI, but questions remain relating to the specific duration and route of therapy. Currently, the efficacy of orally administered treatment is being compared with parenterally administered treatment under controlled conditions. If orally administered therapy is as efficacious as that administered parenterally, concern about variable adherence to a prescribed regimen will remain and influence the decision of whether to hospitalize and whether to administer the antimicrobial(s) parenterally or orally.

As noted in the section "Evaluation: Imaging," ultrasonography is recommended to detect dilatation associated with obstruction and is preferred over other modalities because it is noninvasive and does not expose the child to radiation. Data defining the yield of positive findings were generated before the widespread use of fetal ultrasonography, and it is not clear that they are applicable today. The absence of extensive data from modern studies and variations in the frequency and quality of fetal ultrasonography do not permit a determination of whether ultrasonography can reasonably be omitted. Further complicating the assessment is the changing utilization of fetal ultrasonography under the financial pressures of managed care. Studies in this area will need to be defined carefully so that the generalizability and applicability to individual patients can be assessed.

A study to determine the presence and severity of VUR also is recommended. It is recognized, however, that pyelonephritis (defined by cortical scintigraphy) can occur in the absence of VUR (defined by VCUG or RNC) and that progressive renal scarring (defined by cortical scintigraphy) can occur in the absence of demonstrated VUR. Whether children with pyelonephritis (defined clinically or by cortical scintigraphy) who have normal results on VCUG or RNC benefit from antimicrobial prophylaxis is unknown but is being studied.

The role of cortical scintigraphy in the imaging examination of infants and young children with initial UTI is unclear and requires additional study. The demonstration by cortical scintigraphy of "cold" areas of decreased perfusion has led to the development of alternative imaging techniques, such as enhanced computed tomography and power Doppler ultrasonography. These modalities also can demonstrate hypoperfusion and have advantages, particularly power Doppler ultrasonography, which is noninvasive and does not expose the child to radiation. Studies are now in progress.

References

1. Dolan TF Jr, Meyers A. A survey of office management of urinary tract infections in childhood. *Pediatrics.* 1973;52:21–24
2. Rice DP, Hodgeson TA, Kopstein AN. The economic costs of illness: a replication and update. *Health Care Financ Rev.* 1985;7:61–80
3. Pauker SG, Kassirer JP. The threshold approach to clinical decision making. *N Engl J Med.* 1980;302:1109–1117
4. Hoberman A, Chao HP, Keller DM, et al. Prevalence of urinary tract infection in febrile infants. *J Pediatr.* 1993;123:17–23
5. Roberts KB, Charney E, Sweren RJ, et al. Urinary tract infection in infants with unexplained fever: a collaborative study. *J Pediatr.* 1983;103:864–867
6. Bauchner H, Philipp B, Dahefsky G, Klein JO. Prevalence of bacteriuria in febrile children. *Pediatr Infect Dis J.* 1987;6:239–242
7. Bonadio WA. Urine culturing technique in febrile infants. *Pediatr Emerg Care.* 1987;3:75–78
8. North AF. Bacteriuria in children with acute febrile illnesses. *J Pediatr.* 1963;63:408–411
9. Ginsburg CM, McCracken GH Jr. Urinary tract infections in young infants. *Pediatrics.* 1982;69:409–412
10. Wiswell TE, Smith FR, Bass JW. Decreased incidence of urinary tract infections in circumcised male infants. *Pediatrics.* 1985;75:901–903
11. Wiswell TE, Roscelli JD. Corroborative evidence for the decreased incidence of urinary tract infections in circumcised male infants. *Pediatrics.* 1986;78:96–99
12. Wiswell TE, Hachey WE. Urinary tract infections and the uncircumcised state: an update. *Clin Pediatr.* 1993;32:130–134
13. Craig JC, Knight JF, Sureshjumar P, Mantz E, Roy LP. Effect of circumcision on incidence of urinary tract infection in preschool boys. *J Pediatr.* 1996;128:23–27
14. Winter AL, Hardy BE, Alton DJ, Arbus GS, Churchill BM. Acquired renal scars in children. *J Urol.* 1983;129:1190–1194
15. Smellie JM, Poulton A, Prescod NP. Retrospective study of children with renal scarring associated with reflux and urinary infection. *Br Med J.* 1994;308:1193–1196
16. Jodal U. The natural history of bacteriuria in childhood. *Infect Dis Clin North Am.* 1987;1:713–729
17. Winberg J, Andersen HJ, Bergstrom T, et al. Epidemiology of symptomatic urinary tract infection in childhood. *Acta Paediatr Scand.* 1974;252:1–20. Supplement
18. Tappin DM, Murphy AV, Mocan H, et al. A prospective study of children with first acute symptomatic *E coli* urinary tract infection: early 99 m technetium dimercaptosuccinic acid scan appearances. *Acta Paediatr Scand.* 1989;78:923–929
19. Verboven M, Ingels M, Delree M, Piepsz A. 99 mTc-DMSA scintigraphy in acute urinary tract infection in children. *Pediatr Radiol.* 1990;20:540–542

20. Rosenberg AR, Rossleigh MA, Brydon MP, Bass SJ, Leighton DM, Farnsworth RH. Evaluation of acute urinary tract infection in children by dimercaptosuccinic acid scintigraphy: a prospective study. *J Urol.* 1992;148:1746–1749. Part II

21. McCarthy PL, Sharpe MR, Spiesel SZ, et al. Observation scales to identify serious illness in febrile children. *Pediatrics.* 1982;70:802–809

22. Pryles CV, Atkin MD, Morse TS, Welch KJ. Comparative bacteriologic study of urine obtained from children by percutaneous suprapubic aspiration of the bladder and by catheter. *Pediatrics.* 1959;24:983–991

23. Leong YY, Tan KW. Bladder aspiration for diagnosis of urinary tract infection in infants and young children. *J Singapore Paediatr Soc.* 1976;18:43–47

24. Djojohadipringgo S, Abdul Hamid RH, Thahir S, Karim A, Darsono I. Bladder puncture in newborns—a bacteriological study. *Paediatr Indonesia.* 1976;16:527–534

25. Sorensen K, Lose G, Nathan E. Urinary tract infection and diurnal incontinence in girls. *Eur J Pediatr.* 1988;148:146–147

26. Turck M, Goffe B, Petersdorf RG. The urethral catheter and urinary tract infection. *J Urol.* 1962;88:834–837

27. Lohf J. *Pediatric Outpatient Procedures.* Philadelphia, PA: JB Lippincott Co;1991:142–152

28. Shannon F, Sepp E, Rose G. The diagnosis of bacteriuria by bladder puncture in infancy and childhood. *Aust Paediatr J.* 1969;5:97–100

29. Cohen M. The first urinary tract infection in male children. *Am J Dis Child.* 1976;130:810–813

30. Ellerstein NS, Sullivan TD, Baliah T, Neter E. Trimethoprim/sulfamethoxazole and ampicillin in the treatment of acute urinary tract infections in children: a double-blind study. *Pediatrics.* 1977;60:245–247

31. Khan AJ, Ubriani RS, Bombach E, Agbayani MM, Ratner H, Evans HE. Initial urinary tract infection caused by *Proteus mirabilis* in infancy and childhood. *J Pediatr.* 1978;93:791–793

32. Howard JB, Howard JE. Trimethoprim-sulfamethoxazole vs sulfamethoxazole for acute urinary tract infections in children. *Am J Dis Child.* 1978;132:1085–1087

33. Wientzen RL, McCracken GH Jr, Petruska ML, Swinson SG, Kaijer B, Hanson LA. Localization and therapy of urinary tract infections of childhood. *Pediatrics.* 1979;63:467–474

34. Sullivan TD, Ellerstein NS, Neter E. The effects of ampicillin and trimethoprim/sulfamethoxazole on the periurethral flora of children with urinary tract infection. *Infection.* 1980;8:S339–S341. Supplement 3

35. Fennell RS, Luengnaruemitchai M, Iravani A, Garin EH, Walker RD, Richard GA. Urinary tract infections in children: effect of short course antibiotic therapy on recurrence rate in children with previous infections. *Clin Pediatr.* 1980;19:121–124

36. Shapiro ED, Wald ER. Single-dose amoxicillin treatment of urinary tract infections. *J Pediatr.* 1981;99:989–992

37. Helin I. Short-term treatment of lower urinary tract infections in children with trimethoprim/sulphadiazine. *Infection.* 1981;9:249–251

38. Pitt WR, Dyer SA, McNee JL, Burke JR. Single dose trimethoprim-sulphamethoxazole treatment of symptomatic urinary infection. *Arch Dis Child.* 1981;57:229–231

39. Avner ED, Ingelfinger JR, Herrin JT, et al. Single-dose amoxicillin therapy of uncomplicated pediatric urinary tract infections. *J Pediatr.* 1983;102:623–627

40. Aarbakke J, Opshaug O, Digranes A, Hoylandskjaer A, Fluge G, Fellner H. Clinical effect and pharmacokinetics of trimethoprim-sulphadiazine in children with urinary tract infections. *Eur J Clin Pharmacol.* 1983;24:267–271

41. Stahl G, Topf P, Fleisher GR, Normal ME, Rosenblum HW, Gruskin AB. Single-dose treatment of uncomplicated urinary tract infections in children. *Ann Emerg Med.* 1984;13:705–708

42. Hashemi G. Recurrent urinary tract infection. *Indian J Pediatr.* 1985;52:401–403

43. Rajkumar S, Saxena Y, Rajogopal V, Sierra MF. Trimethoprim in pediatric urinary tract infection. *Child Nephrol Urol.* 1988;9:77–81

44. Madrigal G, Odio CM, Mohs E, Guevara J, McCracken GH Jr. Single dose antibiotic therapy is not as effective as conventional regimens for management of acute urinary tract infections in children. *Pediatr Infect Dis J.* 1988;7:316–319

45. Nolan T, Lubitz L, Oberklaid F. Single dose trimethoprim for urinary tract infection. *Arch Dis Child.* 1989;64:581–586

46. Bailey RR, Abbott GD. Treatment of urinary tract infection with a single dose of trimethoprim-sulfamethoxazole. *Can Med Assoc J.* 1978;118:551–552

47. Bailey RR, Abbott GD. Treatment of urinary tract infection with a single dose of amoxycillin. *Nephron.* 1977;18:316–320

48. Copenhagen Study Group of Urinary Tract Infections in Children. Short-term treatment of acute urinary tract infection in girls. *Scand J Infect Dis.* 1991;23:213–220

49. McKerrow W, Davidson-Lamb N, Jones PF. Urinary tract infection in children. *Br Med J.* 1984;289:299–303

50. Kleinman PK, Diamond DA, Karellas A, Spevak MR, Nimkin K, Belanger P. Tailored low-dose fluoroscopic voiding cystourethrography for the reevaluation of vesicoureteral reflux in girls. *AJR Am J Roentgenol.* 1994;162:1151–1154

51. Kramer MS, Tange SM, Drummond KN, Mills EL. Urine testing in young febrile children: a risk–benefit analysis. *J Pediatr.* 1994;125:6–13

52. Dick PT, Feldman W. Routine diagnostic imaging for childhood urinary tract infections: a systematic overview. *J Pediatr.* 1996;128:15–22

Algorithm

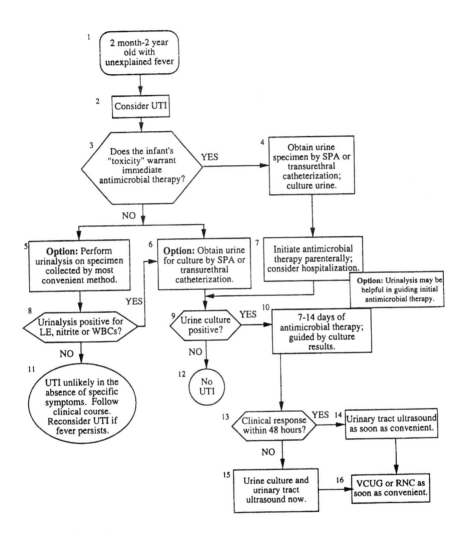

Technical Report Summary:
Urinary Tract Infections in Febrile Infants and Young Children

Authors:

Stephen M. Downs, MD, MS

American Academy of Pediatrics
PO Box 927, 141 Northwest Point Blvd
Elk Grove Village, IL 60009-0927

Abstract

Overview

The Urinary Tract Infection Subcommittee of the American Academy of Pediatrics' Committee on Quality Improvement has analyzed alternative strategies for the diagnosis and management of urinary tract infection (UTI) in children. The target population is limited to children between 2 months and 2 years of age who are examined because of fever without an obvious cause. Diagnosis and management of UTI in this group are especially challenging for these three reasons: 1) the manifestation of UTI tends to be nonspecific, and cases may be missed easily; 2) clean voided midstream urine specimens rarely can be obtained, leaving only urine collection methods that are invasive (transurethral catheterization or bladder tap) or result in nonspecific test results (bag urine); and 3) a substantial number of infants with UTI also may have structural or functional abnormalities of the urinary tract that put them at risk for ongoing renal damage, hypertension, and end-stage renal disease (ESRD).

Methods

To examine alternative management strategies for UTI in infants, a conceptual model of the steps in diagnosis and management of UTI was developed. The model was expanded into a decision tree. Probabilities for branch points in the decision tree were obtained by review of the literature on childhood UTI. Data were extracted on standardized forms. Cost data were obtained by literature review and from hospital billing data. The data were collated into evidence tables. Analysis of the decision tree was used to produce risk tables and incremental cost-effectiveness ratios for alternative strategies.

Results

Based on the results of this analysis and, when necessary, consensus opinion, the Committee developed recommendations for the management of UTI in this population. This document provides the evidence the Subcommittee used in the development of its recommendations.

Conclusions

The Subcommittee agreed that the objective of the practice guideline would be to minimize the risk of chronic renal damage within reasonable economic constraints. Steps involved in achieving these objectives are: 1) identifying UTI; 2) short-term treatment of UTI; and 3) evaluation for urinary tract abnormalities.

Methods

Analysis of the data on UTI consisted of several steps. The Subcommittee met to define the target population, setting, and providers for whom the practice parameter is intended. Subcommittee members identified the outcomes of interest for the analysis. A conceptual evidence model of the diagnosis and management of UTI was developed. The evidence model was used to generate a decision tree. A comprehensive review of the literature determined the probability estimates used in the tree. The tree was used to conduct risk analyses and cost-effectiveness analyses of alternative strategies for the diagnosis and management of UTI. Based on the results of these analyses and consensus when necessary, an algorithm representing the strategies with acceptable risk-benefit trade-offs was developed.

Evidence Model

The overall problem of managing UTI in children between 2 months and 2 years of age was conceptualized as an evidence model. The model depicts the relationships between the steps in the diagnosis and management of UTI. The steps are divided into the following four phases: 1) recognizing the child at risk for UTI, 2) making the diagnosis of UTI, 3) short-term treatment of UTI, and 4) evaluation of the child with UTI for possible urinary tract abnormality.

Phase 1 represents the recognition of the child at risk for UTI. Age and other clinical features define a prevalence or *a priori* probability of UTI, determining whether the diagnosis should be pursued. If children at sufficiently high risk for UTI are not identified for diagnostic evaluation, the potential benefit of treatment will be lost. However, children with a sufficiently low likelihood of UTI should be saved the cost of diagnosis (and perhaps misdiagnosis) of UTI when the potential for benefit is minimal.

Phase 2 depicts the diagnosis of UTI. Alternative diagnostic strategies may be characterized by their cost, sensitivity, and specificity. The result of testing is the division of patients into groups according to a relatively higher or lower probability of having a UTI. The probability of UTI in each of these groups depends not only on the sensitivity and specificity of the test, but also on the prior probability of the UTI among the children being tested. In this way, the usefulness of a diagnostic test depends on the prior probability of UTI established in phase 1. Overdiagnosis of UTI may result in unnecessary treatment and unnecessary imaging evaluation for urinary tract abnormalities. Underdiagnosis will result in missing the opportunity to treat the acute infection and the consequences of possible underlying urinary tract abnormalities.

Phase 3 represents the short-term treatment of UTI. Alternatives for treatment of UTI may be compared, based on their likelihood of clearing the initial UTI (IUTI).

Phase 4 depicts the imaging evaluation of infants with the diagnosis of UTI to identify those with urinary tract abnormalities such as vesicoureteral reflux (VUR). Children with VUR are believed to be at risk for ongoing renal damage with subsequent infections, resulting in hypertension and renal failure. Prophylactic antibiotic therapy or surgical procedures such as ureteral reimplantation may prevent progressive renal damage. Therefore, identifying urinary abnormalities may offer the benefit of preventing hypertension and renal failure. Each alternative strategy for imaging evaluation can be characterized according to its cost, invasiveness, and test characteristics (sensitivity and specificity). The potential yield of an imaging evaluation will be affected by the accuracy of the initial diagnosis of UTI. If the probability of UTI is low because a non-specific test was used to make the diagnosis, the cost of an imaging study will yield little benefit. Therefore, the value of imaging strategies depends on the accuracy of the diagnosis of UTI in phase 2.

Because the consequences of detection and early management of UTI are affected by subsequent evaluation and long-term management and, likewise, long-term management of patients with UTI depends on how they are detected at the outset, the Subcommittee elected to analyze the entire process from detection of UTI to the evaluation for, and consequences of, urinary tract abnormalities.

Decision Tree

The conceptual model was used to develop a decision tree. The tree quantifies the relationship between alternative strategies for the diagnosis and treatment of UTI, the evaluation of children for abnormalities of the urinary tract, and the anticipated consequences of these alternative diagnostic and treatment strategies.

In the diagnosis and treatment of UTI, four alternatives are represented. As anchor points, the alternatives of treating all or treating none of the patients at risk are represented. Two alternative tests are represented in the other branches. The test characteristics and costs of these tests were adjusted to correspond with the tests the Subcommittee chose to evaluate. In this way, the Subcommittee compared alternative testing strategies.

In the decision tree, if a testing strategy is used, the result is positive or negative. A positive result was assumed to lead to a decision to treat and a negative result to a decision to observe without treatment. If treatment is chosen, presumptively or based on the results of a diagnostic test, a treatment complication may result. Rarely, as in the case of anaphylaxis, the complication may result in death.

For all other patients, there is a risk of urosepsis. This risk is the probability of UTI multiplied by the prevalence of urosepsis among infants with UTI. Assuming urosepsis behaves like bacteremia from other sources in infants, the infection may clear spontaneously in those who have urosepsis. The probability of clearing the infection is increased among those who receive antimicrobials. If urosepsis does not clear, hospitalization will result, and the child has a risk of dying.

Once the short-term outcome of the UTI has been resolved, the second decision is whether and how to image the urinary tract for structural and functional abnormalities. The three following options are modeled: 1) a full evaluation, including ultrasonography or an intravenous pyelogram and voiding cystourethrography (VCUG) or radionuclide cystourethrography (RCG); 2) ultrasonography alone; and 3) no evaluation.

The results of the evaluation are determined separately for each patient type. For patients who have no UTI (false-positive diagnosis of UTI), it is assumed that abnormalities are not present and the infant is not at increased risk of renal damage. Patients who have a true UTI may or may not have VUR. Among those with VUR, the reflux may be low grade (1 or 2) or high grade (3, 4, or 5).

The probability of having a positive result when imaging an abnormal urinary tract depends on the sensitivity of the imaging modality for the abnormality. For example, ultrasonography is much more sensitive to high-grade VUR than to low-grade VUR.6 The analysis assumes that all imaging modalities have 100% specificity (ie, no false-positive diagnoses).

The result of the imaging evaluation would be used to select a treatment (surgical correction or antibiotic prophylaxis as appropriate) to prevent recurrent infections. An evaluation with normal results or no evaluation would lead to no therapy. Identifying the optimal therapy for a given urinary tract abnormality is beyond the scope of the present analysis.

Patients may or may not have recurrent UTI, defined as more than three infections in a 5-year period. Recurrent infections lead to progressive renal scarring. The risk of scarring is highest among those with high-grade VUR and lowest among those with no VUR. Therapeutic interventions reduce the risk of renal scarring by reducing VUR in the case of surgery or preventing infection in the case of antimicrobial prophylaxis.

Patients with progressive renal scarring are at increased risk of hypertension and ESRD. Those who do not experience these outcomes may have decreased renal function but will not have clinically important outcomes.

At the terminal nodes of each branch, the outcomes are tabulated as costs and clinical outcomes. Costs considered include the cost of diagnostic testing, treatment, complications of treatment, hospitalization for urosepsis, imaging studies, surgery or prophylaxis, management of hypertension, and ESRD. Clinical outcomes include chronic hypertension, renal failure, and death.

The decision tree was encoded and evaluated using the Decision Maker software Version 6.0 (Sonnenberg and Pauker, New England Medical Center, Boston, MA).

Literature Review

Articles for review were obtained from four sources in two rounds of searching. In the first round, the MEDLINE database was searched using four separate search strategies corresponding with the four phases of the diagnosis and treatment of UTI: recognition, diagnosis, short-term treatment, and imaging evaluation. The titles and abstracts resulting from these searches were distributed among the Subcommittee members who identified those that were definitely or potentially useful. These articles were reproduced in full.

In a second round of searching, articles were identified from three additional sources: the bibliographies of two recent reviews; a survey of the members of the Subcommittee, soliciting the articles they identified as most important and relevant to the analysis; and articles sought specifically to estimate costs for the management of chronic hypertension and ESRD. At each of the two rounds of searching, the articles were reviewed by the epidemiology consultant, and articles with no original data were removed.

The remaining articles were reviewed and data extracted using a data extraction form designed to identify estimates necessary to evaluate the decision model. In addition, the quality of each article was rated on a scale from 0 to 1 by using quality criteria adapted from Sackett and colleagues. Reviewers also provided a subjective rating of "good," "fair," or "poor" to each article. Data extracted were recorded in evidence tables, using an Excel (Microsoft Corporation, Redmond, WA) spreadsheet. A subset of 24 articles was reviewed twice by different reviewers to check interrater reliability. At the time of analysis of the decision models, the articles were reviewed again by the epidemiology consultant.

Results

Literature Review

In the initial MEDLINE search, 1949 articles were identified. The title and abstract of each of these was reviewed by two members of the Subcommittee and identified as "useful," "potentially useful," or "not useful." After this review and elimination of duplicates, 430 articles were reproduced in full for data extraction. Of these, 105 were rejected because they contained no original data relevant to the analysis. In the second round, an additional 133 articles were identified. Twenty-six of these were rejected for lack of original data. A total of 432 articles were reviewed at least once.

The quality of the articles in this area is highly variable, but most articles met 50% or fewer of the quality criteria. Interrater reliability for quality scores was tested using a subset of the articles. Correlation of scores among reviewers was only fair ($r = 0.43$). Correlation among the readers' subjective ratings was less good ($r = 0.29$).

Age and Gender

The data indicate that the probability of finding UTI in febrile male infants is less than half that in females, and just greater than one third for males between 1 and 2 years of age. Findings from two studies report the prevalence of UTI by gender in an unbiased sample of febrile infants younger than 1 year. The studies show inconsistent results among males younger than 1 year. Among females, the prevalence was similar, 7.4% and 8.8%, respectively. Other studies also suggest a lower risk among males in older age groups.

Other studies used to estimate the effect of age and gender on the prevalence of UTI examined only children with confirmed UTI. Relative risk of UTI for a given gender was estimated from these studies using the odds ratio (OR), $P(\text{male}|\text{UTI})/P(\text{female}|\text{UTI})$. Because this prevalence in males and females in the general population is ~50%, the OR is essentially the same as the ratio of the prevalence of UTI among males to the prevalence among females. The prevalence itself can be derived by assuming an overall prevalence of 5% for both genders and a 50% prevalence of males in the population, using the formula, $P(\text{UTI}|\text{male}) = P(\text{male}|\text{UTI}) \cdot P(\text{UTI})/P(\text{male})$. The comparable formula was used for females.

Studies also were stratified by age. These data and the data for prevalence by gender were used to make crude estimates of the effect of age and gender on the prevalence of UTI in four subgroups: males younger than 1 year (3%), males older than 1 year (2%), females younger than 1 year (7%), and females older than 1 year (8%).

Circumcision

Several studies show a dramatic risk reduction among circumcised males. Most (but not all) of these data are retrospective, and the studies are plagued with missing data, but the findings are quite consistent. In all these studies, the probability of circumcision given UTI [$P(\text{circ}|\text{UTI})$] was reported. Relative risk was estimated by the OR, $P(\text{circ}|\text{UTI})/P(\text{no circ}|\text{UTI})$. Estimates of prevalence of UTI given circumcision [$P(\text{UTI}|\text{circ})$] were calculated by assuming the previous probability of UTI regardless of circumcision status [$P(\text{UTI})$] is 5%, and the probability of circumcision (among males) is 70%. Prevalences are calculated using these estimates and Bayes' formula, $P(\text{UTI}|\text{circ}) = P(\text{circ}|\text{UTI}) \cdot P(\text{UTI})/P(\text{circ})$. The results suggest that the prevalence of UTI among febrile male infants who are circumcised would be ~0.2%.

Most data come from studies of infants younger than 1 year, but the effect seems to persist even beyond infancy. Making the (reasonable) assumption that circumcision status is independent of age, circumcised males older than 1 year are at lowest risk.

Interestingly, circumcision could account for the gender differences in prevalence. If one assumes that febrile females and uncircumcised males have a UTI prevalence of 7%, that circumcised males have a prevalence of 0.2%, and that 70% of males are circumcised, then the prevalence of UTI among males would be $(0.3 \cdot 0.07) + (0.7 \cdot 0.002) = 0.022$ or 2%, a figure consistent with the data.

Tests for UTI

When an infant is considered to be at significant risk for UTI, the next step is to make the diagnosis. Choosing diagnostic criteria for UTI involves two competing considerations. A false-negative diagnosis will leave patients with UTI at risk for serious complications. A false-positive diagnosis may lead to unnecessary, invasive, and expensive testing. In evaluating alternative diagnostic tests for UTI, the Subcommittee defined as a "gold standard" any bacterial growth on a culture of urine obtained by suprapubic bladder aspiration (tap), ie, any bacterial growth on a culture of a urine specimen obtained by tap defines a UTI.

For the analysis, a culture of a urine specimen obtained by a tap was considered to have 100% sensitivity and specificity. However, this was not always used for comparisons in studies of other diagnostic strategies. Alternative diagnostic strategies fall into the three following areas: 1) urine analysis (UA) for immediate diagnostic information, 2) culture of a urine specimen obtained by urine bag or transurethral catheterization, and 3) culture of a urine specimen using the dip-slide culture technique.

UA

The various components of the UA include the reagent slide tests, ie, LE, nitrite, blood, and protein, and microscopic examination for leukocytes or bacteria. The diagnostic characteristics of these tests have been evaluated individually and in combination. Tests can be combined serially, meaning all test results must be positive for the combination to be positive or, in parallel, meaning a positive result on any one of the tests defines a positive result for the combination. The serial strategy maximizes specificity at the expense of sensitivity, whereas parallel testing maximizes sensitivity at the expense of specificity.

Perhaps the most commonly used component of the UA used to evaluate a child who may have a UTI is the reagent strip (dipstick). Tests for UTI that are available on most reagent strips include the LE, nitrite, blood, and protein. The LE is the most sensitive single test. Its reported sensitivity ranges from 67% in a screening setting in which symptoms and, therefore, inflammation, would not be expected, to 94% in settings in which UTI is suspected. The specificity of LE generally is not as good. However, because the specificity describes the performance of the test on specimens from patients without a UTI, it is highly dependent on patient characteristics. The reported specificity varies from 63% to 92%.

The test for nitrite has a much higher specificity (90% to 100%) and lower sensitivity (16% to 82%). For this reason, nitrite may be useful for "ruling in" UTI when it is positive, but it has little value in ruling out UTI. Dipstick tests for blood and protein have poor sensitivity and specificity with respect to UTI. Therefore, the use of results for blood or protein from dipstick testing has a high likelihood of being misleading.

Carefully performed microscopic examination of the urine has high sensitivity and specificity in many studies. However, the wide range of reported test characteristics of microscopy for leukocytes or bacteria presumably reflects the difficulty of performing these tests well and the hazards of performing them poorly. In studies that have shown the best test characteristics, tests were performed by on-site laboratory technicians who often used counting chambers.

When examining the urine for bacteria, unstained and Gram-stained specimens seem to be effective. However, centrifugation of the specimen reduces the specificity of the test. The number of bacteria also is important. Using heavy bacterial counts as a diagnostic criterion results in low sensitivity and high specificity. The reverse applies when observation of any bacteria is considered a positive test.

Microscopy for leukocytes is variably sensitive (32% to 100%) and specific (45% to 97%). Studies with accurate results generally used mirrored counting chambers, on-site technicians, or both. Specimens also must be examined shortly after collection. A 3-hour delay results in a 35% drop in sensitivity. Finally, if the number of leukocytes considered abnormal is high, the test will be insensitive, if the number is low, it will be highly sensitive. The reverse is true for specificity.

A number of special tests have been evaluated for the diagnosis of UTI. The first is a modified nitrite test. This involves incubating a urine specimen for several hours with added nitrite before testing for nitrate. The reported sensitivity and specificity are 93% and 88%, respectively. However, comparable results have not been reported. Immunochemical studies for early detection of bacterial growth have not had impressive results.

Obtaining a Urine Specimen

The Subcommittee defined the gold standard definition of a UTI to be growth on a culture of a urine specimen obtained by tap. Often, however, performance of a bladder tap is resisted because it is invasive. Moreover, bladder taps may not yield urine specimens. Success rates for obtaining urine specimens vary between 23% and 90%. Although 100% success has been achieved when using ultrasonographic guidance, practitioners often use transurethral catheterization or urine bags to obtain urine specimens for culture.

Cultures of urine specimens obtained by catheterization have a specificity of 83% to 89% compared with cultures of urine specimens obtained by tap. However, if only cultures yielding >1000 CFU/mL are considered positive, catheterization cultures have a 95% sensitivity with a specificity of 99%.

Cultures of bag urine specimens are 100% sensitive, but they have a specificity between 14% and 84%. Therefore, because UTI is present in a small minority (5%) of patients tested, use of culture results from urine specimens obtained from the bag to rule in UTI is likely to result in large numbers of false-positive results. Specifically, with a prevalence of 5% and specificity of 70%, the positive predictive value of a positive culture of bag urine specimens would be 15%. That is, 85% of positive cultures of urine specimens obtained from a bag would be false-positive results.

Culturing Techniques

The standard culturing technique involves streaking on blood agar and MacConkey media. More recently, dipslide methods have been developed. The few studies of dipslide cultures that were reviewed reported sensitivities between 87% and 100% and specificities between 92% and 98%.

Consequences of a Missed Diagnosis of UTI

If the diagnosis of UTI is not made because it was not suspected or a test of insufficient sensitivity was used, three consequences may result. The first (see "Prevalence of Urinary Tract Abnormalities") is the lost opportunity to find a urinary tract abnormality that could result in renal damage. The second is the formation of new renal scars. Although repeated UTI lead to scarring (see "Progressive Renal Damage") and progressive scarring is associated with hypertension and ESRD, the role of scarring from a single UTI in long-term clinical consequences is unknown. Nevertheless, timely treatment of febrile UTI in children appears to be important in preventing scars.

The third consequence of missing the diagnosis of UTI results from the urosepsis that occurs in a small proportion of febrile infants with UTI. Among patients with febrile UTI, in the age group to which this analysis applies, the risk of concurrent bacteremia is between 2.2% and 9%. The natural history of bacteremia in infants with febrile UTI is not described. Common pediatric experience is that septic shock and death are rarely seen in this situation, suggesting that spontaneous resolution of bacteremia occurs in this situation as it does in others. However, evidence exists that among infants with bacteremia attributable to *Escherichia coli* in the presence of a UTI, fatality rates may be as high as 10% to 12%.

Short-term Treatment of UTI

In studying the short-term treatment of UTI, the two following issues were addressed: 1) What do the data suggest about the duration of outpatient antibiotic therapy? and 2) What is the best choice for presumptive oral antibiotic therapy for the infant with suspected UTI before culture results are available? From the data presented subsequently in this report, it may be reasonable to conclude the following. 1) Single-dose to 3-day therapy is not as effective as therapy of 7 days or longer (perhaps because of more rapid metabolism of antimicrobials in children), but that the minimal acceptable duration of therapy has not been demonstrated. 2) Cotrimoxazole appears to be superior to amoxicillin for presumptive antibiotic therapy of UTI, but local antibiotic susceptibility patterns should ultimately dictate the antibiotic choice.

Duration of Therapy

Several studies have compared treatment of pediatric UTI with varying durations of therapy. The data have been analyzed in two ways. First, studies that directly compared different durations of therapy were examined. Then, data were pooled by antibiotic and duration of therapy, and the pooled values were compared.

None of the studies of duration of therapy compared 7 days with 10 days. In seven studies with 10 comparisons between long duration (7 to 10 days) and short duration (one dose to 3 days), 8 of 10 comparisons showed better results with an attributable improvement in outcome of 5% to 21%.

When the data were pooled by agent and duration, no discernible differences were found in initial cure or relapse among one-dose, 3-day, and 10-day courses of amoxicillin. However, single-dose cotrimoxazole was 10% less effective than 1-, 3-, 7-, or 10-day therapy. Differences among the latter regimens were not discernible.

Agent

The data pooled by agent and duration of therapy were used to compare amoxicillin and cotrimoxazole. For therapies of one dose, 3 to 4 days, or 10 days, cotrimoxazole consistently shows better cure rates (4% to 42%).

Data comparing parenteral and oral therapy were not found. However, intramuscular ceftriaxone (one dose) or gentamicin (10 days) was 100% effective in resolving UTI in children in whom oral therapy had failed. No data are available that clarify the role of oral vs parenteral therapy for bacteremia in association with UTI. Drawing on analyses of unsuspected bacteremia in children without UTI, parenteral antibiotic therapy is 95% effective in clearing bacteremia.

Prevalence of Urinary Tract Abnormalities

UTI in young children is a marker for abnormalities of the urinary tract. By far, the most common abnormality is VUR, which may be present with different degrees of severity that are graded I to V according to whether the reflux reaches the kidney and the degree of dilation of the collecting system. The grade of VUR is important because it determines the likelihood of detecting VUR on radiologic evaluation and the probability of renal damage, hypertension, or renal failure.

VUR

The Subcommittee identified 77 studies that reported the prevalence of VUR among children with UTI. The range of reported values is wide which may be primarily attributed to small sample size. As the sample size grows, the prevalence reported converges at 30% to 40%. The prevalence appears to decrease with age.

Specific studies of the relationship between age and prevalence of VUR show similar results. For example, one study reported a 68% prevalence among boys younger than 1 year and 25% among boys 1 to 3 years. Another study of boys found some type of abnormality in 76% of boys younger than 10 years (~54% of these were VUR) and 15% in boys older than 10 years. A population-based study showed a peak prevalence of VUR among girls 1 to 3 years of age and a rapid drop-off (perhaps by half) by age 5. A much smaller study found VUR in 100% of 9 boys younger than 1 year of age with a UTI and in 74% of 34 boys 1 to 5 years of age.

This relationship was fitted to a third-degree polynomial and a spline. Although the data are insufficient to define a particular functional relationship, they suggest a decline in the prevalence of VUR with age that seems to be most rapid during the first year of life. It levels off somewhat between 1 and 5 years of age, then drops off again after age 5. When studies of children younger than 3 years were pooled, the prevalence was 50%.

For this analysis, grades of VUR were grouped into low grade (grades I and II) and high grade (grades III to V). This grouping reduces the precision of the analysis slightly because higher grade reflux is easier to detect with ultrasonography and poses a greater risk of subsequent renal damage than do the lower grades. However, these effects were represented in this model, making this a more detailed analysis than has been reported previously. Some studies grouped patients in a similar manner, but grade III VUR was variably grouped as high grade or low grade. For classification of results, the classification used in the articles was (by necessity) used in this analysis. Pooling the data gives a 51.1% prevalence of low-grade (grades I to II) VUR among patients with VUR.

Tests for VUR

The Subcommittee identified the gold standard test for detecting VUR as the VCUG or RCG. These studies have, by definition, 100% sensitivity and specificity. The Subcommittee also believed that renal ultrasonography or intravenous pyelography should be performed to identify obstructions or other structural renal abnormalities.

VCUG and RCG are expensive and invasive. Data were collected on the sensitivity and specificity of renal ultrasonography alone in the detection of VUR. Overall, renal ultrasonography has poor sensitivity (30% to 62%) and good specificity (85% to 100%) for VUR. The sensitivity is better, however, for high-grade VUR than for low-grade VUR (82% to 100% vs 14% to 30%). The Subcommittee members believed that renal ultrasonography in young infants was less reliable than this. However, data supporting this point were not found.

Progressive Renal Damage

The evidence that links the presence of VUR to important clinical outcomes can only be assembled in a piecemeal way. The data link VUR to renal scarring in the presence of recurrent infection, and renal scarring is associated with subsequent hypertension and ESRD. The data support this model indirectly. However, there are no longitudinal data that link directly the presence of VUR in infants with febrile UTI and normal kidneys to the subsequent development of hypertension or ESRD. Therefore, it is difficult to quantify the strength of the relationship or the risk to such patients. The following discussion reviews evidence supporting each step in the hypothesized progression to renal damage.

Reflux and Scarring

The data demonstrate an association between VUR and subsequent renal scarring. More than 48 references reviewed reported renal scarring at rates between 1% and 40% in association with febrile UTI and VUR. Higher grades of VUR are associated with higher risk of scar progression. Patients with high-grade VUR are four to six times more likely to have scarring than those with low-grade VUR and eight to 10 times as likely as those without VUR. In one study of 84 consecutive children 2 to 70 months of age with their first recognized febrile UTI, the presence of VUR was 80% sensitive and 74% specific in predicting subsequent scarring in a follow-up period of 2 years or more. Of those with VUR, 30% had progressive renal scarring. Of those without VUR, only 4% did.

Recurrent Infections and Scarring

The association of VUR with renal scarring seems to be mediated through recurrent symptomatic infections. The association between recurrent bouts of febrile UTI and the risk of renal scarring in one study followed an exponential curve.

Patients with no VUR or low-grade VUR and patients with no recurrences of UTI are at low risk for renal scarring. Thus, prophylactic antibiotic treatment of patients with VUR to prevent recurrences or surgical treatment to prevent VUR would be expected to prevent renal scarring.

ESRD and Hypertension

Retrospective examination of the causes of ESRD in registries of patients with renal failure shows that in 36% (of 9250 patients), the cause of ESRD is obstructive uropathy, renal hypoplasia or dysplasia, pyelonephritis, or a combination of these. Unfortunately, it is not possible to determine which patients originally had normal kidneys in whom disease progressed to ESRD because of VUR and recurrent infection. In the North American Renal Transplant Cooperative Study, the fraction of transplant recipients with reflux nephropathy is 102/2033, or 5%. Patients with pyelonephritis or interstitial nephritis make up another 2% of transplant recipients.

Most cohort studies to quantify the risk of ESRD and hypertension among patients with renal scarring and VUR are based on highly selected patients in whom extensive scarring already has occurred. Long-term studies show that ESRD develops in 3% to 10% of these patients. In addition, 10% may require nephrectomy, and 0.4% renal transplantation. One study followed women from their first UTI in childhood and found that abnormal renal function could be documented in 21% of those with severe scarring. However, this study also had a selected population and did not provide data on VUR.

The rate of hypertension in these and similar studies varies between 0% and 50%. It is apparently lowest in those with low-grade VUR and those with the least scarring. However, the quality of the studies relating VUR nephropathy with ESRD and hypertension was rated poor, and quantification of the relationship is weak. One study identified retrospectively a cohort of children 1 month to 16 years of age with VUR and measured blood pressure levels 5 months to 21 years (average, 9.6 years) after VUR was identified. There was an increase in the blood pressure level associated with increasing grades of VUR. However, none of the patients had hypertension.

Effectiveness of Prophylactic Antimicrobials and Surgical Correction

Ultimately the value of identifying VUR depends on the potential to prevent its long-term consequences. This depends on reducing recurrent infections with antibiotic prophylaxis or eliminating VUR surgically. The efficacy of these procedures is not well documented because controlled studies have not been performed. Studies in which patients receiving antibiotic prophylaxis are compared with those not taking antimicrobials suggest a 50% effectiveness whether comparing rates of reinfection or progression of scarring.

Cost Data

Cost data were derived from literature where available, the accounting department of the University of North Carolina (UNC) Hospital, and the physicians' fee schedule from the UNC Physicians and Associates. Estimates used in the decision model are given below.

UA and Culture

Based on the cost data from the UNC Hospital, the cost of a urine culture is $21.53 (charge, $26.00). The cost of a UA is $6.77 (charge, $15.00).

Treatment

The cost of short-term treatment of UTI varies substantially depending on the treatment chosen. Standard oral therapy, such as amoxicillin or trimethoprim-sulfamethoxazole, costs about $10 for a course. Newer, broad-spectrum oral therapy costs about $40 for a 10-day course. If parenteral therapy, such as intramuscular ceftriaxone, is given, the cost of the drug and the injection may be $125.

Complications of Therapy

For the analysis, only complications requiring a return visit to the physician were considered. This visit would cost a $50 clinic fee, plus a $50 professional fee, for a total of $100. Death attributable to anaphylaxis is rare. The additional cost of this complication was not added.

Cost of Urosepsis

It is assumed that sepsis that does not clear spontaneously or with antibiotic therapy will require hospital admission for intravenous antibiotic therapy at a cost of $10 000.

Imaging Evaluation

The two following imaging strategies were considered: 1) a full work-up, including renal ultrasonography and VCUG, and 2) renal ultrasonography alone. The cost of renal ultrasonography includes the hospital cost of $104 and the physician fee of $200, for a total of $304. The cost of the VCUG is the hospital cost of $123 plus the physician fee of $200, totaling $323. Thus, the full work-up costs $627.

Cost of Treatment of VUR

The estimated cost of antibiotic prophylaxis was based on low-dose nitrofurantoin. The weekly cost was $6 for an average of 3 years. The total is $1040. It was assumed that the cost of ureteral reimplantation surgery was similar.

Complications of VUR

Patients with VUR are at increased risk for recurrent UTI, at least until the VUR resolves. The period the child is at risk was assumed to be 3 years. The cost of these recurrences was based on the average cost of a clinic visit related to a diagnosis of UTI or pyelonephritis in infants at UNC, $134, plus the physician fee of $70. This was multiplied by three, the average number of infections expected over 3 years, for a total of $612.

The cost of ESRD was derived from data in previous analyses. Based on a 10-year period, including 10 years of dialysis or a year in which transplantation occurs followed by 8 years with a functioning graft, followed by 1 year of a failed graft, the cost of ESRD is ~$300 000. The cost of managing severe hypertension and its complications was estimated at $100 000 based on $2000 per year for 50 years.

Analysis of the Decision Model

Using data extracted from the literature as described in "Evidence Tables," probabilities and costs were inserted into the decision tree. Using baseline estimates, three types of analysis were conducted. First, a risk analysis was performed to determine the average cost and frequency of outcomes expected with each of four strategies. Next, a cost-effectiveness analysis was used to determine the incremental cost per major clinical outcome averted by the strategies. Finally, sensitivity and threshold analyses were performed to examine alternative strategies for evaluation and management of UTI.

Risk Analysis

Two risk analyses were performed. The first examined the costs and clinical outcomes expected with different strategies for making the diagnosis of UTI. The second compared alternative strategies for imaging the urinary tract of patients with UTI.

Diagnosis of UTI

The risk analysis of diagnostic strategies examines two anchor states. The first, "treat all," is presumptive antibiotic therapy for occult infection without testing. The second, "observe," is clinical observation without testing or treatment. Neither of these anchor strategies involves subsequent imaging of the urinary tract. Three testing strategies are evaluated. The first is the gold standard, culture of urine specimens obtained by suprapubic tap or transurethral catheter. The second is using a culture of the urine specimen obtained from the urine bag. Culture of bag urine specimens has 100% sensitivity and 70% specificity in the baseline analysis. The third strategy uses the cheaper but less reliable reagent strip as a test for UTI. A positive LE test result, a positive nitrite test result, or both, is considered a positive test result. The sensitivity and specificity of this strategy are 92% and 70%, respectively, based on median values. All three testing strategies include antibiotic therapy and imaging of the urinary tract of patients with positive test results.

The results of the risk analysis are presented as the number of outcomes expected per 100 000 infants treated by using each strategy. To observe patients without testing or treatment is the least expensive strategy. However, it results in inferior clinical outcomes, including death and hospitalization from urosepsis, hypertension, and ESRD. Presumptive treatment of all infants without testing costs slightly more than observing, but prevents hospitalization and death from urosepsis. Under the treat all strategy, it is impossible to select patients for imaging, and it is unreasonably expensive to image the urinary tracts of all patients (see "Cost-effectiveness Analysis"). Therefore, no patient in the treat all strategy undergoes imaging evaluation. As a result, there is no improvement in the rates of hypertension or ESRD.

Using culture of urine specimens obtained by catheterization or tap offers the lowest risk of death, because all children at risk for urosepsis are identified and there are no unnecessary treatments or treatment-related deaths. Moreover, because all children with UTI are identified for imaging evaluation, this strategy minimizes the risk of hypertension and ESRD.

Using a culture of bag urine specimens as a criterion for the diagnosis of UTI also identifies correctly all children with UTI. However, its poor specificity also results in many false-positive results. As a consequence, there are slightly more deaths (3 per million) attributable to unnecessary antibiotic treatment and many more imaging work-ups. This means an additional $47.2 million per 100 000 febrile infants with no improvement in clinical outcomes.

Using LE and nitrite as diagnostic criteria for UTI leaves a small number of UTIs undiagnosed and results in $2\frac{1}{2}$ times as many imaging work-ups compared with a culture of urine specimens obtained by catheterization or tap. The result is poorer clinical outcomes at greater expense despite the lower cost of UA.

A fourth diagnostic strategy also was evaluated that used a full UA (reagent strip and microscopy) as an initial diagnostic test and treated any positive UA component as a positive result. A positive result would lead to presumptive treatment. However, positive results would be confirmed by a culture of urine specimens obtained by tap or catheterization before imaging was performed. This strategy has a sensitivity of virtually 100% and a specificity of 60% for making a treatment decision. Because positive results are confirmed with a culture of urine specimens obtained by catheterization or tap, the specificity is 100% for imaging. The cost of testing is higher for positive results because UA and culture are performed. Also, the false-positive results lead to more unnecessary treatment and the resulting costs and complications. However, there is a cost saving for patients with negative results of the UA because the UA costs less than the culture. Compared with a culture of specimens from all patients, there is a small net decrease in cost using UA followed by a culture of positive results. Moreover, this strategy has the advantage of allowing immediate treatment of patients at risk of UTI. The benefit of early treatment is difficult to quantify, but evidence suggests it reduces the risk of renal scarring. Although this strategy appears to be nearly as effective as (or perhaps more than) the culture of urine specimens obtained by catheterization or tap, its effectiveness depends on the accuracy of the urine microscopy. As noted above, the accuracy of urine microscopy is highly variable and apparently depends on the presence of an on-site technician. In many settings, this may be impossible or so expensive as to offset the benefits.

Imaging Strategies

Three imaging alternatives were evaluated by risk analysis. The first strategy was renal ultrasonography and VCUG. The second was renal ultrasonography alone, and the third was no imaging evaluation at all. The total cost associated with each strategy includes the cost of the imaging studies, the cost of treating abnormalities identified, and the cost of any complications incurred. Together, renal ultrasonography and VCUG will identify all cases of renal abnormalities. Renal ultrasonography alone detects ~42% of all abnormalities. However, most abnormalities (87%) missed by renal ultrasonography alone are low-grade VUR, which carries a lower risk of renal scarring. As a result, the differences in clinical outcomes (cases of hypertension and ESRD) are smaller between renal ultrasonography alone and the full evaluation.

Cost-effectiveness Analysis

Cost-effectiveness analysis was used to quantify the trade-offs between cost and clinical effect when moving from one clinical strategy to another. When one strategy offers a better clinical effect at a lower cost, it is said to be a dominant strategy. However, in most cases, the strategy with better clinical effect also has a higher cost. Cost-effectiveness analysis depicts the additional cost per unit of improvement in clinical effect. For this analysis, the units of effect were defined as cases of death, ESRD, or hypertension prevented.

Strategies were compared using the incremental (or marginal) cost-effectiveness ratio, ie, the difference in cost among strategies divided by the difference in effect. The mathematical term is as follows:

$$\frac{Cost_b - Cost_a}{Effect_b - Effect_a}.$$

Diagnosis of UTI

The least expensive strategy for the diagnosis of UTI is to do nothing. This also is the least effective strategy. By comparison, treating all febrile 2-month to 2-year-olds for UTI without diagnostic testing or urinary tract imaging improves clinical effect at a cost of $61 000 per death prevented. However, it does not prevent ESRD or hypertension.

As an alternative, one could obtain a dipstick UA on all patients, culturing specimens from those for whom the results of UA were positive. Because UA costs less than culture, this strategy has the potential to save money. However, because UA does not have perfect sensitivity, a few cases will be missed. In addition, patients for whom the results of UA are positive will incur the costs of UA and culture. To evaluate this strategy, a new branch was added to the decision tree. The new branch is a dipstick UA. If results are positive, it is linked to the "test" branch; if results are negative, it is linked to the "observe" branch. Positive results involve the cost of the UA plus culture; negative results, only the cost of the UA. This strategy prevents an additional two cases of death or serious complication per 10 000 at a cost of $261 000 per case.

Culturing catheterization or tap urine specimens on all patients and then treating and imaging the urinary tracts of all patients with positive results is the most effective and most expensive strategy. It prevents an additional 2.5 cases of death or serious complication per 100 000 over culture-confirmed positive dipstick results at an additional cost of $434 000 per case prevented. Compared with the no testing strategy, culturing specimens from all patients prevents three cases of death or serious complication per 10 000 at a cost of $200 000 per case prevented.

The optimal strategy depends on the decision-maker's willingness to pay for each additional case prevented. For example, if that willingness to pay is between $261 000 and $434 000, then the positive results of the dipstick confirmed by culture is the best strategy. Culturing specimens from all patients will prevent a few additional cases, but the cost to prevent each of these additional cases exceeds the decision-maker's willingness to pay. If the decision-maker is willing to pay >$434 000 to prevent a case of death or serious complication, then culturing specimens from all patients is the right strategy.

Imaging Strategies

The cost-effectiveness of the alternative imaging strategies also was calculated. The least expensive alternative is to perform no evaluation. Renal ultrasonography alone will prevent almost three cases of ESRD or hypertension per 1000 studies done at a cost of $260 000 per case prevented. A VCUG prevents an additional one case of ESRD or hypertension per 1000 studies over renal ultrasonography at a cost of $353 000 per case.

Again, the optimal strategy depends on the decision-maker's willingness to pay for each additional case prevented. For example, if that willingness to pay is between $260 000 and $353 000, then renal ultrasonography alone is the best strategy. A VCUG will prevent a few additional cases, but the cost to prevent each of these additional cases exceeds the decision-maker's willingness to pay. If the decision maker is willing to pay >$353 000 to prevent a case, then renal ultrasonography and VCUG is the right strategy.

Sensitivity and Threshold Analysis

Choosing one alternative over another from the risk analyses involves striking a balance between the cost of an intervention and the improvement in clinical outcomes. When comparing alternatives, if one alternative provides better clinical outcomes at lower costs, it is the dominant alternative and is the obvious choice. However, in most circumstances, choosing an alternative requires a trade-off between costs and clinical benefit. For example, obtaining a urine specimen for culture by catheterization or tap on all febrile infants, treating those with positive cultures, and imaging their urinary tracts with VCUG and renal ultrasonography improve clinical outcome but at a substantially higher cost than doing none of these evaluations.

To select the optimal alternative and, moreover, to identify different clinical circumstances in which different alternatives may be better, it is first necessary to make explicit the trade-off between costs and clinical outcomes. This means identifying a "willingness to pay" for each untoward clinical outcome avoided. For the following analyses, a value of $700 000 was placed on each case of ESRD or hypertension prevented. This figure is based loosely on the lifetime productivity of a healthy, young adult. Once this cost is assigned to each untoward clinical outcome, it is possible to use the threshold method of decision-making.

The threshold approach to decision-making involves changing the value of a variable in the decision analysis to determine the value at which one alternative becomes too expensive and another would be preferred. In the case of UTI, if the prior probability of UTI is sufficiently high, it costs <$700 000 to prevent a case of ESRD or hypertension by screening all febrile children. However, if the probability that a particular patient has a UTI is sufficiently low, the yield of a urine culture will be extremely low and a positive result of a UA will almost certainly be a false-positive. Under these circumstances, a strategy involving the evaluation of this child's urinary tract would cost >$700 000 per case of ESRD or hypertension prevented. Threshold analysis identifies the threshold probability of UTI above which evaluation would be cost-effective and below which it would not. A number of threshold analyses follow.

Prevalence of UTI and Prevalence of VUR

Because fever without an obvious cause is common in pediatric practice, culturing the urine of all febrile 2-month to 2-year-old children represents a substantial investment. The Subcommittee was interested in determining whether there were some clinical subpopulations in which the prevalence of UTI was low enough that culture was unnecessary. A threshold analysis was used to examine this question.

Cost of Culturing Urine Obtained by Urine Bag

Many practitioners prefer to culture urine specimens obtained by urine bag rather than by transurethral catheter or suprapubic tap because the urine bag is less invasive. However, culture of a urine specimen obtained by bag has low specificity. When the prevalence of UTI is low, as it is in febrile infants, the result is a large number of false-positive urine cultures. False-positive cultures lead to unnecessary antibiotic treatment and urinary tract evaluation. The result is additional costs with no clinical benefit. To examine these additional costs, the difference in costs between a strategy involving urine specimens obtained by catheterization or tap and a strategy involving specimens from bag urine was calculated at different levels of specificity for the urine bag. Results of the analysis imply that culturing urine specimens from bag urine in this setting can only be justified if one is willing to pay between $293 and $1340 per patient to use a urine bag rather than to obtain urine specimens by catheterization or tap.

Sensitivity and Specificity for UA

As an alternative to obtaining urine specimens for culture from all febrile children between 2 months and 2 years of age, one could use a UA to make the diagnosis of UTI. As noted previously, a carefully performed UA has high sensitivity and specificity. Two-way sensitivity analysis was used to determine the minimal sensitivity and specificity that would be necessary to justify the use of UA rather than culture. The results imply that a test must have a sensitivity >92% and a specificity >99% to be preferred over urine culture. This level of sensitivity and specificity is unlikely to be obtained in most clinical settings. Alternatively, several studies demonstrated that combinations of LE, nitrite, microscopy of fresh urine, in which any abnormality constituted a positive test result, yielded a sensitivity of >92%. If one of these tests were used to rule out UTI, and culture of urine specimens obtained by catheterization or tap were used to confirm UTI in positive results, the requisite sensitivity and specificity would be obtained.

Probability of UTI and Urinary Tract Imaging

The decision to image the urinary tracts of infants with documented UTI presumes that the diagnosis of UTI is certain. If an imperfect test (eg, using a bag urine specimen) is used to make the diagnosis of UTI, a substantial number of these patients in fact may not have had a UTI and, therefore, the yield of the imaging will be lower. Threshold analysis was used to determine the minimal probability of UTI that justified a full imaging evaluation. The analysis indicates that if the probability of UTI is <49%, imaging becomes too expensive. Bayes's theorem shows that among patients with a prevalence of UTI that is 5%, those who have a positive urine culture obtained by bag have a probability (positive predictive value) of UTI that is 15%, well below 49%. This implies that if the best evidence of the UTI available in a given patient is a positive culture of urine obtained by bag, additional imaging of the urinary tract is not justified.

Sensitivity of Renal Ultrasonography for VUR

Because VCUG is invasive and expensive, a threshold analysis was used to explore the possible use of renal ultrasonography alone in evaluating the urinary tracts of children with UTI. Renal ultrasonography has low sensitivity for low-grade VUR, but relatively higher sensitivity for high-grade VUR. Based on the professional opinion of the UTI Subcommittee, a sensitivity of 14% for low-grade VUR and 82% for high-grade VUR is a better reflection of the situation in children 2 months to 2 years of age. This implies that renal ultrasonography alone is an inadequate imaging evaluation for infants with UTI.

Risk of Renal Scarring With UTI

One area of relative uncertainty, in which quality data are lacking, is the risk of scarring in undetected or untreated VUR. This risk is higher for children with high-grade VUR than for those with low-grade VUR. Threshold analysis was used to explore how this risk of scarring affects the decision to culture urine specimens from all children 2 months to 2 years of age with fever and no obvious cause for the fever. Figure 14 plots the risk of scar progression given low-grade VUR on the x-axis and the risk of scar progression given high-grade VUR on the y-axis. For values that plot above and to the right of the threshold line, culture of urine specimens from all febrile infants is the preferred strategy. For values that plot below and to the left of the threshold line, no urine culture is the preferred strategy. The baseline estimates used in the analysis, 14% for low-grade VUR and 53% for high-grade VUR, are plotted on the graph. The risk of scarring because of untreated VUR seems to be high enough to justify culturing specimens from all febrile infants.

Risk of Hypertension and ESRD

The weakest probability estimates in the present analysis relate to the risk of ESRD and hypertension among patients who have progressive renal scarring attributable to VUR. Two-way sensitivity analysis was used to determine the effect of varying these estimates on the results of the analysis. Our best estimate of the risk of hypertension and ESRD justifies culturing urine specimens from febrile infants as a strategy to prevent these complications. However, the quality of evidence about the future risks of ESRD and hypertension among infants with UTI later found to have VUR is tenuous at best. This is an area that needs additional investigation.

Recommendations

Who Should Be Evaluated for UTI?

Under the assumptions of the analysis, all febrile children between the ages of 2 months and 24 months with no obvious cause of infection should be evaluated for UTI, with the exception of circumcised males older than 12 months.

Minimal Test Characteristics of Diagnosis of UTI

To be as cost-effective as a culture of a urine specimen obtained by transurethral catheter or suprapubic tap, a test must have a sensitivity of at least 92% and a specificity of at least 99%. With the possible exception of a complete UA performed within 1 hour of urine collection by an on-site laboratory technician, no other test meets these criteria.

Performing a dipstick UA and obtaining a urine specimen by catheterization or tap for culture from patients with a positive LE or nitrite test result is nearly as effective and slightly less costly than culturing specimens from all febrile children.

Treatment of UTI

The data suggest that short-term treatment of UTI should not be for <7 days. The data do not support treatment for >14 days if an appropriate clinical response is observed. There are no data comparing intravenous with oral administration of medications.

Evaluation of the Urinary Tract

Available data support the imaging evaluation of the urinary tracts of all 2- to 24-month-olds with their first documented UTI. Imaging should include VCUG and renal ultrasonography. The method for documenting the UTI must yield a positive predictive value of at least 49% to justify the evaluation. Culture of a urine specimen obtained by bag does not meet this criterion unless the previous probability of a UTI is >22%.

Pediatric Vesicoureteral Reflux Guidelines Panel Summary Report on the Management of Primary Vesicoureteral Reflux in Children

The following guideline for management of primary vesicoureteral reflux in children, developed by the American Urological Association, has been endorsed by the American Academy of Pediatrics.

Pediatric Vesicoureteral Reflux Guidelines Panel Summary Report on the Management of Primary Vesicoureteral Reflux in Children

Authors:

Jack S. Elder, Craig A. Peters, Billy S. Arant, Jr., David H. Ewalt,
Charles E. Hawtrey, Richard S. Hurwitz, Thomas S. Parrott,
Howard M. Snyder, III, Robert A. Weiss, Steven H. Woolf,
and Vic Hasselblad

Abstract

Purpose: The American Urological Association convened the Pediatric Vesicoureteral Reflux Guidelines Panel to analyze the literature regarding available methods for treating vesicoureteral reflux diagnosed following a urinary tract infection in children and to make practice policy recommendations based on the treatment outcomes data insofar as the data permit.

Materials and Methods: The panel searched the MEDLINE data base for all articles from 1965 to 1994 on vesicoureteral reflux and systematically analyzed outcomes data for 7 treatment alternatives: 1) intermittent antibiotic therapy, 2) bladder training, 3) continuous antibiotic prophylaxis, 4) antibiotic prophylaxis and bladder training, 5) antibiotic prophylaxis, anticholinergics and bladder training, 6) open surgical repair and 7) endoscopic repair. Key outcomes identified were probability of reflux resolution, likelihood of developing pyelonephritis and scarring, and possibility of complications of medical and surgical treatment.

Results: Available outcomes data on the various treatment alternatives were summarized in tabular form and graphically, and the relative probabilities of possible outcomes were compared for each alternative. Treatment recommendations were based on scientific evidence and expert opinion. The panel concluded that only a few recommendations can be derived purely from scientific evidence of a beneficial effect on health outcomes.

Conclusions: For most children the panel recommended continuous antibiotic prophylaxis as initial treatment. Surgery was recommended for children with persistent reflux and other indications, as specified in the document.

Key Words: vesico-ureteral reflux, kidney, ureter, bladder, outcome assessment (health care)

Vesicoureteral reflux refers to the retrograde flow of urine from the bladder into the upper urinary tract. Reflux is a birth defect but it may also be acquired. Vesicoureteral reflux predisposes an individual to renal infection (pyelonephritis) by facilitating the transport of bacteria from the bladder to the upper urinary tract. The immunological and inflammatory reaction caused by a pyelonephritic infection may result in renal injury or scarring. Extensive renal scarring causes decreased renal function and it may result in renal insufficiency, end stage renal disease, renin mediated hypertension, decreased somatic growth and morbidity during pregnancy.

The primary goal of treatment in children with reflux is preventing renal injury, symptomatic pyelonephritis and other complications of reflux. Medical therapy is based on the principle that reflux often resolves with time, and antibiotics maintain urine sterility and prevent infections while the patient awaits spontaneous resolution. The basis for surgical therapy is that, in select situations, ongoing vesicoureteral reflux has caused or has a significant potential for causing renal injury or other reflux related complications and elimination of the reflux condition will minimize their likelihood. Although reflux is common in children with a urinary tract infection, there is disagreement even among specialists regarding optimal management.[1] Because of the lack of consensus regarding management of this common condition, the American Urological Association (AUA) convened the Pediatric Vesicoureteral Reflux Guidelines Panel.

The tasks of this panel were to conduct a comprehensive survey and meta-analysis of published outcomes data on the available methods of treating pediatric vesicoureteral reflux diagnosed following a urinary tract infection, analyze the limitations in the treatment literature, make practice policy recommendations based on the data insofar as the evidence permits, use expert opinion when necessary and make recommendations for further research.[2] The full report, which contains all studies, data and references, is available from the AUA.[3]

Methodology

The AUA Pediatric Vesicoureteral Reflux Guidelines Panel developed recommendations for managing reflux in children following an explicit approach to the development of practice policies. The panel review of the outcomes evidence concerning treatment of reflux in children began with MEDLINE literature searches encompassing the years 1965 through December 1994. The search strategy was all-inclusive, using "vesico-ureteral-reflux" as the major or minor MESH heading. All peer reviewed journal articles in the English literature related to primary vesicoureteral reflux in children younger than age 10 years were retrieved.

Outcomes were identified as criteria by which effectiveness of treatment would be analyzed (table 1). The review of evidence was organized around this framework. Outcomes included health outcomes (effects directly perceived in some way by patient or family), intermediate outcomes (those not

TABLE 1. Outcomes in pediatric vesicoureteral reflux

Health outcomes:	Harms of medical therapy:
Pyelonephritis	Adverse drug reactions
Cystitis	Hospitalization
Hypertension	Adverse effects of surveillance testing
Uremia	Harms of surgical therapy:
Somatic growth	Obstruction
Morbidity during pregnancy	Bleeding/transfusion
Death	Infection
Intermediate outcomes:	Contralateral reflux
Reflux resolution	Bladder injury
Reflux duration	Pain
Renal scarring	Hospitalization
Renal growth	Adverse effects of surveillance
Renal function	testing.

directly perceived by the patient or family but that are associated with or precede health outcomes) and harms of various forms of management. Each article was accepted or rejected on the basis of the treatment outcome data it contained and it was verified by 2 panel members in consultation with the panel chairman. Two panel members extracted data from each accepted article and the data were tabulated on the data retrieval form developed by the panel. Each data retrieval sheet was reviewed by the panel chairman, providing a triple review for each article. The panel reviewed the evidence and focused attention on randomized controlled studies when possible. The total number of articles retrieved was 3,207 of which 413 were selected for initial panel review. Final panel review yielded 168 articles, which formed the basis for the panel analysis of reflux.

The panel synthesized the evidence using techniques described by Eddy et al,[4] and Cooper and Hedges.[5] Evidence from randomized controlled trials was combined using meta-analytical techniques and the FAST*PRO computer package.[6] Data from single arm studies were combined using random effects models and adjusting for risk factors, such as initial grade of reflux and patient age. The methodology of these analyses was described by Hasselblad,[7] and calculations were done using EGRET software.[8]

Evidence on some outcomes was reviewed from select articles that were not collected and analyzed systematically. These areas included the impact of reflux on pregnancy, hospitalization due to antireflux surgery or pyelonephritis, adverse drug reactions, adverse effects of surveillance testing and other surgical harms.

The panel considered 7 modalities as treatment alternatives, including 1) no treatment (intermittent antibiotic therapy); 2) bladder training (regular, volitional, low pressure voiding and complete bladder emptying); 3) continuous antibiotic prophylaxis; 4) antibiotic prophylaxis and bladder training; 5) antibiotic therapy, bladder training and anticholinergics for dysfunctional voiding; 6) open surgical repair, and 7) endoscopic repair.

Limitations of the Literature

The panel attempted to rely on published evidence when possible. Many studies that addressed a particular issue were not used quantitatively in the various syntheses because of inconsistent reporting of data, limited followup, incomplete description of treatments or poorly defined patient populations. Analyses were also complicated by the existence of at least 5 methods used for grading reflux, nonuniformity in characterizing reflux grade and patient population, and lack of a standard method of reporting outcomes. Only 3 prospective randomized controlled trials compared medical to surgical therapy (the Birmingham Reflux Study,[9] the International Reflux Study in Children[10,11] and a study by Scholtmeijer from Rotterdam, The Netherlands[12]). The literature on certain issues, such as complication rates of surgery and adverse drug reactions, was limited and in some cases so sparse that judgments were made on the basis of expert opinion.

Outcomes Analysis

The following represents a brief summary of the statistical analysis that formed the basis of the treatment recommendations.

Health outcomes. Urinary Tract Infection: The panel reviewed 41 articles that described the incidence of urinary tract infection in children with vesicoureteral reflux treated with antibiotic prophylaxis or reimplantation. In grades III to IV reflux the incidence of pyelonephritis was approximately 2.5 times higher in patients treated with antibiotic prophylaxis than in those treated surgically. The incidence of cystitis in patients with vesicoureteral reflux was not significantly different in those treated medically or surgically. In children treated medically recurrent symptomatic urinary tract infections were more common in those with voiding dysfunction than in those with normal bladder function.

Hypertension: The panel reviewed 10 reports that described blood pressure measurements after reimplantation surgery. No statistically significant difference was found in the risk of hypertension related to treatment modality. However, these studies indicated that renal scarring increases the relative risk of hypertension to 2.92 (95% confidence interval 1.2 to 7.1) compared to the risk without renal scarring.

Uremia: It was impossible to determine whether even optimal treatment of reflux and urinary tract infection can prevent progressive renal failure and ultimately uremia after severe bilateral reflux nephropathy has been diagnosed.

Somatic Growth: No evidence substantiated an effect of reflux treatment on somatic growth.

Morbidity During Pregnancy: The panel performed a limited search of the pertinent literature on reflux, renal insufficiency and adverse outcomes of pregnancy. The morbidity of persistent reflux during pregnancy has not been studied extensively. Martinell et al reported that pyelonephritis occurred during pregnancy in 3 of 8 women with but only 2 of 33 without reflux.[13] In this series reflux was generally grade I or II. Although the data suggest a greater risk of morbidity from pyelonephritis in women who have persistent reflux during pregnancy, the sample size was small and only limited conclusions can be based on this evidence. The panel reviewed 5 studies that demonstrated that women with renal insufficiency have an increased incidence of toxemia, preterm delivery, fetal growth retardation, fetal loss and deteriorating renal function.

Intermediate outcomes. Reflux Resolution—Medical Therapy (Continuous Antibiotic Prophylaxis): The data base included 26 reports with data pertaining to reflux resolution after medical therapy, comprising 1,987 patients (1,410 girls and 304 boys or a girl-to-boy ratio of 4.3:1) and 2,902 ureters. The panel used the individual data bases of Skoog et al[14] and Arant,[15] and the data reported by the International Reflux Study, European Branch,[10] to estimate the probability of reflux resolution with continuous antibiotic

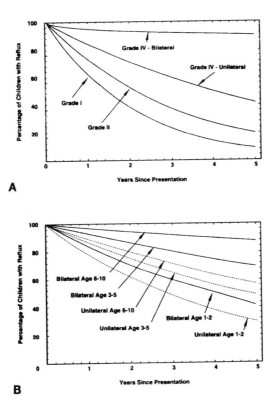

Percent chance of reflux persistence for 1 to 5 years following presentation.[10,13,14] *A*, grades I, II and IV reflux. *B*, grade III reflux by patient age at presentation.

prophylaxis (see figure). In general, a lower reflux grade correlated with a better chance of spontaneous resolution. Data for grades I and II reflux showed no differences in regard to patient age at presentation or laterality (unilateral versus bilateral). For grade III reflux age and laterality (unilateral versus bilateral) were important prognostic factors with increasing age at presentation and bilateral reflux decreasing the probability of resolution. Bilateral grade IV reflux had a particularly low chance of spontaneous resolution. All estimates are subject to 2 restrictions: 1) estimates are only valid for up to 5 years after diagnosis, and 2) for grade IV disease estimates only apply to the time of diagnosis and they are not age specific. No data were available for reflux resolution with intermittent antibiotic therapy. In children with reflux and voiding dysfunction (frequency, urgency, urge incontinence and incomplete bladder emptying) available results from series with control groups suggested that the reflux resolution rate increased with anticholinergic therapy and bladder training.

Reflux Resolution—Surgical Therapy: The panel reviewed 86 reports outlining open surgical success, including 6,472 patients (8,563 ureters). Overall surgical success was reported in 959 of 1,008 patients (95.1%) and 7,731 of 8,061 ureters (95.9%). Surgical success was achieved in 108 of 109 ureters (99%) with grade I, 874 of 882 (99.1%) with grade II, 993 of 1,010 (98.3%) with grade III, 386 of 392 (98.5%) with grade IV and 155 of 192 (80.7%) with grade V reflux.

For endoscopic therapy most reports in the literature describe results of the use of polytetrafluoroethylene (Teflon). Overall reflux was corrected in 77.1% of ureters after a single injection. Reflux resolved after initial treatment in only 6 of 19 ureters (32%) with grade V disease. Currently no injectable substance has been approved for endoscopic antireflux surgery by the Food and Drug Administration.

Renal Scarring: The panel believed that relevant data pertaining to renal scarring should be analyzed primarily from studies with a minimum of 5 years of followup. Four prospective trials comparing the outcomes of medical and surgical management included analysis of new renal scarring. None of these trials showed a statistically significant difference in the rate of new renal scarring. In the European arm of the International Reflux Study the rate of scarring was similar in patients receiving antibiotic prophylaxis and those treated surgically.[10] However, 80% of new renal scars in the surgical group appeared by 10 months after randomization, whereas new renal scars appeared throughout the 5-year period in the group managed medically. The Birmingham Reflux Study identified new scars after 5 years in only 6 and 5.2% of patients treated medically and surgically, respectively, with no additional scars detected after 2 years of followup.[9] In the prospective study of the Southwest Pediatric Nephrology Study Group of children younger than age 5 years with grade I, II or III reflux and normal kidneys at entry, new scars developed in 16% with continuous antibiotic prophylaxis.[14] On the other hand, the International

Reflux Study noted new scars in 15.7 and 17.2% of children with reflux in Europe, and in 21.5 and 31.4% of those in North America undergoing medical and surgical treatment, respectively. Few data were available to analyze the relationship between bacteriuria and new renal scarring in children with reflux.

Renal Growth and Function: On the basis of studies available to date there is no evidence that renal growth is impaired in unscarred kidneys exposed to sterile reflux of any grade or surgical correction of reflux facilitates growth of the kidney postoperatively. Surgical correction of reflux stabilizes the glomerular filtration rate but it has not been shown to lead to long-term improvement.

Harms of medical treatment (adverse drug reactions). Potential adverse reactions to antimicrobial prophylaxis include minor effects, such as nausea/vomiting, abdominal pain, a bad taste, increased antibiotic resistance and marrow suppression as well as more serious side effects. Few studies dealing with the medical management of reflux included information on any drug reaction.

Harms of surgery. Obstruction: A total of 33 studies provided rates of obstruction after ureteral reimplantation for reflux. The likelihood of obstruction in the 33 series ranged from 0 to 9.1% with a combined rate of 2% in studies published after 1986. The reoperation rate ranged from 0.3 to 9.1% with an overall prevalence of 2%. There was no difference among various surgical techniques.

A total of 15 series provided detailed information on post-operative ureteral obstruction following endoscopic treatment of reflux. The 15 series included 1,741 refluxing ureters treated using polytetrafluoroethylene (1,437) or collagen (304) as the injected substance. Seven persistent obstructions (0.4% of cases) were reported.

Contralateral Reflux: The development of contralateral reflux after unilateral ureteral surgery has been reported in numerous series. Of 1,566 ureters considered at risk there was an overall incidence of 142 reported new cases (9.1%) of contralateral reflux. The surgical method of reimplantation did not influence the likelihood of new contralateral reflux. Ross et al reported a high incidence of contralateral reflux in ureters with previously demonstrated vesicoureteral reflux.[16] Contralateral reflux generally resolves with time and surgical intervention usually was not performed for at least 1 year.

Recommendations

The recommendations that follow and those listed in tables 2 and 3[3] are intended to assist physicians specifically in the treatment of vesicoureteral reflux in children diagnosed following a urinary tract infection. They apply only to children 10 years old or younger at presentation with unilateral or bilateral reflux and with or without scarring. The recommendations assume that the patient has uncomplicated reflux (for example no voiding dysfunction, neuropathic bladder, posterior urethral valves, bladder exstrophy or fixed anatomical abnormalities).

The panel generated its practice policy recommendations on the basis of evidence based outcomes and panel opinion, reflecting its clinical experience in pediatric urology and pediatric nephrology. In the guidelines report statements based on opinion are explicitly identified and evidence based recommendations are accompanied by appropriate references.[3] Only a few recommendations could be derived purely from scientific evidence of a beneficial effect on health outcomes.

Recommendations were derived from a panel survey of preferred treatment options for 36 clinical categories of children with reflux. Treatment recommendations were classified as guidelines, preferred options and reasonable alternatives. Treatment options selected by 8 or 9 of the 9 panel members were classified as guidelines. Treatment options that received 5 to 7 votes were designated as preferred options and treatment options that received 3 to 4 votes were designated as reasonable alternatives. Treatments that received no more than 2 votes were designated as having no consensus.

Treatment recommendations. Treatment recommendations that derived from this methodology are summarized in tables 2 and 3. See the complete AUA report for more details.[3]

Other management recommendations. In children with vesicoureteral reflux, urethral dilation and internal urethrotomy are not beneficial. In addition, cystoscopic examination of the ureteral orifices does not appear to aid in predicting whether reflux will resolve. In children with symptoms of voiding dysfunction urodynamic evaluation may be helpful but evocative cystometry is unnecessary in those with reflux and a normal voiding pattern. In children with reflux who are toilet trained, regular and volitional low pressure voiding with complete bladder emptying should be encouraged. If it is suspected that the child is experiencing uninhibited bladder contractions, anticholinergic therapy may be beneficial.

The clinician should provide parents with information about the known benefits and harms of available options, including continuous antibiotic prophylaxis, surgery and intermittent antibiotic therapy. The clinician should indicate to what extent the estimates of benefits and harms are based on scientific evidence or on opinion and clinical experience. Given the general lack of direct evidence that any treatment option is superior to another (especially when total benefits, harms, costs and inconvenience are considered), parent and patient preferences regarding treatment options should generally be honored.

In children in whom antireflux surgery is elected the panel does not recommend the endoscopic form of therapy because of the lack of proved long-term safety and efficacy of most materials used for injection and the lack of approval of such materials by the Food and Drug Administration.

TABLE 2. Treatment recommendations: boys and girls with primary vesicoureteral reflux and no renal scarring[3]

Clinical Presentation		Treatment					
		Initial (antibiotic prophylaxis or open surgical repair)			Followup (continued antibiotic prophylaxis, cystography or open surgical repair[*])		
Reflux Grade/Laterality	Pt. Age (yrs.)	Guideline	Preferred Option	Reasonable Alternative	Guideline[†]	Preferred Option[‖]	No Consensus[‡]
I–II/Unilat. or bilat.	Younger than 1	Antibiotic prophylaxis					Boys and girls
	1–5	Antibiotic prophylaxis					Boys and girls
	6–10	Antibiotic prophylaxis					Boys and girls
III–IV/Unilat. or bilat.	Younger than 1	Antibiotic prophylaxis			Bilat.: surgery if persistent	Unilat.: surgery if persistent	
	1–5	Unilat.: antibiotic prophylaxis	Bilat.: antibiotic prophylaxis			Surgery if persistent	
	6–10		Unilat.: antibiotic prophylaxis Bilat.: surgery	Bilat.: antibiotic prophylaxis		Surgery if persistent	
V/Unilat. or bilat.	Younger than 1		Antibiotic prophylaxis		Surgery if persistent		
	1–5		Bilat.: surgery Unilat.: antibiotic prophylaxis	Bilat.: antibiotic prophylaxis Unilat.: surgery	Surgery if persistent		
	6–10	Surgery					

* For patients with persistent uncomplicated reflux after extended treatment with continuous antibiotic therapy.

† See Duration of Reflux regarding the time that clinicians should wait before recommending surgery.

‡ No consensus was reached regarding the role of continued antibiotic prophylaxis, cystography or surgery.

TABLE 3. Treatment recommendations: boys and girls with primary vesicoureteral reflux and with renal scarring[3]

Clinical Presentation		Treatment					
		Initial (antibiotic prophylaxis or open surgical repair)			Followup (continued antibiotic prophylaxis, cystography, or open surgical repair*)		
Reflux Grade/Laterality	Pt. Age (yrs.)	Guideline	Preferred Option	Reasonable Alternative	Guideline[†]	Preferred Option[†]	No Consensus[‡]
I–II/Unilat. or bilat.	Younger than 1	Antibiotic prophylaxis					Boys and girls
	1–5	Antibiotic prophylaxis					Boys and girls
	6–10	Antibiotic prophylaxis					Boys and girls
III–IV/Unilat.	Younger than 1	Antibiotic prophylaxis			Girls: surgery if persistent	Boys: surgery if persistent	
	1–5	Antibiotic prophylaxis			Girls: surgery if persistent	Boys: surgery if persistent	
	6–10		Antibiotic prophylaxis		Surgery if persistent		
III–IV/Bilat.	Younger than 1	Antibiotic prophylaxis			Surgery if persistent		
	1–5		Antibiotic prophylaxis	Surgery	Surgery if persistent		
	6–10	Surgery			Surgery if persistent		
V/Unilat. or bilat.	Younger than 1		Antibiotic prophylaxis	Surgery	Surgery if persistent		
	1–5	Bilat: surgery	Unilat: surgery			Surgery if persistent	
	6–10	Surgery				Surgery if persistent	

* For patients with persistent uncomplicated reflux after extended treatment with continuous antibiotic therapy.
† See Duration of Reflux regarding the time that clinicians should wait before recommending surgery.
‡ No consensus was reached regarding the role of continued antibiotic prophylaxis, cystography or surgery.

Followup evaluation should be performed at least annually, at which time patient height and weight should be recorded and urinalysis should be done. If the child has renal scarring, blood pressure should be measured. When deciding how often to obtain followup cystography in children treated medically the clinician should consider the risk of continued antibiotic prophylaxis, the risks of radiological study and the likelihood of spontaneous resolution (see figure). In general, cystography does not need to be performed more than once yearly.

Rationale for treatment recommendations. The panel recommendations to offer continuous antibiotic prophylaxis as initial therapy are based on limited scientific evidence. To our knowledge controlled studies comparing the efficacy of continuous antibiotic prophylaxis and intermittent therapy on health outcomes in children with reflux have not been performed. However, the opinion of the panel is that maintaining continuous urine sterility is beneficial for decreasing the risk of renal scarring and this benefit outweighs the potential adverse effects of antibiotics.

Recommendations to proceed to surgery in children with reflux that has not resolved spontaneously are supported by limited scientific evidence: open antireflux surgery is 95 to 98% effective for correcting reflux, and in grades III to IV reflux the risk of clinical pyelonephritis is 2 to 2.5 times higher in children treated with continuous prophylaxis than in those treated surgically. Nevertheless, randomized controlled trials with such children have shown that a urinary tract infection does not develop in most while they are receiving prophylaxis.

Recommendations for more aggressive treatment of girls than boys (for example for persistent grades III to IV reflux in children 1 to 5 years old) are based on epidemiological evidence that girls have a higher risk of urinary tract infection than boys. Recommendations for more aggressive treatment of grade V reflux (for example surgical repair as initial therapy) are based on panel opinion that such reflux is unlikely to resolve spontaneously with time, surgery is effective for resolving severe reflux and these benefits outweigh the potential harms of surgery. More aggressive recommendations for children who have renal scarring at diagnosis are based on panel opinion that such patients have a higher risk of progressive scarring and decreased renal functional reserve.

An important variable in the scope of treatment is the presence of voiding dysfunction, a common occurrence in children with reflux. Such children may require more aggressive treatment with anticholinergics and bladder training in addition to antibiotic prophylaxis. Surgical repair of reflux is slightly less successful in children with voiding dysfunction and, thus, a higher threshold is necessary before surgery is recommended in such patients. Consequently children with reflux should be assessed for voiding dysfunction as part of the initial evaluation.

Research Priorities

The panel identified many research areas as needing further investigation. Presently there is little information regarding health outcomes pertaining to reflux (table 1). A significant priority should be to continue to acquire this information.

Basic research into the pathogenesis as well as genetics of vesicoureteral reflux is needed. Further randomized controlled trials studying the role of medical and surgical therapy using dimercapto-succinic acid renal scan for evaluation of renal scarring are indicated. Future studies should stratify results by patient gender, age and reflux grade, reporting reflux resolution by rate of ureteral and case resolution. Confirmation of the panel finding that reflux resolution depends on patient age and laterality (unilateral versus bilateral) in grade III disease but not in grades I and II reflux would be worthwhile.

The extent to which reflux increases the risk of renal scarring associated with urinary tract infection and the mechanism of this effect deserve investigation. Comparison of the efficacy of intermittent and continuous antibiotic therapy would be beneficial. The role of voiding dysfunction in the pathogenesis of reflux and its risk on reflux complications, such as renal scarring, and the complications of surgery also deserve further investigation. Matched controlled studies of anticholinergic therapy and bladder training on reflux related outcomes in children with voiding dysfunction are necessary.

Less traumatic methods of determining whether reflux is present should be developed as well as techniques of voiding cystourethrography that result in less radiation exposure. Analysis of the costs of reflux treatment and surveillance is important, particularly comparing those associated with medical and surgical therapy. The impact of screening populations at risk and early medical or surgical intervention on reflux related outcomes in such patients should be analyzed. The development of minimally invasive techniques of antireflux surgery is indicated. Newer materials that can be used for endoscopic subureteral injection and that are safe in children should be studied. The natural history of vesicoureteral reflux in women with persistent reflux deserves investigation, including an analysis of the morbidity of persistent reflux, and need for and efficacy of prophylaxis in pregnant and nonpregnant women.

Gail J. Herzenberg, Project Director, Michael D. Wong, Information Services Director, and Joan A. Saunders, Writer/ Editor, of Technical Resources International, Inc., assisted in the preparation of this report. Regina O'Donnell, Washington, D. C., assisted in obtaining the original data of Skoog et al.[14]

References

1. Elder, J. S., Snyder, H. M., III, Peters, C., Arant, B., Hawtrey, C. E., Hurwitz, R. S., Parrott, T. S. and Weiss, R. A.: Variations in practice among urologists and nephrologists treating children with vesicoureteral reflux. J. Urol., part 2. **148**: 714, 1992.

2. Eddy, D. M.: A Manual for Assessing Health Practices and Designing Practice Policies: The Explicit Approach. Philadelphia: American College of Physicians, 1992.

3. Elder, J. S., Peters, C. A., Arant, B. S., Jr., Ewalt, D. H., Hawtrey, C. E., Hurwitz, R. S., Parrott, T. S., Snyder, H. M., III, Weiss, R. A., Woolf, S. H. and Hasselblad, V.: Report on the management of primary vesicoureteral reflux in children. Baltimore: American Urological Association, Inc., 1997.

4. Eddy, D. M., Hasselblad, V. and Shachter, R. D.: The Statistical Synthesis of Evidence: Meta-Analysis by the Confidence Profile Method. Boston: Academic Press, 1992.

5. Cooper, J. H. and Hedges, L. V.: The Handbook of Research Synthesis. New York: Russell Sage Foundation, 1994.

6. Eddy, D. M. and Hasselblad, V.: FAST*PRO Software for Meta-Analysis by the Confidence Profile Method. Boston: Academic Press, 1992.

7. Hasselblad, V.: Meta-analysis of multi-treatment studies. Med. Decis. Making, submitted for publication.

8. EGRET Reference Manual, revision 4. Seattle: Statistics and Epidemiology Research Corp., 1993.

9. Prospective trial of operative versus non-operative treatment of severe vesicoureteric reflux in children: five years' observation. Birmingham Reflux Study Group. Brit. Med. J., **295**: 237, 1987.

10. Tamminen-Möbius, T., Brunier, E., Ebel, K. D., Lebowitz, R., Olbing, H., Seppänen, U. and Sixt, R. on behalf of the International Reflux Study in Children: Cessation of vesicoureteral reflux for 5 years in infants and children allocated to medical treatment. J. Urol., **148**: 1662, 1992.

11. Weiss, R., Duckett, J. W. and Spitzer, A.: Results of a randomized clinical trial of medical versus surgical management of infants and children with grades III and IV primary vesicoureteral reflux (United States). J. Urol., **148**: 1667, 1992.

12. Scholtmeijer, R. J.: Treatment of vesicoureteric reflux: results after 3 years in a prospective study. Child. Nephrol. Urol., **11**: 29, 1991.

13. Martinell, J., Jodal, U. and Lidin-Janson, G.: Pregnancies in women with and without renal scarring after urinary infections in childhood. Brit. Med. J., **300**: 840, 1990.

14. Skoog, S. J., Belman, A. B. and Majd, M.: A nonsurgical approach to management of primary vesicoureteral reflux. J. Urol., **138**: 941, 1987.

15. Arant, B. S., Jr.: Medical management of mild and moderate vesicoureteral reflux: followup studies of infants and young children. A preliminary report of the Southwest Pediatric Nephrology Study Group. J. Urol., part 2, **148**: 1683, 1992.

16. Ross, J. H., Kay, R. and Nasrallah, P.: Contralateral reflux after unilateral ureteral reimplantation in patients with a history of resolved contralateral reflux. J. Urol., **154**: 1171, 1995.